First Aid
Manual

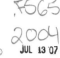

American College of Emergency Physicians®

First Aid
Manual

Medical editor
Jon R. Krohmer, MD, FACEP

LONDON, NEW YORK, MUNICH, MELBOURNE, DELHI

**THIS BOOK IS THE OFFICIAL, AUTHORIZED MANUAL OF THE
AMERICAN COLLEGE OF EMERGENCY PHYSICIANS.**

DK PUBLISHING, INC.

SENIOR EDITOR	Jill Hamilton
EDITORIAL ASSISTANT	Madeline Farbman
ASSISTANT MANAGING ART EDITOR	Michelle Baxter
DESIGN ASSISTANT	Miesha Tate
DTP DESIGNER	Milos Orlovic
PRODUCTION MANAGER	Chris Avgherinos
PROJECT MANAGER	Sharon Lucas
CREATIVE DIRECTOR	Tina Vaughan
PUBLISHER	Chuck Lang

DORLING KINDERSLEY LTD.

SENIOR EDITOR	Janet Mohun
EDITOR	Katie John
PROJECT ART EDITOR	Janice English
ART EDITOR	Sara Freeman
DESIGN ASSISTANT	Iona Hoyle
DTP DESIGNER	Julian Dams
MANAGING EDITOR	Jemima Dunne
MANAGING ART EDITOR	Louise Dick
PRODUCTION CONTROLLER	Rita Sinha
PRODUCTION MANAGER	Michelle Thomas
ILLUSTRATOR	Richard Tibbitts
PHOTOGRAPHER	Gary Ombler

AMERICAN COLLEGE OF EMERGENCY PHYSICIANS

MEDICAL EDITOR	Jon R. Krohmer, MD, FACEP

ASSOCIATE EXECUTIVE DIRECTOR, EDUCATION AND PROFESSIONAL PUBLICATIONS	Thomas Werlinich

Second American Edition, 2004
06 07 08 10 9 8 7 6 5

Published in the United States by DK Publishing, Inc.
375 Hudson Street, New York, New York 10014

Illustration copyright © 2002 by Dorling Kindersley Limited, except as listed in acknowledgments, p.288
Text copyright © 2002 by St. John Ambulance; St. Andrew's Ambulance Association; The British Red Cross Society

A Cataloging-in-Publication record for this book is available from the Library of Congress

ISBN 0-7566-0195-9

Reproduced in Singapore by Colourscan
Printed and bound in China by Leo Paper Products Ltd.

Discover more at
www.dk.com

FOREWORD

The goal of the American College of Emergency Physicians (ACEP) is to support high-quality emergency care in our country. This extends from the care provided in emergency departments, to the care provided by the emergency medical services (EMS) systems around the country, and to the care provided by bystanders in the community. Either directly or indirectly, every family is affected by injury or illness almost on a daily basis. It is important for all of us to have skills in the recognition of emergency medical events and to be able to provide care until additional care resources can be obtained. That is the goal of this manual.

More than 100 million persons come to hospital emergency departments every year, seeking care for everything from mild illnesses and injuries to life-threatening conditions. The emergency department is part of the continuum of care that starts with the bystander who first recognizes a problem and begins treatment. It is vital for all of us to know the steps to follow in a medical emergency.

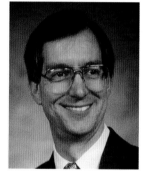

JON R. KROHMER, MD, FACEP

This manual shows you what to do for the common, mild, serious, and life-threatening situations with which you will be faced, in a step-by step-manner, using illustrations and photographs to help you understand the problem at hand. Although it is designed to provide you with a good knowledge base, I encourage you to take a formal first aid course from one of the organizations in your community that provides such training. These organizations include the American Red Cross, the American Heart Association, EMS agencies, and hospitals in the area.

The American College of Emergency Physicians was founded by physicians who realized that a unique body of medical knowledge was needed to provide appropriate emergency care. This led to the development of emergency medicine as a medical specialty, with its own residency training programs and board certification process. Today, more than 22,000 emergency physicians have an ever-expanding role in meeting emergency health care needs, including antiterrorism response. They are also integral to supporting the EMS systems around the country.

On behalf of ACEP and emergency medicine specialists throughout the United States, it is my pleasure to bring this second edition of the ACEP *First Aid Manual* to you. Thanks for joining the emergency care team!

CONTENTS

INTRODUCTION   10

1 FIRST-AID ESSENTIALS   11

Being a first aider................................12
Looking after yourself........................14
Regulations and legislation..............17
Action at an emergency....................18
Telephoning for help.........................20
Multiple victims.................................21
Road incidents...................................22
Fires...24
Electrical injuries...............................26
Water rescue.....................................28
Assessing a victim.............................29
Primary survey...................................29
Secondary survey...............................30
Symptoms and signs.........................32
Examining a victim............................34
Treatment and aftercare...................36
Passing on information......................37
Using observation charts...................38

2 TECHNIQUES AND EQUIPMENT   39

Removing clothing.............................40
Removing headgear...........................41
Monitoring vital signs........................42
First-aid materials..............................44
Dressings...46
Sterile dressings...........................47
Nonsterile dressings.....................48
Adhesive dressings.......................49

Cold compresses................................49
Principles of bandaging.....................50
Roller bandages.................................52
Elbow and knee bandages.................54
Hand and foot bandages....................55
Tubular bandages...............................56
Triangular bandages..........................57
Square knots......................................58
Scalp bandage...................................59
Arm sling...60
Elevation sling...................................61
Improvised slings..............................62
Victim handling..................................63
Assisting a walking victim..................65
Controlling a fall................................66
Moving from chair to floor.................67
Moving a collapsed victim.................68
Moving equipment.............................69
Stretchers and boards........................70

3 LIFE-SAVING PROCEDURES   71

Breathing and circulation...................72
Life-saving priorities..........................73
Adult resuscitation chart....................75
Unconscious adult..............................76
Child resuscitation chart....................86
Unconscious child (1–7 years)...........87
Infant resuscitation chart...................94
Unconscious infant (under 1 year).....95
Choking summary charts....................99
Choking adult...........................100
Choking child (1–7 years).............101
Choking infant
   (under 1 year)......................102

4 RESPIRATORY PROBLEMS 103

The respiratory system...........104
Hypoxia..........106
Airway obstruction..........107
Hanging and strangulation..........108
Drowning..........109
Inhalation of fumes..........110
Penetrating chest wound..........112
Hyperventilation..........114
Asthma..........115
Croup..........116

5 HEART AND CIRCULATORY PROBLEMS 117

The heart and blood vessels..........118
Shock..........120
Internal bleeding..........122
Anaphylactic shock..........123
Angina pectoris..........124
Acute heart failure..........124
Heart attack..........125
Fainting..........126

6 WOUNDS AND BLEEDING 127

Bleeding and types of wounds..........128
Severe bleeding..........130
Impalement..........132
Amputation..........132
Crush injury..........133
Cuts and abrasions..........134
Foreign object in a cut..........135
Bruising..........136
Infected wound..........136
Scalp and head wounds..........137
Eye wound..........138

Bleeding from the ear..........138
Nosebleed..........139
Bleeding from the mouth..........140
Knocked-out tooth..........140
Wound to the palm..........141
Wound at a joint crease..........141
Abdominal wound..........142
Vaginal bleeding..........143
Bleeding varicose vein..........144

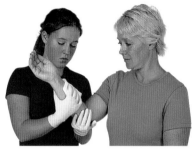

7 BONE, JOINT, AND MUSCLE INJURIES 145

The skeleton..........146
Bones, muscles, and joints..........148
Fractures..........150
Dislocated joint..........153
Strains and sprains..........154
Major facial fracture..........156
Cheekbone and nose fractures..........157
Lower jaw injury..........157
Fractured collarbone..........158
Shoulder injury..........159
Upper arm injury..........160
Elbow injury..........161
Forearm and wrist injuries..........162
Hand and finger injuries..........163
Injury to the ribcage..........164
Spinal injury..........165
Back pain..........168
Fractured pelvis..........169
Hip and thigh injuries..........170
Knee injury..........172
Lower leg injury..........173
Ankle injury..........174
Foot and toe injuries..........174

8 NERVOUS SYSTEM PROBLEMS   175

The nervous system............................176
Impaired consciousness......................178
Head injury...179
Concussion..180
Cerebral compression.........................181
Skull fracture......................................182
Stroke...183
Seizures in adults...............................184
Absence seizures.................................185
Seizures in children.............................186
Meningitis...187
Headache..188
Migraine...188

Prickly heat...202
Heat exhaustion..................................203
Heatstroke..204
Frostbite..205
Hypothermia.......................................206

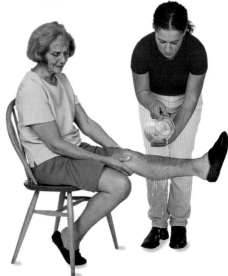

10 FOREIGN OBJECTS   209

The sensory organs..............................210
Splinter...212
Embedded fishhook.............................213
Foreign object in the eye.....................214
Foreign object in the ear.....................215
Foreign object in the nose...................215
Inhaled foreign object.........................216
Swallowed foreign object.....................216

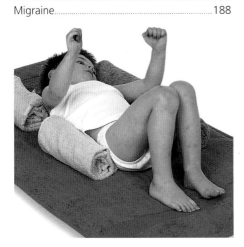

9 ENVIRONMENTAL INJURIES   189

The skin...190
Assessing a burn.................................192
Severe burns and scalds......................194
Minor burns and scalds.......................196
Burns to the airway.............................197
Electrical burn.....................................198
Chemical burn.....................................199
Chemical burn to the eye.....................200
Flash burn to the eye..........................201
Tear gas or pepper spray injury...........201
Sunburn..202

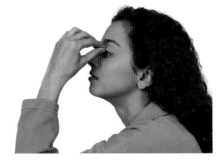

11 POISONING, BITES, AND STINGS 217

How poisons affect the body...........218
Swallowed poisons...........220
Chemicals on the skin...........221
Inhaled gases...........221
Poisons in the eye...........221
Drug poisoning...........222
Alcohol poisoning...........223
Food poisoning...........224
Poisonous plants and fungi...........225
Insect sting...........226
Other bites and stings...........227
Tick bite...........227
Snake bite...........228
Stings from sea creatures...........229
Marine puncture wound...........229
Animal bite...........230

12 CHILDBIRTH AND MEDICAL PROBLEMS 231

Childbirth...........232
Childbirth: first stage...........233
Childbirth: second stage...........234
Childbirth: third stage...........236
Miscarriage...........237
Allergy...........238
Hiccups...........238
Fever...........239
Vertigo...........239
Diabetes mellitus...........240
Hyperglycemia...........240
Hypoglycemia...........241
Panic attack...........242
Disturbed behavior...........242

Earache...........243
Toothache...........244
Sore throat...........244
Abdominal pain...........245
Hernia...........246
Vomiting and diarrhea...........247
Stitch...........247
Cramp...........248
Overseas travel health...........249

13 EMERGENCY FIRST AID 252

Action in an emergency...........252
Unconscious adult...........254
Unconscious child (1–7 years)...........258
Unconscious infant (under 1 year)...........262
Choking adult...........264
Choking child (1–7 years)...........265
Choking infant (under 1 year)...........266
Asthma attack...........267
Shock...........268
Anaphylactic shock...........269
Severe bleeding...........270
Heart attack...........271
Head injury...........272
Spinal injury...........273
Seizures in adults...........274
Seizures in children...........275
Broken bones...........276
Burns...........277
Eye injury...........278
Swallowed poisons...........279
Observation charts...........280

INTRODUCTION

The American College of Emergency Physicians First Aid Manual uses photographs to give you clear and comprehensive step-by-step guidance. However, first-aid techniques are constantly being reviewed to ensure that the victim is getting the best possible care. This revised edition includes the latest guidelines for all conditions, first-aid treatments, and resuscitation techniques that have been agreed upon and updated both in the US and internationally. To help you to understand why and how first-aid techniques work, great emphasis has been placed on how people are structured (anatomy) and how we function (physiology). A clearer understanding of what is normal should help you decide what may be wrong or abnormal, and enable you to provide the correct treatment.

There is a chapter on Emergency First Aid that gives you at-a-glance, life-saving action plans for all emergency situations. This quick-reference guide has been placed at the end of the Manual for easy access.

Wherever you use it, at home, at work, or in your car or boat, this indispensable Manual is the only guide to first aid that you will need.

HOW TO USE THIS BOOK

Color bars help you to find relevant sections quickly

Introductory text describes likely causes and effects of condition

"Your aims" box summarizes purposes of treatment

Annotated photographs show details of particular techniques

Steps explain each stage of first aid action

List of recognition features provides quick-reference guide to help you identify condition

Cross-references direct you to articles on related conditions or further treatment

"Special case" box highlights instances in which alternative action may be needed

"Warning" box advises how to deal with dangers and avoid further risks to victims or yourself

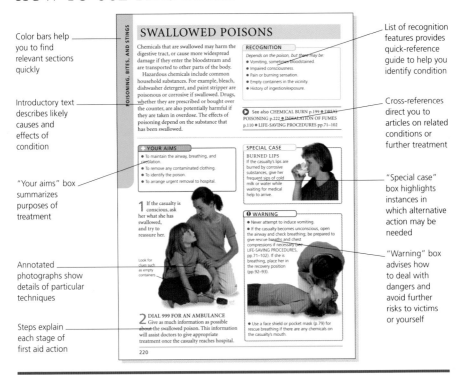

1

FIRST AID is the initial assistance or treatment given to someone who is injured or suddenly taken ill. This chapter describes the sequence of priorities for giving first aid, providing essential information on how to deal with emergencies and how to look after yourself. It also covers the steps involved in assessing and treating a victim.

LEARNING FIRST-AID SKILLS
By following the guidance in this book, most people can give effective first aid. However, to become a fully competent rescuer you should complete a first-aid course to acquire the necessary practical skills, and gain an appropriate certificate. The American Red Cross and many EMS organizations give a variety of first-aid courses at different levels. Contact a local group for a course specific to your needs.

CONTENTS

Being a first aider........................ 12

Looking after yourself............... 14

Regulations and legislation......... 17

Action at an emergency............. 18

Telephoning for help................. 20

Multiple victims.......................... 21

Traffic incidents......................... 22

Fires.. 24

Electrical injuries....................... 26

Water rescue............................. 28

Assessing a victim...................... 29

Primary survey........................... 29

Secondary survey....................... 30

Symptoms and signs.................. 32

Examining a victim..................... 34

Treatment and aftercare............ 36

Passing on information.............. 37

Using observation charts........... 38

+ FIRST-AID PRIORITIES

- Assess the situation quickly and calmly.
- Protect yourself and the victims from danger.
- Assess the conditions of all victims.
- Comfort and reassure the victims.
- Deal with any life-threatening conditions first.
- Obtain medical aid if necessary. Dial 9•1•1 or call EMS if you suspect a serious illness or injury.

BEING A FIRST AIDER

The first aid learned from a manual or study program is not really like reality. Most of us feel apprehensive when dealing with "the real thing." By accepting these feelings, we are better able to cope with the unexpected.

DOING YOUR BEST

First aid is not an exact science and is open to human error. Even with appropriate treatment, and however hard you try, a victim may not respond as you hoped. Some conditions are inevitably fatal, even with the best medical care. If you do your best, your conscience can be clear.

ASSESSING RISKS

The golden rule is, "First do no harm," while applying the principle of "calculated risk." You should use the treatment that is most likely to be of benefit to an injured person, but do not use a treatment that you are not sure about just for the sake of doing something.

The principle of the "Good Samaritan" supports those performing first aid to the best of their abilities, but not those who act in gross negligence. The exact law varies from state to state, and you should check on the law in your area.

Your responsibilities

The first aider's responsibilities are clearly defined. They are as follows:
● To assess a situation quickly and safely, and summon appropriate help.
● To protect victims and others at the scene from possible danger.
● To identify, as much as possible, the injury or nature of the illness affecting a victim.
● To give each victim early and appropriate treatment, treating the most serious conditions first.

● To arrange for the victim's transport to a hospital, into the care of a doctor, or to his home as necessary.
● If medical aid is needed, to remain with a victim until further care is available.
● To report your observations to those taking over care of the victim, and to give further assistance if required.
● To prevent cross-infection between yourself and the victim as much as possible (p.15).

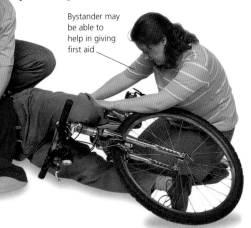

Talk to victim to reassure him and obtain information about his condition

Bystander may be able to help in giving first aid

Treat victim in position found

Assess the situation
Ask the victim and any bystanders what has happened. Try to identify his injuries and treat urgent ones first. Do not move him unless it is absolutely necessary.

Giving care with confidence

Every victim needs to feel secure and in safe hands. You can create an air of confidence and assurance by:
● Being in control both of your own reactions and of the problem.
● Acting calmly and logically.
● Being gentle, but firm.
● Speaking to the victim kindly but in a clear and purposeful way.

BUILDING UP TRUST
While performing your examination and treatment, talk to the victim throughout.
● Explain what you are going to do.
● Try to answer questions honestly to allay fears as best you can. If you do not know the answer, say so.
● Continue to reassure the victim, even when the treatment is finished. In addition, find out about the next of kin, or anyone else who should be contacted about the incident. Ask if you can help to make arrangements so that any responsibilities the victim may have, such as collecting a child from school, can be taken care of.
● Do not leave someone whom you believe to be dying, seriously ill, or badly injured. Continue to talk to the victim, and hold his hand; never allow the person to feel alone.

TALKING TO RELATIVES
The task of informing relatives of a death is usually the job of the police or EMS personnel on duty. However, it may well be that you have to tell relatives or friends

that someone has been injured or taken ill. Always make sure that you are speaking to the right person first. Then explain, as simply and honestly as you can, what has happened and, if appropriate, where the victim has been taken. Do not be vague or exaggerate because this may cause unnecessary alarm. It is better to admit ignorance than to give someone misleading information about an injury or illness.

COPING WITH CHILDREN
Young children are extremely perceptive and will quickly detect any uncertainty on your part. Gain an injured or sick child's confidence by talking first to someone he trusts – a parent if possible. If the parent accepts you and believes you will help, this confidence will be conveyed to the child. Always explain simply to a child what is happening and what you intend to do; do not talk over his head. You should not separate a child from his mother, father, or other trusted person.

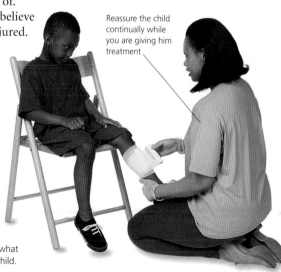

Reassure the child continually while you are giving him treatment

Giving first aid to a child
Try to make a child feel comfortable and confident with your treatment. Always explain what you are doing, no matter what the age of the child.

LOOKING AFTER YOURSELF

When carrying out first aid, it is important for you to protect yourself from injury and infection. One of the primary rules of first aid is to ensure that the situation is safe before treating a victim. Bear in mind that infection may be a risk, even with relatively minor injuries, so you need to take steps to avoid contracting an infection from a victim or passing on any infection that you have. In addition, you need to look after your psychological health and try to deal with stress effectively (p.16).

Personal safety

Do not attempt heroic rescues in hazardous circumstances. If you put yourself at risk, you are unlikely to be able to help victims effectively. Always assess the situation first and make sure that the situation you are entering is safe for you (p.18).

THE "FIGHT OR FLIGHT RESPONSE"
In an emergency, your body responds by releasing certain hormones in the "fight or flight" response. When you experience this response, your heart beats faster, and your breathing is deeper and more rapid. You may also notice that you are sweating more than usual and that you are more alert.

STAYING CALM
Sometimes too great a rush of hormones may affect your ability to cope with a situation. Taking slow, deep breaths will help you calm down, leaving you better able to remember your first-aid procedures.

Protection from infection

An important part of first aid is preventing "cross infection" (either transmitting germs to a victim or contracting an infection yourself). This is a particular concern if you are treating open wounds.

Simple measures, such as washing your hands and wearing disposable gloves, may provide sufficient protection. Infection with blood-borne viruses such as hepatitis B or C is a risk, but these viruses can only be transmitted by blood-to-blood contact – if an infected person's blood makes contact with yours through, for example, a cut. There is no known evidence of hepatitis or HIV being transmitted during resuscitation, but they are transmitted by blood or other bodily fluids.

Protection from hepatitis B
All first aiders should be protected by immunization against hepatitis B. The vaccine is given as a series of three injections in the upper arm.

IMMUNIZATION
It is recommended that all first aiders are immunized against hepatitis B. Currently, there is no vaccine against hepatitis C or HIV. If you think you have been exposed to any infection after giving first aid, seek medical aid immediately.

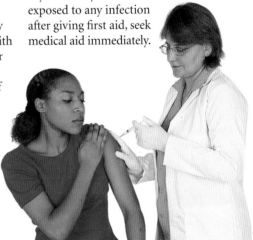

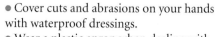

Guidelines for preventing cross infection

Following good practice guidelines will help prevent the spread of infection.

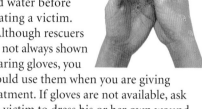

- If facilities are available, wash your hands thoroughly with soap and water before treating a victim.
- Although rescuers are not always shown wearing gloves, you should use them when you are giving treatment. If gloves are not available, ask the victim to dress his or her own wound, or enclose your hands in clean plastic bags.

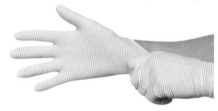

- Cover cuts and abrasions on your hands with waterproof dressings.
- Wear a plastic apron when dealing with large quantities of body fluids, and wear plastic glasses to protect your eyes.
- Avoid touching a wound or touching any part of a dressing that will come into contact with a wound.
- Try not to breathe, cough, or sneeze over a wound while you are treating a victim.
- Take care not to prick yourself with any needle found on or near a victim or cut yourself on glass.
- If a face shield or pocket mask is available, use it when giving rescue breaths (p.79).
- Dispose of all waste safely (below).

> **⚠ WARNING**
>
> If you accidentally prick or cut your skin or splash your eyes, wash the area thoroughly and seek medical help immediately.

Dealing with waste

Once you have finished treatment, dispose of all waste material carefully to prevent the spread of infection. Place soiled items and used gloves in a plastic bag; ideally, use a special red bag called a biohazard bag. To dispose of sharp objects, such as needles, you should use a specially designed plastic container called a sharps container. Seal the bag or container tightly, and label it to show that it contains clinical waste.

Biohazard bags should be destroyed by burning (incineration). If you do not have access to incineration facilities, ask your local ambulance service or local environmental health department how to deal with this type of waste.

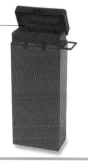

Lid can be locked or sealed after use

Sharps container
This is a plastic box designed to hold used needles and other sharp items for safe disposal. Sharps containers are usually red.

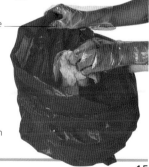

Keep gloves on until you have finished disposing of waste, then dispose of gloves

Using a biohazard bag
If you have a red biohazard bag available, you should use the bag to dispose safely of waste items such as soiled dressings. The bag should then be sealed and incinerated.

LOOKING AFTER YOURSELF (continued)

Dealing with stress

It is natural to feel stressed when you are called upon to administer first aid and to be very emotional once you have finished treating the victim. Stress can interfere with a person's physical and mental well-being. Some people are more susceptible to stress than others. It is important to learn how to deal with stress to maintain your own health and effectiveness as a first aider.

FEELINGS AFTER AN INCIDENT

For all first aiders, an emergency is an emotional experience. Emotional reactions can include satisfaction or even elation, but it is more common to feel upset. After you have treated a victim – depending on the type of incident and the outcome – you might experience:

- Satisfaction and pleasure.
- Confusion and doubt.
- Anger and sadness.

Never reproach yourself or try to hide your feelings. It is much more helpful to talk over your experience with a colleague, your supervisor, your first-aid trainer, or your own doctor. By doing so you will probably find that your feelings about the incident resolve quickly. Ideally, speak to someone else who was present at the incident because both of you may be having similar feelings.

DELAYED REACTIONS

Involvement in an incident can lead to a delayed stress reaction once you have returned to your everyday environment. The extent of the effect may depend on the level of your first-aid experience and the nature of the incident. In the longer term, stress can manifest itself in many different ways, including:

- Tremor of the hands and stomach.
- Excessive sweating.
- Flashbacks of the incident.
- Nightmares or disturbed sleep.
- Tearfulness.
- Tension and irritability.
- Withdrawal and isolation.

These symptoms should pass in time. Exercise or relaxation techniques, such as meditation or yoga, may help. In fact, doing any activity that you enjoy is a good way to relax and may help you to relieve tension.

SEVERE STRESS REACTIONS

If you have witnessed or experienced a serious threat to life, you may find yourself suffering from severe feelings of stress for some time after the incident. You might be:

- Reliving the event.
- Avoiding situations, people, and places associated with the event.
- Feeling hyperactive and restless.

If you experience intrusive or persistent symptoms associated with a stressful incident, it is important that you seek medical help from your doctor or possibly from a counselor.

Talking to a friend
Face up to what has happened by confiding in a friend or relative. Ideally, talk to someone who also attended the incident; he or she may have the same feelings as you.

REGULATIONS AND LEGISLATION

First aid may be practiced in any situation where accidents or illnesses have occurred. In many cases, the first person on the scene is an ordinary citizen who wants to help, rather than someone who is medically trained. The United States has no laws governing the administration of first aid in such cases, although it is important to be aware that giving first aid to others involves certain ethical and legal considerations.

Good Samaritan principles

People are encouraged to help those in distress by an acceptance in all 50 states of the Good Samaritan principles. If you assist someone during an emergency, acting in good faith with neither compensation nor gross negligence, the law will generally grant you immunity.

In any circumstances where help may be needed, you must first identify yourself and get permission from the victim to provide assistance. An individual has the right to refuse your offer of help and, should he do so, this must be respected.

In some circumstances, obtaining consent from the afflicted individual is not possible. In the case of a young child, obtain consent from the immediate family or parent, if they are present. Consent is implied with an unconscious person in a life-threatening condition, because it is assumed that an unresponsive victim would consent to lifesaving interventions. Consent is also implied when the first-aider begins care and the victim does not resist. Some people do not wish to be resuscitated, and such information may be visible on a Medic Alert bracelet or on a card in the victim's wallet. You must always honor this request.

Provide any first-aid assistance to the best of your abilities. Once you have accepted the responsibility of assisting someone in need, do not abandon that person until other appropriate help has arrived, you are too exhausted to continue, or your life is in danger. If you are unsure of yourself, call for help or do what you know, and wait for someone more experienced to take over.

Providing first-aid assistance to someone in need is a humanitarian act supported by society. As long as you respect the wishes of the individual and provide care to the very best of your ability, your first-aid skills will be appreciated by those you assist, and valued by your community.

Taking first-aid courses

Reading this manual is an important first step in familiarizing yourself with first-aid principles and practices. Learning the contents of this book will equip you with the confidence and knowledge to provide first aid to acutely ill and injured people.

However, knowledge of first aid must be combined with the practical skills necessary to administer physical care and assistance. You can best acquire these skills by taking a course from a qualified first-aid instructor.

First-aid courses are provided by the American Red Cross, National Safety Council, and various other organizations. Ask friends who have trained in first aid to recommend a suitable course, or call providers listed in your telephone directory under "First-Aid Services."

With the information and skills you acquire, you should be comfortable providing first aid and confident in your ability to assist someone in need.

ACTION AT AN EMERGENCY

In any emergency, you must follow a clear plan of action. This will enable you to prioritize the demands that may be made on you and help you decide on your response. The principal steps are: Assess the situation, Make the area safe, Give emergency aid, and Get help from others (below).

Before taking any action, try to control your feelings and take a moment to think. It is important to avoid placing yourself in danger, so do not rush into a potentially risky situation. Be aware of hazards such as gas or chemicals. In addition, do not attempt to do too much by yourself.

FIRST-AID PRIORITIES
- Assess the situation. Quickly and calmly, observe what has happened, and look for dangers to yourself and to the victim. Never put yourself at risk.
- Make the area safe. Protect the victim from danger as far as you can, but be aware of your limitations.
- Give emergency aid. Assess all victims to determine treatment priorities, and treat those with life-threatening conditions first.
- Get help from others. Quickly make sure that any necessary medical aid or other expert help has been called and is on its way.

Assess the situation

Your approach should be brisk but calm and controlled. Your priorities are to identify any risks to yourself, to the victim, and to bystanders, then to assess the resources available to you and the kind of help you may need. When offering your help, state that you have first-aid skills. If there are no doctors, nurses, EMS personnel, or more experienced people present, calmly take charge. First, ask yourself these questions:
- Is there any continuing danger?
- Is anyone's life in immediate danger?
- Are there any bystanders who can help?
- Do I need specialized help?

Make the area safe

The conditions that gave rise to the incident may still be presenting a danger. Remember that you must put your own safety first. Often, simple measures, such as turning off a switch, are enough to make the area safe. If you cannot eliminate a life-threatening hazard, you should try to put some distance between it and the victim and minimize the danger if possible. As a last resort, you should remove the victim from the danger (*see* VICTIM HANDLING, pp.63–64). Usually, you will need specialized help and equipment to move a victim.

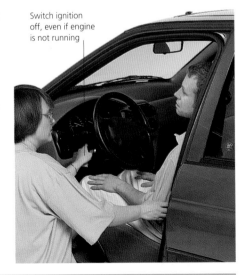

Switch ignition off, even if engine is not running

Making a vehicle safe
The first priority, when dealing with a victim who is inside a vehicle, is to switch the ignition off. This action will reduce the risk of a spark causing a fire.

Give emergency aid

Once the area has been made safe, quickly carry out an initial assessment, or primary survey, of each victim (p.29) so that any victim needing emergency first aid is treated immediately. However, do not delay in summoning necessary help; if possible, ask a bystander to do this.

For each victim, establish the following:
- Is he conscious?
- Is his airway open?
- Is he breathing?
- Does he have signs of circulation?

Your findings dictate your priorities and when and how much help is needed.

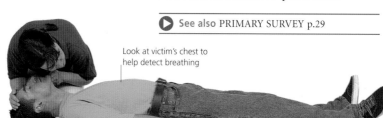

See also PRIMARY SURVEY p.29

Carrying out emergency aid
As soon as it is safe to do so, carry out a primary survey: check that the victim has an open airway, is breathing, and has signs of circulation.

Look at victim's chest to help detect breathing

Get help from others

You may be faced with several tasks: to maintain safety, to call for help (overleaf), and to start first aid. Other people can be asked to perform the following functions:
- Make the area safe.
- Telephone for assistance.
- Fetch first-aid equipment.
- Control traffic and onlookers.
- Control bleeding or support a limb.
- Maintain the victim's privacy.
- Transport the victim to a safe place.

CONTROLLING BYSTANDERS
The reactions of bystanders may cause you concern or even anger. They may have had no first-aid training and may feel helpless or frightened. If they have witnessed or been involved in the incident themselves, they too may be injured and will certainly be distressed. Bear this in mind if you need to ask a bystander to help you in some way. Use a firm but gentle manner.

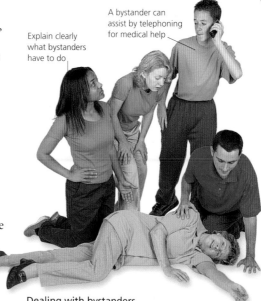

A bystander can assist by telephoning for medical help

Explain clearly what bystanders have to do

Dealing with bystanders
People at the scene of an incident may be able to help you in several ways, such as getting equipment or controlling other onlookers. Tell them that you have first-aid training, and be clear in what you ask.

TELEPHONING FOR HELP

You can summon help by telephone from a number of sources.

● **Emergency services (dial 9·1·1):** In most areas, dialing 9·1·1 will connect you to a dispatcher who contacts the police, fire department, or EMS. Some areas in the US do not have 9·1·1 service. If you are in such an area, you must dial the number of your local emergency service. Carry this telephone number with you at all times.

Emergency calls are free and can be made from any telephone, including most car phones and cellular phones.

Most large companies have special arrangements for calling for assistance, and you should try to ensure that you are familiar with all of them.

If it is necessary to leave an injured person alone to telephone for help, minimize the risk to the victim by taking any vital action first (*see* PRIMARY SURVEY, p.29). Make your call short but detailed and accurate. If you ask someone else to make the call, always ask this person to come back after the call has been made to confirm that help is on the way.

Making a call

When you dial 9·1·1, you will be asked which service you require and will be put through to the appropriate dispatcher. Whenever there are injured people involved, ask for the emergency medical services. If you are unsure of your location, do not panic – in many municipalities your call can be traced. Stay on the telephone until the dispatcher has hung up. You may be asked to remain by the telephone to "lead in" the emergency services. If you delegate this task, make sure the person understands how important it is, and that he reports back to you.

WHAT TO TELL EMERGENCY SERVICES
State your name and the location and nature of the incident clearly. The following details are essential:

● Your telephone number.
● The exact location of the incident; give a road name or number, if possible, and mention any intersections or landmarks.
● The type and gravity of the emergency; for example, "Traffic incident, two cars, road blocked, three people are trapped."
● The number, sex, and approximate ages of the victims, and anything you know about their condition; for example, "Man, early fifties, suspected heart attack, cardiac arrest."
● Details of any hazards such as gas, toxic substances, power-line damage, or relevant weather conditions, such as fog or ice.

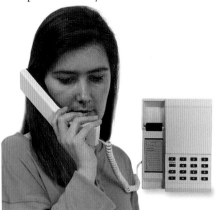

Phoning the emergency services
Try to stay calm so that you can give all the information the emergency services need. Do not hang up until the dispatcher has cleared the line.

MULTIPLE VICTIMS

In situations such as major traffic accidents, you may find yourself having to deal with several victims at the same time. You may be on your own, working with other first aiders, or assisting professionals. Whatever the situation, a systematic, calm approach is crucial in the initial chaos. Identify and attend to all unconscious victims first, and conduct a primary survey (p.29) to find and treat any life-threatening injuries.

Dealing with the incident

Major incidents involving a large number of victims can place overwhelming demands on rescuers. The most experienced first aider present should take charge.

The first task is to make sure that the emergency services are contacted and given accurate information about the incident. The next priority is to assess the scene and, if possible, to make it safe. Then, if it is safe to do so, start giving emergency first aid. If other first aiders come forward, give them as much information as possible.

When the emergency services arrive, they will take control of the situation. It is essential not to disturb any evidence at the site of the incident because there may be a legal inquiry later.

THE ROLE OF THE FIRST AIDER
At major public events, the first aiders constitute the on-site medical team until EMS arrives. When they do arrive, your role in dealing with the incident will obviously diminish.

At any major incident, you must leave the scene if you are asked to do so by a member of the emergency services. However, you may be asked to assist the medical team by performing simple tasks – for example, holding drips or supporting injured limbs. Always do as you are asked; your help will be greatly appreciated.

HOW YOU CAN HELP
● Identify the serious victims and mark them for immediate treatment. Move all victims with minor injuries quickly from the site to allow access to serious cases; minor injuries can be treated when time allows. This process is called triage.
● Leave any victims who are obviously dead so that you can give effective help to those who need it.
● Label all victims, and write down their names and the details about their condition, to provide accurate records for medical personnel.
● Alert workers or residents near the site of a disaster to any further hazards.

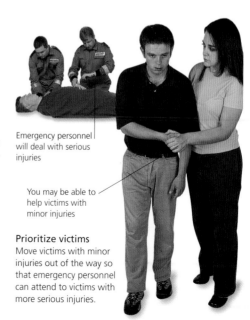

Emergency personnel will deal with serious injuries

You may be able to help victims with minor injuries

Prioritize victims
Move victims with minor injuries out of the way so that emergency personnel can attend to victims with more serious injuries.

ROAD INCIDENTS

The severity of road incidents can range from a fall from a bicycle to a major vehicle crash that involves many victims. Often, the incident site will present serious risks to safety, largely because of passing traffic.

It is essential to make the incident area safe before attending to any victims. This measure enables you to protect yourself, the victims, and other road users. Once the area is safe, quickly assess the victims and prioritize treatment. Help those who need emergency aid before treating anyone else.

▶ **See also** ● CRUSH INJURY p.133 ● PRIMARY SURVEY p.29 ● SPINAL INJURY pp.165–167

Make the area safe

First, ensure your own safety and do not do anything that might put you in danger.
● Park safely, well clear of the incident site, and turn on your flashing hazard lights.
● Do not run across a busy highway.
● At night, wear or carry something light or reflective, and use a flashlight.
Then take these general precautions:
● Have a helper warn drivers to slow down.
● Set up warning triangles or lights at least 50yds (45m) from the site in each direction.
● Switch off the ignition of any damaged vehicle and, if you can, disconnect the battery. Switch off the fuel supply on diesel vehicles and motorcycles if possible.
● Stabilize the vehicle. If it is upright, apply the handbrake and put it in gear, or place blocks just in front of the wheels. If a vehicle is on its side, do not attempt to right it, but try to prevent it from rolling over.
● Look out for physical dangers. Make sure that no one smokes. Alert EMS to damaged power lines, spilled fuel, or vehicles displaying hazardous substance symbols.

HAZARDOUS SUBSTANCES

Incidents may be complicated by spills of dangerous substances or the escape of toxic vapors. Keep bystanders away, bearing in mind that poisonous fumes may be released and travel some distance. Stand upwind of the accident. Note any hazardous substance symbols on vehicles and inform EMS. If in doubt about your safety or the meaning of a symbol, keep your distance and take particular care if there is a spill.

Hazardous substance symbols

The symbols shown here warn that a vehicle is carrying a hazardous substance. The numbers are coded and will be understood by EMS, so make a note of the numbers and pass them on when telephoning for help.

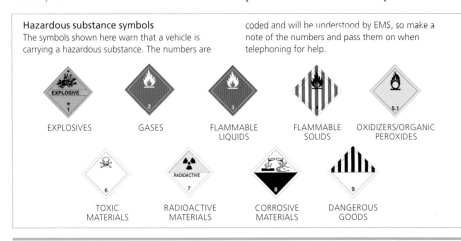

EXPLOSIVES   GASES   FLAMMABLE LIQUIDS   FLAMMABLE SOLIDS   OXIDIZERS/ORGANIC PEROXIDES

TOXIC MATERIALS   RADIOACTIVE MATERIALS   CORROSIVE MATERIALS   DANGEROUS GOODS

Check the victims

Quickly assess all victims. If there is more than one victim, deal first with those who may have life-threatening injuries, such as severe wounds or burns. If possible, treat victims in the position in which you find them; move them only if they are in danger or to provide life-saving treatment.

Search the area thoroughly, so that you do not overlook any victim who has been thrown clear or who has wandered away from the site while confused.

If a victim is trapped inside or under a vehicle, you will need the help of the fire and rescue services, so call them at once.

When dealing with a victim, first carry out a primary survey (p.29) and deal with any life-threatening injuries if possible. Always assume that there is a neck (spinal) injury in any victim who has been injured in a traffic accident, and support the head with your hands until help arrives.

Monitor and record the victim's vital signs while waiting for specialized help: level of response, pulse, and breathing (pp.42–43).

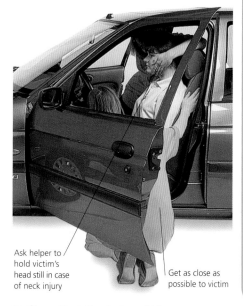

Ask helper to hold victim's head still in case of neck injury

Get as close as possible to victim

Dealing with victims in the vehicle
Bystanders can help by supporting the victim's head while you check her for any injuries that may be potentially life-threatening.

Dealing with victims on the road
Once you are sure that the situation is safe, check the victim for life-threatening injuries. Move the victim only if absolutely necessary.

> **⚠ WARNING**
>
> ● Do not move the victim unless it is absolutely necessary.
>
> ● If it is essential to move the victim, the method you use will depend on the victim's condition and whether help is available (*see* VICTIM HANDLING, pp.63–64).
>
> ● Ask a bystander to mark the position of the vehicle and the victim to provide information for the police.

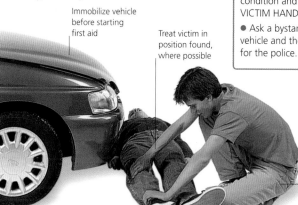

Immobilize vehicle before starting first aid

Treat victim in position found, where possible

Place warning triangles at least 50 yds (45 m) away to alert other road users before they reach incident site

Make sure that you are not in danger

FIRES

Rapid, clear thinking at a fire is vital. Fire spreads very quickly, so your first priority is to warn any people at risk. If in a building, activate the nearest fire alarm. You should also alert the emergency services at once, but do not put your safety at risk if this action will delay your escape from the area.

Panic spreads fast among people trapped in a fire. As a first aider, you may be able to reduce panic by trying to calm anyone whose behavior is likely to increase alarm in others. Encourage and assist people to evacuate the area. Do not delay or re-enter a burning building to collect personal possessions. Do not return to a building until cleared to do so by a fire officer.

▶ **See also** BURNS TO THE AIRWAY p.197
● INHALATION OF FUMES pp.110–111
● SEVERE BURNS AND SCALDS pp.194–195

Dealing with fire

A fire needs three components to start and maintain it: ignition (an electric spark or open flame); a source of fuel (gasoline, wood, or fabric); and oxygen (air). Remove any one of these to break this "triangle of fire." For example:
● Switch off a car's ignition, or pull the fuel cut-off on a large diesel vehicle.

● Remove from the path of a fire any combustible materials, such as paper or cardboard, that may fuel the flames.
● Shut a door on a fire in order to cut off its oxygen supply.
● Smother flames with a fire blanket or other impervious substance to prevent oxygen from reaching them.

Leaving a burning building

If you see or suspect a fire in a building, activate the first fire alarm you see. Try to help people out of the building without putting yourself at risk. Close doors behind you to help prevent the fire from spreading. Look for fire exits and assembly points.

You should already know the evacuation procedure at your workplace. If you are visiting other premises, follow the signs for escape routes and obey any instructions.

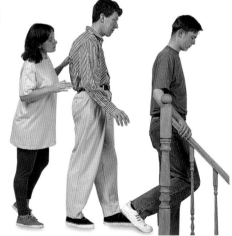

Helping escape from a burning building
Encourage people to leave the building calmly but quickly by the nearest safe exit. If you need to use stairs, make sure that people do not rush and risk falling.

Clothing on fire

Always follow this procedure: Stop, Drop, and Roll. If possible, wrap the victim in heavy fabric before rolling him.

- Stop the victim from panicking, running around, or going outside; any movement or breeze will fan the flames.
- Drop the victim to the ground.
- If possible, wrap the victim tightly in a coat, curtain, blanket (not a nylon or cellular type), rug, or other heavy fabric.
- Roll the victim along the ground until the flames have been smothered.
- If water or another nonflammable liquid is readily available, lay the victim down with the burning side uppermost and cool the burn with the liquid.

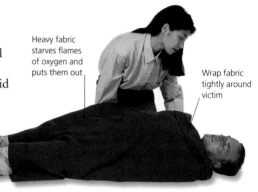

Heavy fabric starves flames of oxygen and puts them out

Wrap fabric tightly around victim

Smoke and fumes

Fire in a confined space creates a dangerous atmosphere that is low in oxygen and may be polluted by carbon monoxide and toxic fumes. Never enter a burning or smoke-filled building or open a door leading to a fire. Let the fire department do this.

WHAT YOU CAN DO
- If trapped in a burning building, go into a room with a window and shut the door. If you have to cross a smoke-filled room, stay low: air is clearest at floor level.
- If you have to escape through a window, go out feet first; lower yourself to the full length of your arms before dropping down.

Avoiding smoke and fumes
Take measures to avoid inhaling harmful smoke and fumes if you are in a burning building. Block any gaps under the door, and stay down close to the floor where you are less likely to encounter smoke.

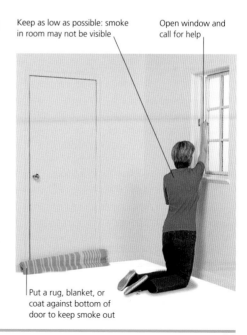

Keep as low as possible: smoke in room may not be visible

Open window and call for help

Put a rug, blanket, or coat against bottom of door to keep smoke out

ELECTRICAL INJURIES

When a person is electrocuted, the passage of electrical current through the body may stun him, causing his breathing and even his heartbeat to stop. The electrical current may cause burns both where it enters the body and where it exits the body to go to "earth." In some cases, the current also causes muscular spasms that may prevent a victim from breaking contact with it, so the person may still be electrically charged ("live") when you come on the scene.

Electrical injuries usually occur in the home or workplace, due to contact with sources of low-voltage current (opposite). They may also result from contact with sources of high-voltage current (below), such as fallen power lines. People who are electrocuted by a high-voltage current rarely survive.

▶ See also ELECTRICAL BURN p.198
● LIFE-SAVING PROCEDURES pp.71–102

Lightning

A natural burst of electricity discharged from the atmosphere, lightning forms an intense trail of light and heat. The lightning seeks contact with the ground through the nearest tall feature in the landscape and,

possibly, through anyone standing nearby. A lightning strike may set clothing on fire, knock the victim down, or even cause instant death. Clear everyone from the site of a lightning strike as soon as possible.

High-voltage current

Contact with high-voltage current, found in power lines and overhead high-tension (HT) cables, is usually immediately fatal. Anyone who survives will have severe burns. In addition, the shock produces a muscular spasm that may propel the victim some distance, causing injuries such as fractures.

High-voltage electricity may jump ("arc") up to 20yds (18m). Materials such as dry wood or clothing will not protect you. Do not put yourself in danger. Before you approach the victim, it is essential to ensure that the power is cut off and isolated.

The victim is likely to be unconscious. Once it is safe to do so, open the airway and check breathing; be ready to begin rescue breaths and chest compressions if necessary (see LIFE-SAVING PROCEDURES, pp.71–102). If the victim is breathing, place him in the recovery position. Regularly monitor and record vital signs – level of response, pulse, and breathing (pp.42–43).

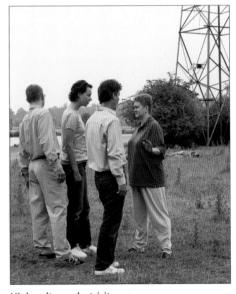

High-voltage electricity
Keep any bystanders away from any incident involving high-voltage current. A safe distance is more than 20 yds (18 m) from the source of the electricity.

Low-voltage current

Domestic current, used in homes and workplaces, can cause serious injury or even death. Incidents are usually due to faulty switches, frayed insulation, or defective appliances. Young children are particularly at risk – they may put fingers or other objects into electrical wall sockets.

Water, which is a dangerously efficient conductor of electricity, presents additional risks. Handling an otherwise safe electrical appliance with wet hands, or when standing on a wet floor, greatly increases the risk of an electric shock.

WHAT YOU CAN DO
Break the contact between the victim and the electrical supply by switching off the current at the main switch or fuse box if it can be reached easily. Otherwise, unplug or disconnect the appliance.

If you cannot reach the plug or main switch, do the following:
● To protect yourself, stand on some dry insulating material such as a wooden box, a plastic mat, or a telephone book.
● Using something made of wood (such as a broom), push the victim's limbs away from the electrical source or push the source away from the victim.

Removing the source of electricity
If you cannot switch off the electric current, stand on dry insulating material, such as a telephone book, and use a broom handle to move the electrical source away from the victim. Do not touch the victim directly.

> **❶ WARNING**
>
> ● Do not touch the victim if he is in contact with the electrical current; he will be "live" and you risk electrocution.
>
> ● Do not use anything metallic to break the electrical contact. Stand on some dry insulating material and use a wooden object.
>
> ● If the victim stops breathing, be prepared to give rescue breaths and chest compressions (see LIFE-SAVING PROCEDURES, pp.71–102) until emergency help arrives.

● If it is not possible to break the contact with a wooden object, loop a length of rope around the victim's ankles or under the arms, taking great care not to touch him, and pull him away from the source of the electrical current.
● If absolutely necessary, pull the victim free by pulling at any articles of loose, dry clothing. Do this only as a last resort because the victim may still be "live."

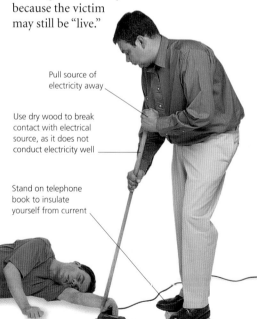

Pull source of electricity away

Use dry wood to break contact with electrical source, as it does not conduct electricity well

Stand on telephone book to insulate yourself from current

Victim may still be "live"

WATER RESCUE

Incidents around water may involve people of any age. Young children are at risk around even very shallow water. However, most cases of drowning involve people who have been swimming in strong currents or very cold water, or who have been swimming or boating after drinking alcohol.

DANGERS OF COLD WATER

Open water in the US is often very cold, even in summer. Ocean temperatures range from 41°F (5°C) to 59°F (15°C); inland waters may be even colder.

Cold water increases the dangers to both the victim and the rescuer because it may cause the following:

• Uncontrollable gasping when the person enters the water, with the consequent risk of water inhalation.

• A sudden rise in blood pressure, which can precipitate a heart attack.

• Sudden inability to swim.

• Hypothermia if the person is immersed in the water for a prolonged period or is exposed to the wind.

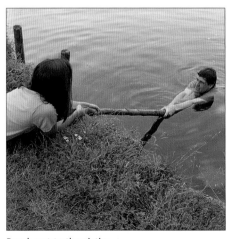

Reach out to the victim
If possible, avoid entering the water yourself to rescue a victim. Instead, hold out a long object such as a stick for the victim to grasp, then pull him toward land.

> **❶ CAUTION**
>
> If the victim is unconscious, lift her clear of the water, and carry her with her head lower than her chest to protect the airway if she vomits.

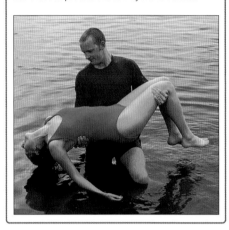

WHAT YOU CAN DO

Your first priority is to get the victim onto dry land with the minimum of danger to yourself. The safest way to rescue a victim is to stay on land and pull him from the water with your hand, a stick, a branch, or a rope; alternatively, throw him a float. If you are a trained life-saver, or if the victim is unconscious, you may have to wade or swim to the victim and tow him to dry land. It is safer to wade than to swim.

Once the victim is out of the water, try to shield him from the wind, if possible, to prevent his body from being chilled any further, and then treat him for drowning (p.109) and the effects of severe cold (*see* HYPOTHERMIA, pp.206–208).

Arrange to take or send the victim to a hospital, even if he seems to have recovered well. If necessary, or if you are at all concerned, dial 9·1·1 or call EMS.

 See also DROWNING p.109
• HYPOTHERMIA pp.206–208

ASSESSING A VICTIM

Your first duty when attending a victim is to assess him or her for life-threatening conditions that need emergency first aid. This initial assessment is called the primary survey. Once the victim is out of immediate danger, you should carry out a secondary survey (pp.30–31). For information on when to dial 9·1·1 or call EMS, see p.74.

PRIMARY SURVEY

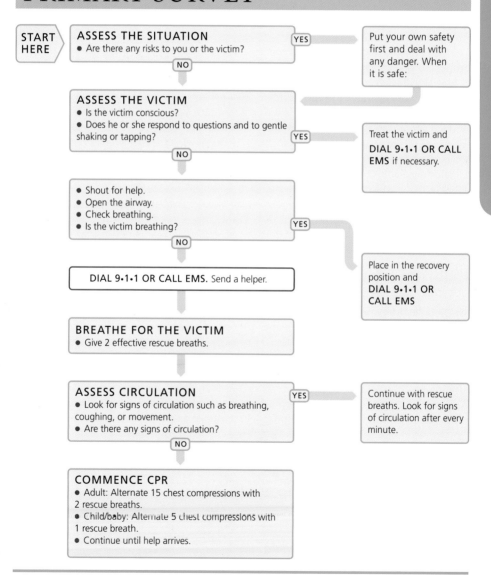

START HERE

ASSESS THE SITUATION
- Are there any risks to you or the victim?

YES → Put your own safety first and deal with any danger. When it is safe:

NO ↓

ASSESS THE VICTIM
- Is the victim conscious?
- Does he or she respond to questions and to gentle shaking or tapping?

YES → Treat the victim and **DIAL 9·1·1 OR CALL EMS** if necessary.

NO ↓

- Shout for help.
- Open the airway.
- Check breathing.
- Is the victim breathing?

YES → Place in the recovery position and **DIAL 9·1·1 OR CALL EMS**

NO ↓

DIAL 9·1·1 OR CALL EMS. Send a helper.

↓

BREATHE FOR THE VICTIM
- Give 2 effective rescue breaths.

↓

ASSESS CIRCULATION
- Look for signs of circulation such as breathing, coughing, or movement.
- Are there any signs of circulation?

YES → Continue with rescue breaths. Look for signs of circulation after every minute.

NO ↓

COMMENCE CPR
- Adult: Alternate 15 chest compressions with 2 rescue breaths.
- Child/baby: Alternate 5 chest compressions with 1 rescue breath.
- Continue until help arrives.

SECONDARY SURVEY

Once you have made sure that the victim is out of immediate danger, and you have completed the primary survey (previous page), carry out a secondary survey. This action involves finding out what happened (taking a history) and performing a physical examination (pp.34–35). Circumstances determine how detailed the examination will be. For example, in cold, wet conditions, when help is on its way, only major injuries need attention; the priority is to keep the victim warm and dry. If a person can describe any of the symptoms (p.32), concentrate on treating these problems.

Taking a history

The history is the story of how an incident happened, how any injury was sustained, or how any illness began and continued. To take the history, question the victim and talk to any bystanders who witnessed the incident. Try to form a full picture of the situation. For example:

● When did the victim last have something to eat or drink?
● Does the victim have any illness, and is he taking any medication?
● How much force was involved in an injury, and how was it exerted (opposite)?

● Ask about the environment – was the victim in a hot and stuffy, or cold, room, or exposed to wind or rain?
● Find out the victim's age and state of health: a young, fit adult who trips may sprain a wrist or an ankle, but an elderly woman who does the same is more likely to break her arm or her hip.
● Establish who the victim is and, if possible, where he lives.

Make a note of this information, including the time of injury and your examination, to give to a doctor or emergency services.

External clues

If the victim is unable to cooperate, or is unconscious, look for external clues about his or her condition. (Beware needles and syringes if you suspect drug abuse.) You may find an appointment card for a hospital or clinic, or a card indicating a history of allergy, diabetes, or epilepsy. Horseback-riders or cyclists may carry such a card inside a riding hat or helmet.

Medication or food may also give valuable clues about an incident; for example, people with diabetes may carry sugar lumps. In addition, a person with a known disorder may have medical warning information on a special necklace or bracelet (such as a "MedicAlert") or on a wallet card. Keep any such item with the victim or give it to the emergency services.

  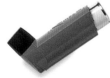 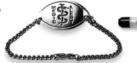 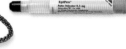

Medicines
Nitroglycerin is taken for angina and phenytoin for epilepsy.

"Puffer" inhaler
The presence of an inhaler usually indicates that the victim has asthma.

Warning bracelet
May give diagnosis and a phone number for more on victim's medical history.

Auto-injector
This contains epinephrine (adrenaline), for people at risk of anaphylactic shock.

Mechanics of injury

You can gain further clues about possible injuries and their extent by looking at the circumstances in which the injury was sustained and the forces involved. This information is useful because it can help people predict the type and severity of injury. In many cases, this vital information can only be obtained by those people who deal with the victim at the scene or at the time of injury – often first aiders.

CIRCUMSTANCES OF INJURY

The extent and type of injuries sustained due to impact – for example, falls from a height or the impact of a car crash – can be predicted if you know exactly how the incident happened. For example, a car occupant is more likely to sustain serious injuries in a side impact collision than in a frontal collision at the same speed. This is because the side of the car provides less protection and cannot absorb as much energy as the front of the vehicle.

In a driver who is wearing a seat-belt and whose vehicle is struck head-on or from behind, a specific pattern of injuries can be suspected. The body is suddenly propelled one way, but the head lags behind for a moment before moving. This results in a "whiplashing" movement of the neck (right). The victim may also have injuries due to seat belt restraint, such as bruising or fracture of the breastbone and possibly bruising of the heart or lungs. There may be injuries to the face due to contact with the steering wheel or an inflated air bag.

FORCES EXERTED ON THE BODY

The energy forces exerted during an impact are another important indicator of the type or severity of any injury. For example, if a man falls from a height of 3 ft (1 m)

onto hard ground, he will probably suffer bruising but no serious injury. A fall from a height greater than 6 ft (2 m), however, is likely to produce more serious injuries, such as rib and pelvic fractures and internal bleeding from injury to internal organs.

QUESTIONS TO ASK

When you are attending a victim, ask the victim, or any witnesses, questions to try to find out the mechanics of the injury. Possible questions include the following:
- Was the victim ejected from a vehicle?
- Was the victim wearing a correctly adjusted seat belt?
- Did the vehicle roll over?
- Was the victim wearing a helmet?
- How far did the victim fall?
- What type of surface did he land on?
- Is there evidence of body contact with a solid object, such as the floor or a vehicle's windscreen or dashboard?

Such questions are especially important if victims are unable to provide you with the information themselves. Pass on all the information that you have gathered to the emergency services (p.37).

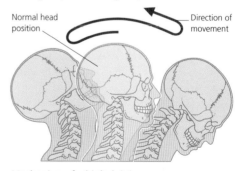

Normal head position

Direction of movement

Mechanism of whiplash injury
The head may be whipped backward and then rapidly forward, or vice versa, due to the sudden forces on the body in a car crash. This produces a whiplash injury, with strained muscles and stretched ligaments in the neck.

SYMPTOMS AND SIGNS

Injuries and illnesses usually manifest themselves as groups of distinctive features. There are two types of feature: symptoms (below), which the victim may report, and signs (opposite), which you may detect. Some features will be obvious, but others may be missed unless you examine the victim thoroughly (pp.34–35).

Wherever possible, examine a conscious victim in the position in which he is found, and with any obvious injury supported.

If the victim is unconscious, the airway must first be cleared and kept open. Do not remove items of clothing unnecessarily, and do not leave the victim exposed to cold any longer than required. Use your senses – look, listen, feel, and smell.

Be quick and alert but thorough, and do not make unjustified assumptions. You should handle the victim gently, but your touch must be sufficiently firm for you to detect any swelling, irregularity, or tender spot. If he is conscious, ask him to describe any sensations that your touch causes.

Feel along and compare both sides of body at same time

Watch victim's face for expressions of pain or anxiety

Looking for signs
A head-to-toe examination of the victim will help you detect signs of injury or illness and identify the condition.

Examine feet last of all

Assessing symptoms

Symptoms are sensations that the victim experiences and may be able to describe. Ask if she has had any abnormal sensations. If there is pain, ask where she feels it, what type of pain it is, what makes it better or worse, and how it is affected by movement and breathing. If the pain did not follow an injury, ask how and where it began. Ask if there are other symptoms, such as nausea, giddiness, heat, cold, weakness, or thirst. If appropriate, confirm the symptoms by an examination for signs of injury or illness.

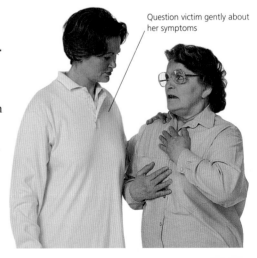

Question victim gently about her symptoms

Asking about symptoms
A victim may be able to tell you about any symptoms that she is experiencing. These details may help you determine the nature of the injury or illness.

Looking for signs

Signs are details of a victim's condition that you can see, feel, hear, or smell. Many are obvious, but others may be discovered only by means of a thorough examination (pp.34–35). Assess the victim's level of response (p.42). If she is unconscious or unable to speak clearly, you may have to make a diagnosis purely on the history of the incident, information obtained from any onlookers, and the signs that you find.

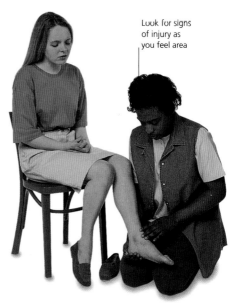

Look for signs of injury as you feel area

APPLY YOUR SENSES

Look for features such as swelling, bleeding, discoloration, or deformity. Feel the rhythm and strength of the pulse (p.42). Listen to breathing, and check for any abnormal sounds, such as crackling due to air trapped in skin tissues. Gently feel areas that are painful; note any tenderness over bones and changes in alignment. Check if the victim is unable to perform normal functions, such as moving the limbs. Use your sense of smell to search for further clues.

Feeling for signs of injury
When examining an injured part of the body, feel for tenderness, and look for deformity or color changes around the site of the injury. Keep the part well supported while you examine it.

SYMPTOMS AND SIGNS OF ILLNESS OR INJURY

Method of identification	Symptoms or signs
The victim may tell you of these symptoms	Pain ● Anxiety ● Heat ● Cold ● Loss of sensation ● Abnormal sensation ● Thirst ● Nausea ● Tingling ● Pain on touch or pressure ● Faintness ● Stiffness ● Momentary unconsciousness ● Weakness ● Memory loss ● Dizziness ● Sensation of broken bone ● Sense of impending doom
You may see these signs	Anxiety and painful expression ● Unusual chest movement ● Burns ● Sweating ● Wounds ● Bleeding from orifices ● Response to touch ● Response to speech ● Bruising ● Abnormal skin color ● Muscle spasm ● Swelling ● Deformity ● Foreign bodies ● Needle marks ● Vomit ● Incontinence ● Loss of normal movement ● Containers and other circumstantial evidence
You may feel these signs	Dampness ● Abnormal body temperature ● Swelling ● Deformity ● Irregularity ● Grating bone ends
You may hear these signs	Noisy or distressed breathing ● Groaning ● Sucking sounds (chest injury) ● Response to touch ● Response to speech ● Grating bone (crepitus)
You may smell these signs	Acetone ● Alcohol ● Burning ● Gas or fumes ● Solvents or glue ● Urine ● Feces ● Cannabis

EXAMINING A VICTIM

Once you have taken the history (p.30) and asked about any symptoms that the victim has (p.32), you should carry out a detailed examination of the person. During this procedure you may have to move or remove clothing (pp.40–41), but ensure that you do not move the victim more than is strictly necessary. Always start at the head and work down; this "head-to-toe" routine is both easily remembered and thorough.

Head-to-toe survey

1 Run your hands carefully over the scalp to feel for bleeding, swelling, or depression, which may indicate a possible fracture. Be careful not to move the victim if you suspect that she may have injured her neck.

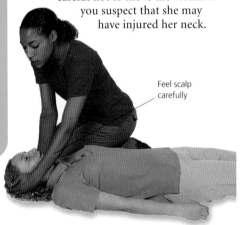

Feel scalp carefully

2 Speak clearly to the victim in both ears to find out if she responds or if she can hear. Look for blood or clear fluid (or both) coming from either ear. These discharges may be signs of damage inside the skull.

3 Examine both eyes. Note whether the eyes are open. Check the size of the pupils, whether the pupils are equal in size (as they should be), and whether they react to light (the pupils should shrink when light falls on them). Look for any foreign object, blood, or bruising in the whites of the eyes.

4 Check the nose for discharges as you did for the ears. Look for blood or clear fluid (or a mixture of both) coming from either nostril. Any of these discharges might indicate damage inside the skull.

5 Note the rate, depth, and nature (easy or difficult, noisy or quiet) of the breathing. Note any odor on the breath. Look inside the mouth for anything that might obstruct the airway. If the victim is wearing dentures, and these are intact and fit firmly, leave them in place. Look for any wound in the mouth or irregularity in the line of the teeth. Check the lips for burns.

6 Note the color, temperature, and state of the skin: is it pale, flushed, or gray-blue (cyanosis); is it hot or cold, dry or damp? For example, pale, cold, sweaty skin suggests shock; a flushed, hot face suggests fever or heatstroke. A blue tinge indicates lack of oxygen; look for this sign especially in the lips, ears, and face.

7 Loosen clothing around the neck, and look for signs such as a medical warning medallion (p.30) or a hole (stoma) in the windpipe left by a surgical operation. Run your fingers gently along the spine from the base of the skull downward as far as possible, without disturbing the victim's position; check for any irregularity, swelling, or tenderness.

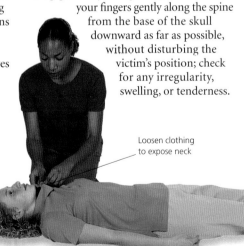

Loosen clothing to expose neck

8 Ask the victim to breathe deeply, and note whether the chest expands evenly, easily, and equally on both sides. Feel the rib cage to check for deformity, irregularity, or tenderness. Ask if the victim feels grating sensations on breathing, and listen for unusual sounds. Observe whether breathing causes any pain. Look for bleeding.

11 If there is any impairment in movement or loss of sensation in the limbs, do not move the victim to examine the spine, because these signs suggest spinal injury. Otherwise, gently pass your hand under the hollow of the back and feel along the spine, checking for swelling and tenderness.

12 Gently feel the victim's abdomen to detect any evidence of bleeding, and to identify any rigidity or tenderness of the abdomen's muscular wall.

Feel gently with your whole hand

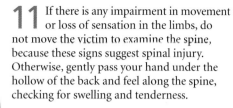
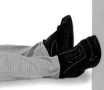

9 Gently feel along both the collarbones and the shoulders for any deformity, irregularity or tenderness.

13 Feel both sides of the hips, and gently move the pelvis to look for signs of fracture. Check the clothing for any evidence of incontinence or bleeding from orifices.

10 Check the movements of the elbows, wrists, and fingers by asking the victim to bend and straighten the arm and hand at each of the joints. Check that the victim can

Support the arm while checking movement

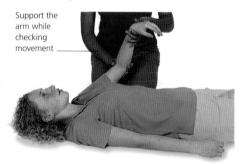

14 Ask the victim to raise each leg in turn, and to move her ankles and knees. Look and feel for bleeding, swelling, deformity, or tenderness.

15 Check the movement and feeling in the toes. Look at their skin color: gray-blue skin may indicate a circulatory disorder or an injury due to cold.

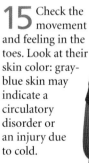
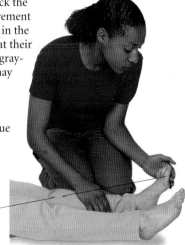

feel normally with her fingers and that there are no abnormal sensations in the limbs. Note the color in the fingers: if the fingertips are pale or gray-blue, this may indicate a problem with the circulation. Look for any needle marks on the forearms, and for a medical warning bracelet (p.30). Take the pulse at the wrist or neck (p.42).

Check toes once you have removed shoes and socks

TREATMENT AND AFTERCARE

Treat each condition methodically and calmly. Reassure and listen to the victim. Do not let people crowd the scene. Avoid moving the victim unnecessarily. If necessary, ensure that someone contacts his family. Call EMS to evaluate the patient except in the most minor of situations.

TREATMENT PRIORITIES
The order of priorities is as follows:
- Carry out a primary survey (p.29) and act on your findings, making sure that the victim's airway is kept open and clear.
- Control bleeding.
- Carry out a secondary survey.
- Treat large wounds and burns.
- Immobilize bone and joint injuries.
- Give appropriate treatment for other injuries and conditions found.
- Regularly monitor and record vital signs (pp.42–43). Deal with any problems.

ARRANGING AFTERCARE
Decide whether the victim needs medical aid. If help is needed, send someone else to summon help if possible. Stay with the victim until help arrives, in case his condition alters or worsens. According to your assessment of the victim's condition, you may need to:
- Call a doctor for advice.
- Dial 9·1·1 or call EMS for help.
- Pass care of the victim to a doctor, nurse, or ambulance crew.
- Take the victim to a nearby house or shelter to await medical help.
- Allow the victim to go home, ensuring that he is accompanied if possible. Ask if someone will be at home to meet him.
- Advise the victim to see a doctor.

> **❶ CAUTION**
> - Any victim who has impaired consciousness, serious injuries, severe breathing difficulties, or signs of shock (p.120) must not be allowed to go home. Stay with the victim until help arrives.
> - Do not give anything by mouth to any victim who may have internal injuries or to anyone who needs hospital care.
> - Do not allow the victim to smoke.

Care of personal belongings

If you have to search a victim's belongings for identification or clues to his condition, do so in front of a reliable witness. Make sure that all of the victim's clothing and personal belongings go with him to the hospital or are handed over to the police.

Searching belongings
In some cases, the only way of finding clues to a victim's identity or condition is by searching belongings.

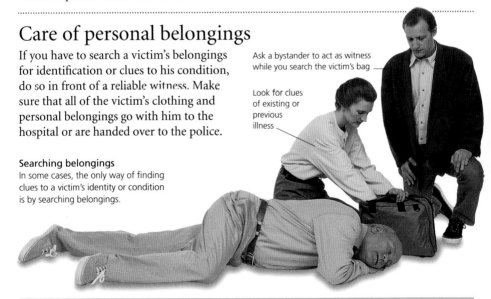

Ask a bystander to act as witness while you search the victim's bag

Look for clues of existing or previous illness

The use of medication

In first aid, administering medication is largely confined to relieving general aches and pains. It usually involves simply helping a victim take acetaminophen, as described in the relevant sections of this book.

A wide variety of medications can be bought without a doctor's prescription, and you may know and have used many of them. However, when treating a victim, you must not buy or borrow medication to administer yourself, even if the victim has forgotten his own medication or you have the type he might normally expect to use.

If you administer, or advise taking, any medication other than those stipulated in this manual when giving first aid, the victim may be put at risk, and you could face legal or civil action as a consequence.

Whenever a victim takes medication, it is essential to make sure that:
- It is appropriate for the condition.
- It is not out of date.
- It is taken as advised.
- Any precautions are strictly followed.
- The recommended dose is not exceeded.
- A record is kept of the name and dose and the time and method of administration.

❶ CAUTION

If the necessary medication is not available, seek medical help. The only exception to this principle occurs where there are clear protocols laid down by an employer or volunteer organization. Such protocols allow trained staff or members to administer medication in specific circumstances, such as giving antidotes to industrial poisons.

PASSING ON INFORMATION

Having summoned medical aid, try to make notes on the incident and on the victim so that you can pass on this information to medical personnel. The charts overleaf show examples of specific observations, such as level of response, pulse, and breathing. You should make a brief written report to accompany your observations.

A written record of the timing of events is particularly valuable to medical personnel. Note, for example, the length of a period of unconsciousness, the duration of a seizure, the time of any changes in the victim's condition, and the time of any intervention or treatment. Hand over your report or a copy to medical staff or emergency services.

Record your observations
While waiting for help to arrive, make a note of your observations. The records you keep will be important for the medical staff who take over the care of the victim.

MAKING A REPORT
Your report should include:
- Victim's name and address.
- History of the incident or illness.
- Brief description of any injuries.
- Any unusual behavior.
- Any treatment given, and when.
- Level of response, pulse, and breathing.

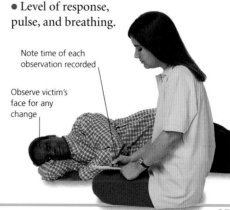

Note time of each observation recorded

Observe victim's face for any change

USING OBSERVATION CHARTS

Every time you attend to a victim, you should monitor and record vital signs – level of response, pulse, and breathing (pp.42–43). This information is important for medical personnel. Note the details on observation charts at regular intervals. Completed charts are shown below; blank charts for use by first aiders are provided on p.280.

On the levels of response chart, place a dot opposite the appropriate score at each time interval. For example, if the victim does not respond to speech at the first check, place a dot opposite 1 in the first column.

On the pulse and breathing check chart, indicate the relevant rates at each time interval; in addition, record the quality of the pulse and breathing as shown.

▶ **See also** MONITORING VITAL SIGNS pp.42–43 ● OBSERVATION CHARTS p.280

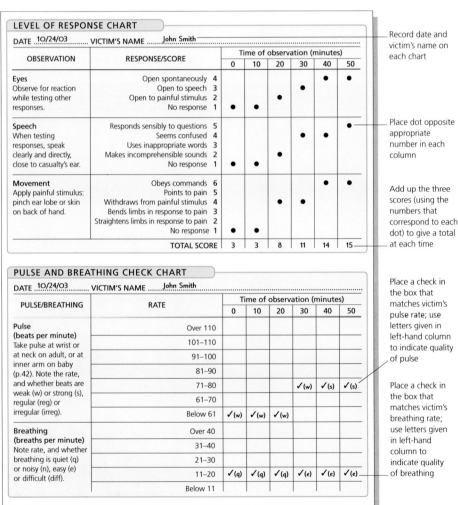

LEVEL OF RESPONSE CHART

DATE 10/24/03   VICTIM'S NAME John Smith

OBSERVATION	RESPONSE/SCORE		0	10	20	30	40	50
		Time of observation (minutes)						
Eyes Observe for reaction while testing other responses.	Open spontaneously	4					●	●
	Open to speech	3				●		
	Open to painful stimulus	2			●			
	No response	1	●	●				
Speech When testing responses, speak clearly and directly, close to casualty's ear.	Responds sensibly to questions	5						●
	Seems confused	4				●	●	
	Uses inappropriate words	3			●			
	Makes incomprehensible sounds	2						
	No response	1	●	●				
Movement Apply painful stimulus: pinch ear lobe or skin on back of hand.	Obeys commands	6					●	●
	Points to pain	5						
	Withdraws from painful stimulus	4				●		
	Bends limbs in response to pain	3			●			
	Straightens limbs in response to pain	2						
	No response	1	●	●				
	TOTAL SCORE		3	3	8	11	14	15

Record date and victim's name on each chart

Place dot opposite appropriate number in each column

Add up the three scores (using the numbers that correspond to each dot) to give a total at each time

PULSE AND BREATHING CHECK CHART

DATE 10/24/03   VICTIM'S NAME John Smith

PULSE/BREATHING	RATE	0	10	20	30	40	50
		Time of observation (minutes)					
Pulse (beats per minute) Take pulse at wrist or at neck on adult, or at inner arm on baby (p.42). Note the rate, and whether beats are weak (w) or strong (s), regular (reg) or irregular (irreg).	Over 110						
	101–110						
	91–100						
	81–90						
	71–80				✓(w)	✓(s)	✓(s)
	61–70						
	Below 61	✓(w)	✓(w)	✓(w)			
Breathing (breaths per minute) Note rate, and whether breathing is quiet (q) or noisy (n), easy (e) or difficult (diff).	Over 40						
	31–40						
	21–30						
	11–20	✓(q)	✓(q)	✓(q)	✓(e)	✓(e)	✓(e)
	Below 11						

Place a check in the box that matches victim's pulse rate; use letters given in left-hand column to indicate quality of pulse

Place a check in the box that matches victim's breathing rate; use letters given in left-hand column to indicate quality of breathing

2

THIS CHAPTER outlines the core procedures that underpin first aid. Techniques that help a first aider to assess a victim are outlined first. These are followed by a guide to the materials that make up a useful first-aid kit, and how to use them. Applying dressings and bandages is an essential part of first aid: wounds usually require a dressing, and almost all injuries benefit from the support that bandages can give.

Usually, a first aider is not expected to move an injured person, but in some circumstances – for example, when a person is in immediate danger – it may be necessary. Some of the key principles and techniques for handling and moving victims are described here.

FIRST-AID PRIORITIES

- Assess the victim's condition.
- Comfort and reassure the victim.
- Remove clothing if necessary.
- Use a first-aid technique relevant to the injury.
- Use dressings and bandages as needed.
- Monitor and record level of response, pulse, and breathing.
- Apply good handling techniques if moving a victim.
- Obtain medical aid if necessary. Call 9•1•1 or EMS if you suspect a serious illness or injury.

CONTENTS

Removing clothing......................40

Removing headgear.....................41

Monitoring vital signs................42

First-aid materials........................44

Dressings......................................46

Sterile dressings.........................47

Nonsterile dressings.................48

Adhesive dressings.....................49

Cold compresses.........................49

Principles of bandaging.............50

Roller bandages..........................52

Elbow and knee bandages.........54

Hand and foot bandages...........55

Tubular bandages.......................56

Triangular bandages..................57

Square knots...............................58

Hand and foot cover..................58

Scalp bandage............................59

Arm sling....................................60

Elevation sling............................61

Improvised slings.......................62

Victim handling.........................63

Assisting a walking victim..........65

Controlling a fall........................66

Moving from chair to floor.........67

Moving a collapsed victim.........68

Moving equipment.....................69

Stretchers and boards................70

TECHNIQUES AND EQUIPMENT

REMOVING CLOTHING

To make a thorough examination of a victim, obtain an accurate assessment, or give treatment, you may have to remove some of his or her clothing. This should only be done if there will be a delay in EMS arriving. Remove as little clothing as possible and do not damage clothing unless it is absolutely necessary. If you need to cut a garment off a victim, try to cut along the seams of trousers or sleeves. Try to maintain the victim's privacy as much as possible and prevent exposure to cold. Stop if removing clothing increases the victim's discomfort or pain.

REMOVING CLOTHING IN LOWER BODY INJURIES

1 Support the ankle and carefully remove the shoe. Do not try to remove long boots yourself - wait until EMS arrives.

2 Remove socks by pulling them off gently. If this is not possible, lift each sock away from the leg and cut the fabric with scissors.

3 Gently pull up the trouser leg to expose the calf and knee. Pull trousers down from the waist to remove them or expose the thigh.

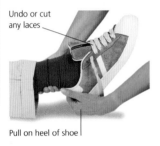
Undo or cut any laces

Pull on heel of shoe

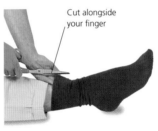
Cut alongside your finger

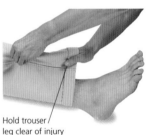
Hold trouser leg clear of injury

REMOVING CLOTHING IN UPPER BODY INJURIES

1 Undo any fastenings on the garment, such as buttons or zippers. Gently pull the garment off the victim's shoulders.

2 Remove the arm on the uninjured side from its sleeve. Pull the garment round to the injured side.

3 Support the injured arm and ease the garment off, keeping the arm as still as possible.

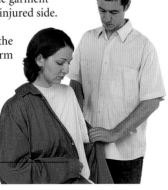
Support injured arm on lap

> ### SPECIAL CASE
>
> **SWEATERS AND SWEATSHIRTS**
> With clothing that cannot be unfastened, begin by easing the arm on the uninjured side out of its sleeve. Next, roll up the garment and stretch it over his head. Finally, slip off the other sleeve of the garment, taking care not to disturb the arm.
>
>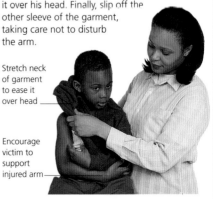
> Stretch neck of garment to ease it over head
>
> Encourage victim to support injured arm

REMOVING HEADGEAR

Protective headgear, such as a bicycle helmet, riding hat, or motorcyclist's crash helmet, is best left on; it should be removed only if strictly necessary (for example, to maintain an open airway). If the item does need to be removed, the victim should do this himself if possible; otherwise, you and a helper should remove it. Take care to support the head and neck at all times and keep the head aligned with the spine.

▶ **See also** SPINAL INJURY, pp.165–167

FOR AN OPEN-FACE HELMET

> **❶ CAUTION**
>
> Do not remove the helmet unless it is absolutely necessary.

1 Unfasten or cut through the chinstrap. Support the victim's head and neck, keeping them aligned with the spine.

2 Ask a helper to grip the sides of the helmet from above, and pull them apart to take pressure off the head. He should then gently lift the helmet upward and backward.

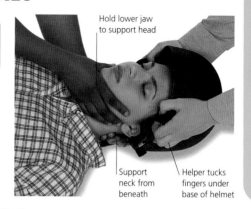

Hold lower jaw to support head

Support neck from beneath

Helper tucks fingers under base of helmet

FOR A FULL-FACE HELMET

> **❶ CAUTION**
>
> Do not remove the helmet unless it is absolutely necessary.

1 Undo or cut the straps. Support the neck with one hand and hold the lower jaw firmly. Working from the base of the helmet, ease your fingers underneath the rim. Ask a helper to hold the helmet with both hands.

2 Ask the helper, working from above, to tilt the helmet backward (try not to move the head at all) and gently lift the front clear of the victim's chin.

3 Continue to support the victim's neck and lower jaw. Ask your helper to tilt the helmet forward slightly so that it will pass over the base of the skull, and then lift it straight off the victim's head.

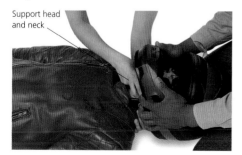

Support head and neck

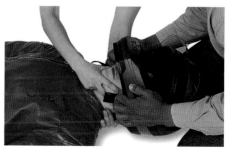

MONITORING VITAL SIGNS

When treating a victim, you may need to assess and monitor his level of response, pulse, and breathing. You may also need to monitor temperature. These vital signs may help you identify specific problems and indicate changes in a victim's condition.

Monitoring should be repeated regularly and your findings recorded on an observation chart and handed over to the medical assistance taking over (p.37).

 See also OBSERVATION CHARTS p.280

CHECKING LEVEL OF RESPONSE

You will need to monitor a victim's level of response to assess consciousness. Any injury or illness that affects the brain may affect consciousness, and any deterioration is potentially serious.

Assess the victim's level of response using the AVPU code:

A – Is the victim *Alert*? Does the victim open his eyes and respond to questions?

V – Does the victim respond to *Voice*? Does he answer simple questions and obey commands?

P – Does the victim respond to *Pain*? Does he open his eyes or move if pinched?

U – Is the victim *Unresponsive* to any stimulus?

Using this code, you can check whether there is any change in the victim's condition.

CHECKING PULSE

Each heartbeat creates a wave of pressure as blood is pumped along the arteries (*see* THE HEART AND BLOOD VESSELS, pp.116–117). In places where arteries lie just under the skin surface, such as on the inside of the wrist and at the neck, this pressure wave can be felt as a pulse. The normal pulse rate in adults is 60–100 beats per minute. The rate is faster in children and may be slower in very fit adults. An abnormally fast or slow pulse may be a sign of certain illnesses.

The pulse may be measured at the neck (carotid pulse) or the wrist (radial pulse). In babies, the pulse in the upper arm (brachial pulse) may be easier to find.

When checking a pulse, use your fingers rather than your thumb (which has its own pulse), and press lightly until you can feel the pulse. Record the following points:
- Rate (number of beats per minute).
- Strength (strong or weak).
- Rhythm (regular or irregular).

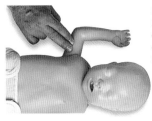

Brachial pulse
Place two fingers on the inner side of the infant's upper arm.

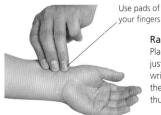

Use pads of your fingers

Radial pulse
Place three fingers just below the wrist creases at the base of the thumb.

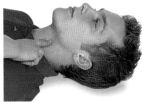

Carotid pulse
Place two fingers on the side of the neck, in the hollow between the windpipe and the large neck muscle.

CHECKING BREATHING

When assessing a victim's breathing, check the rate of breathing and listen for any breathing difficulties or unusual noises.

The normal breathing rate in adults is 12–16 breaths per minute; in babies and young children it is 20–30 breaths per minute. To check breathing, listen to the breathing and watch the victim's chest movements. For a baby or young child, it might be easier to place your hand on the chest and feel for breathing. Record the following information:

- Rate (number of breaths per minute).
- Depth (deep or shallow breaths).
- Ease (easy, difficult, or painful breaths).
- Noise (quiet or noisy breathing, and types of noise).

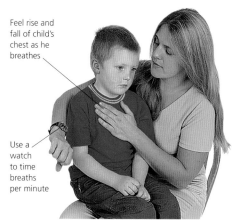

Feel rise and fall of child's chest as he breathes

Use a watch to time breaths per minute

Assessing breathing rate
Watch the chest move and count the number of breaths per minute. For a baby or young child, it may be easier if you place your hand on the chest.

CHECKING TEMPERATURE

To assess body temperature, feel exposed skin and use a thermometer to obtain an accurate reading. Normal body temperature is 98.6°F (37°C). A high temperature (fever) is usually caused by infection. A low body temperature (hypothermia) may result from exposure to cold and/or wet conditions. There are several types of thermometers, including the traditional glass mercury thermometer and digital thermometers. Make sure that you know how to use the particular type of thermometer.

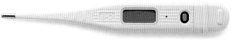

Digital thermometer
This can be used to measure temperature under the tongue or under the armpit. It should be left it in place until it makes a beeping sound (about 30 seconds), then the temperature should be read from the display.

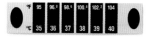

Forehead thermometer
This small heat-sensitive strip is useful for a young child, but it is not as accurate as the digital thermometer. Hold the strip in place against the child's forehead for about 30 seconds. The color indicates the temperature.

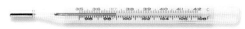

Mercury thermometer
Before using this thermometer you should check that the mercury level is below 98.6°F (37°C). Leave the thermometer in position (under the tongue or in the armpit) for 2–3 minutes before reading.

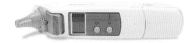

Ear sensor
Place the tip of this thermometer inside the ear; it will give a reading within 1 second. The sensor is easy to use and can be used for a sick child or a sleeping child. However, it is not as accurate as a digital thermometer.

FIRST-AID MATERIALS

All workplaces, sports centers, homes, and cars should have first-aid kits. The kits for workplaces or sports centers must conform to legal requirements; they should also be clearly marked and easily accessible. For a home or a car, you can either buy a kit or assemble first aid items yourself and keep

them in a clean, waterproof container. Any first-aid kit must be kept in a dry place, and checked and replenished regularly, so that the items are always ready for use.

The items on these pages are the basis of a first-aid kit for the home. You may wish to add items such as acetaminophen.

DRESSINGS

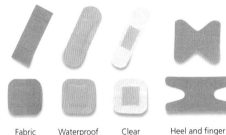

| Fabric dressings | Waterproof dressings | Clear dressings | Heel and finger dressings |

Adhesive dressings
These are applied to small cuts and abrasions and are made of fabric or waterproof plastic. Use waterproof adhesive bandages for hand wounds, and hypoallergenic dressings for people who are allergic to the normal adhesive.

Sterile dressings
These consist of a dressing pad attached to a roller bandage, and are sealed in a protective wrapping. They are easy to apply, so are ideal in an emergency. Various sizes are available.

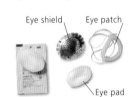

Medium dressing   Large dressing   Extra-large dressing

Sterile eye pads
Eye pads are dressings to protect injured eyes. Some eye pads have straps attached so that they can be secured to a victim's head.

Eye shield   Eye patch

Eye pad

BANDAGES

Self-adhesive roller bandage   Crêpe roller bandage   Open-weave roller bandage

Triangular bandages
Made of cloth, these items can be used as bandages and slings. If they are sterile and individually wrapped, they may also be used as dressings for large wounds and burns.

Folded cloth triangular bandage

Elasticized roller bandage   Conforming roller bandage   Crêpe conforming roller bandage

Roller bandages
These items are used to give support to injured joints, restrict movement, secure dressings in place and maintain pressure on them, and limit swelling.

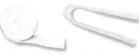

Elasticated tubular bandage   Gauze tubular bandage   Tubular gauze applicator

Tubular bandages
These bandages are seamless tubes of gauze or strong, elasticized material. They are used on joints and on toes or fingers. Gauze types are used with a special applicator.

USEFUL ADDITIONAL ITEMS

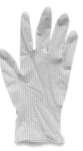

Disposable gloves
Wear disposable gloves, if available, whenever you dress wounds or when you handle body fluids or other waste materials to prevent cross-infection.

Bandage clip

Safety pins

Pins and clips
These items can be used to secure the ends of bandages.

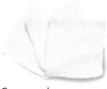

Gauze pads
Use these as dressings, as padding, or as swabs to clean around wounds.

Face protection
Use a plastic face shield (left) or a pocket mask (right) whenever possible to protect you and the victim from cross-infection when giving rescue breaths.

Face shield

Pocket mask

Cleansing wipes
Alcohol-free wipes can be used to clean skin around wounds, or to clean your hands if water and soap are not available.

Cotton padding
This material can be used as padding or an absorbent layer over a dressing. Never place it directly on a wound.

Items for use outdoors
A blanket can protect a victim from complications caused by the cold, such as hypothermia. A flashlight improves visibility, and a whistle can be used to attract attention and summon help.

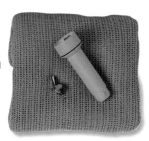

Blanket, flashlight, and whistle

Adhesive tape
Use tape to secure dressings or the ends of bandages. Some people are allergic to the adhesive, so check first. Hypoallergenic tape is available.

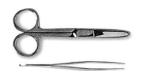

Scissors and tweezers
Choose items that are blunt-ended so that they will not cause injuries.

MATERIALS FOR A HOME FIRST-AID KIT

BASIC MATERIALS
- Easily identifiable watertight box.
- 20 adhesive dressings in assorted sizes.
- Six medium sterile dressings.
- Two large sterile dressings.
- Two extra-large sterile dressings.
- Two sterile eye pads.
- Six triangular bandages.
- Six safety pins.
- Disposable gloves.

USEFUL ADDITIONS
- Two roller bandages.
- Scissors.
- Tweezers.
- Cotton padding.
- Alcohol-free wound cleansing wipes.
- Adhesive tape.
- Plastic face shield or pocket face mask.
- Notepad and pencil.
- Blanket, flashlight, whistle.

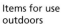

DRESSINGS

You should always cover a wound with a dressing because this helps prevent infection. With severe bleeding, dressings are used to aid the blood-clotting process by exerting pressure on the wound.

Use a prepacked sterile dressing (opposite) whenever possible. If no sterile dressing is available, any clean, nonfluffy material can be used to improvise a dressing (p.48). Small cuts and abrasions can be protected by an adhesive dressing (p.49).

▶ **See also** CUTS AND ABRASIONS p.134
● FIRST-AID MATERIALS pp.44–45 ● SEVERE BLEEDING p.130

RULES FOR USING DRESSINGS

When handling or applying a dressing, there are a number of rules to follow. These enable you to apply dressings correctly; they also protect both the victim and yourself from infection (*see* GUIDELINES FOR PREVENTING CROSS INFECTION, p.15).
● Always wear disposable gloves, if these are available, before handling any dressing other than an adhesive dressing.

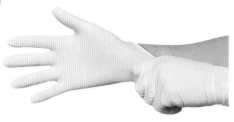

● Always use a dressing that is large enough to cover the wound and extend beyond the wound's edges.
● Hold the dressing at the edges, keeping your fingers well away from the area that will be in contact with the wound.

● Place the dressing directly on top of the wound; do not slide it on from the side.
● Remove and replace any dressing that slips out of position.
● If there is only one sterile dressing, use this to cover the wound, and apply other clean materials on top of the dressing.
● If blood seeps through the dressing, do not remove it; instead, apply another dressing over the top. If blood seeps through a second dressing, remove both dressings completely and then apply a fresh dressing, making sure that you apply pressure over the bleeding point.
● After treating a wound, dispose of gloves, used dressings, and soiled items in a suitable plastic bag. Always keep disposable gloves on until you have finished handling any other contaminated materials.

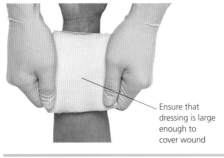

Ensure that dressing is large enough to cover wound

Use a red biohazard bag if possible

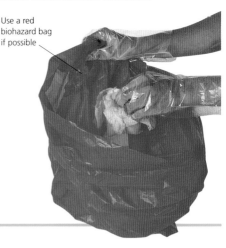

STERILE DRESSINGS

This type of dressing is a sterilized bandage sold in a sealed package. The one illustrated below consists of a dressing pad attached to a roller bandage. You can make a similar bandage using separately packaged sterile pads and roller bandages. Once the seal on a sterile dressing has been broken, the dressing is no longer sterile and should not be used.

> **⊘ CAUTION**
>
> ● If the dressing slips out of place, remove it and apply a new dressing.
>
> ● If bleeding appears through the dressing, apply another on top of the original one. If blood seeps through the second dressing as well, take both dressings off and apply a fresh dressing.
>
> ● Take care not to impair the circulation beyond the dressing.

1 Break the seal and remove the wrapping. Unwind the bandage, taking care not to drop the roll or touch the dressing pad.

2 Unfold the dressing pad, holding the bandage on each side of it. Lay the pad directly on the wound.

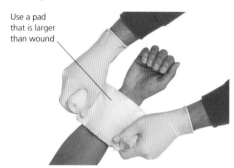

Use a pad that is larger than wound

3 Wind the short end (tail) of the bandage once around the limb and the dressing to secure the pad.

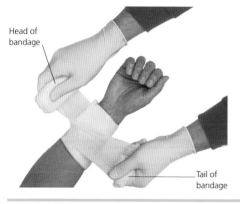

Head of bandage

Tail of bandage

4 Wind the other end (head) of the bandage around the limb to cover the whole pad. Leave the tail of the bandage hanging free.

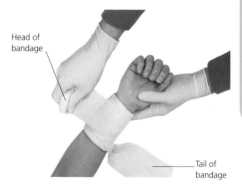

Head of bandage

Tail of bandage

5 To secure the bandage, tie the ends in a square knot (p.58). Tie it directly over the pad to exert firm pressure on the wound.

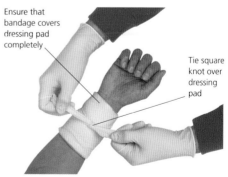

Ensure that bandage covers dressing pad completely

Tie square knot over dressing pad

6 Once you have secured the bandage, check the circulation in the limb beyond it (p.51). Loosen the bandage if it is too tight.

NONSTERILE DRESSINGS

If a sterile dressing is not available, you can use items such as gauze pads or any clean, nonfluffy material and apply cotton padding on top to absorb blood or other fluids. When using a nonsterile dressing, make sure the item is clean. Wear disposable gloves if possible, and keep your fingers away from the surface of the dressing that will be touching the wound. In order to apply pressure to a wound, secure the dressing with tape or a bandage.

> **! CAUTION**
>
> - Never apply adhesive tape all the way around a limb or digit, since this can impair circulation.
> - Check that the victim is not allergic to the adhesive before using adhesive tape; if there is any allergy, use a bandage.

▶ **See also** ROLLER BANDAGES pp.52–53

GAUZE DRESSINGS

1 Holding the gauze pad by the edges, place it directly on the wound.

2 Add a layer of cotton padding on top of the gauze dressing.

3 Secure the gauze and padding with adhesive tape or a roller bandage.

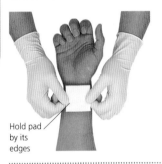

Hold pad by its edges

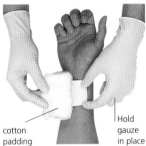

cotton padding

Hold gauze in place

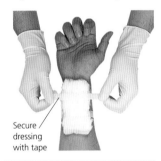

Secure dressing with tape

IMPROVISED DRESSINGS

1 Hold the material by the edges. Open it out and refold it so that the inner surface faces outward.

2 Place the pad of cloth directly on the wound. If necessary, cover the pad with more material.

3 Secure the pad with a bandage or a clean strip of cloth, such as a scarf. Tie the ends in a square knot (p.58).

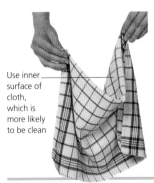

Use inner surface of cloth, which is more likely to be clean

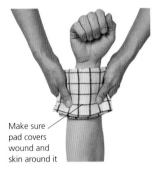

Make sure pad covers wound and skin around it

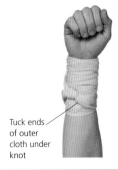

Tuck ends of outer cloth under knot

ADHESIVE DRESSINGS

Adhesive dressings are useful for small cuts and abrasions. They consist of a gauze or cellulose pad and an adhesive backing, and are often wrapped singly in sterile packs. There are several sizes and special shapes for use on fingertips, heels, and elbows; some types are waterproof. Before you apply an adhesive dressing, check that the

> **❶ CAUTION**
> Always ask whether the victim is allergic to adhesive dressings.

victim is not allergic to the adhesive. People who work with food must cover wounds on their hands with waterproof, easily visible, blue adhesive dressings.

1 Clean and dry the skin around the wound. Unwrap the adhesive dressing and hold it by the protective strips over the backing, with the pad side facing downward.

2 Peel back the strips to expose the pad, but do not remove them. Without touching the pad surface, place the pad on the wound.

3 Carefully pull away the protective strips, then press the edges of the dressing down.

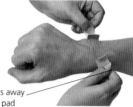

Keep fingers away from sterile pad

COLD COMPRESSES

Cooling an injury such as a bruise or sprain can reduce swelling and pain, although it will not relieve the injury itself. There are two types of compress: cold pads, which are made from material dampened with cold water; and ice packs, which are cold items (such as ice cubes or bags of frozen peas or other vegetables) wrapped in a dry cloth.

COLD PAD

1 Soak a cloth or towel in cold water. Wring it out lightly and fold it into a pad, then place it firmly on the injury.

2 Re-soak the pad in cold water every 3–5 minutes to keep it cold. Cool the injury for at least 10 minutes.

ICE PACK

1 Partly fill a plastic bag with small ice cubes or crushed ice, or use a pack of frozen vegetables. Wrap the bag in a dry cloth.

> **❶ CAUTION**
> To prevent cold injuries, always wrap an ice pack in a cloth; and do not use it for more than 10 minutes at one application.

2 Hold the pack firmly on the area. Cool for 10 minutes, replacing the pack as needed.

Cover injury and surrounding area with pack

PRINCIPLES OF BANDAGING

There are a number of different first aid uses for bandages: they can be used to secure dressings, control bleeding, support and immobilize limbs, and reduce swelling in an injured part. There are three main types of bandage. Roller bandages secure dressings and support injured limbs. Tubular bandages hold dressings on fingers or toes or support injured joints. Triangular bandages can be used as large dressings; as slings; to secure dressings; or to immobilize limbs. If you have no bandage available, you can improvise one from an everyday item; for example, you can fold a square of fabric, such as a headscarf, diagonally to make a triangular bandage (p.57).

▶ **See also** ROLLER BANDAGES pp.52–55 ● TUBULAR BANDAGE p.56 ● TRIANGULAR BANDAGES pp.57–62

RULES FOR APPLYING A BANDAGE

● Before applying a bandage, reassure the injured person and explain clearly what you are going to do.
● Make the person comfortable, in a suitable sitting or lying position.
● Keep the injured part supported while you are working on it. Ask the victim or a helper to do this.
● Always work at the front of the person, and from the injured side where possible.

● If the injured person is lying down, pass the bandages under the body's natural hollows at the ankles, knees, waist, and neck, then slide the bandages into position by easing them back and forth under the body. For example, to bandage the head or upper trunk, pull a bandage through the hollow under the neck.

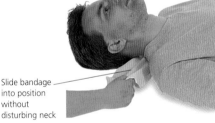

Slide bandage into position without disturbing neck

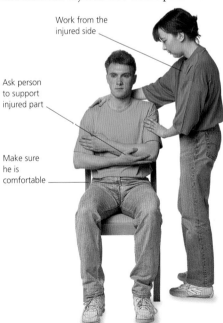

Work from the injured side

Ask person to support injured part

Make sure he is comfortable

● Apply bandages firmly, but not so tightly that they interfere with circulation to the area beyond the bandage (opposite).
● Leave the fingers or toes on a bandaged limb exposed, if possible, so that you can check the circulation afterward.
● Use square knots to tie bandages. Ensure that the knots do not cause discomfort, and do not tie the knot over a bony area. Tuck loose ends under a knot if possible.
● Regularly check the circulation in the area beyond the bandage (opposite). If necessary, unroll the bandage until the blood supply returns, and reapply it more loosely.

IMMOBILIZING A LIMB

When applying bandages to immobilize a limb, you also need to use soft, bulky material, such as towels or clothing, as padding. Place the padding between the legs, or between an arm and the body, so that the bandaging does not displace broken bones or press bony areas against each other. Tie the bandages at intervals along the limb, avoiding the injury site. Secure with square knots (p.58) on the uninjured side. If both sides of the body are injured, you should tie knots in the middle or where there is least chance of causing further damage.

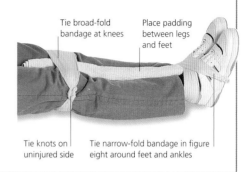

Tie broad-fold bandage at knees

Place padding between legs and feet

Tie knots on uninjured side

Tie narrow-fold bandage in figure eight around feet and ankles

CHECKING CIRCULATION AFTER BANDAGING

When bandaging a limb or using a sling, you must check the circulation in the hand or foot immediately after you have finished bandaging, and every 10 minutes thereafter. These checks are essential because limbs swell after an injury, and a bandage can rapidly become too tight and interfere with blood circulation to the area beyond it. The symptoms of impaired circulation change as first the veins and then the arteries become constricted.

If circulation is impaired there may be:
- A swollen and congested limb.
- Blue skin with prominent veins.
- A feeling that the skin is painfully distended.

Later there may be:
- Pale, waxy skin.
- Cold numbness.
- Tingling, followed by deep pain.
- Inability to move affected fingers or toes.

1 Briefly press one of the nails (inset), or the skin, until it turns pale, then release the pressure. If the color does not return, or returns slowly, the bandage may be too tight.

2 Loosen a tight bandage by unrolling just enough turns for warmth and color to return to the skin. The person may feel a tingling sensation. Reapply the bandage.

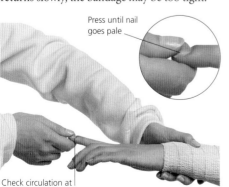

Press until nail goes pale

Check circulation at ends of fingers or toes

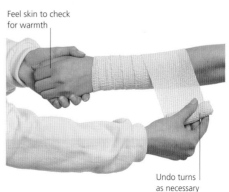

Feel skin to check for warmth

Undo turns as necessary

ROLLER BANDAGES

These bandages are made of cotton, gauze, elasticized fabric, or linen, and are wrapped around the injured part in spiral turns. There are three main types of roller bandage:

- Open-weave bandages, which are used to hold dressings in place. Because of their loose weave they allow good ventilation, but they cannot be used to exert direct pressure on the wound or to give support to joints.
- Elasticized bandages, which mold to the body shape. These are used to secure dressings and support soft tissue injuries.
- Tensor bandages, which are used to give firm support to injured joints.

SECURING ROLLER BANDAGES

There are several ways to fasten the end of a roller bandage. Safety pins or adhesive tape are usually included in first-aid kits. Specialized kits may contain bandage clips. If you do not have any of these, a simple tuck should keep the bandage end in place.

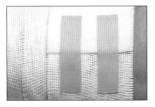

Adhesive tape
The ends of bandages can be folded under and then stuck down with small strips of adhesive tape.

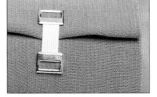

Bandage clip
Metal clips are sometimes supplied with elasticized and tensor roller bandages for securing the ends.

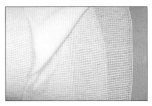

Tucking in the end
If you have no fastening, secure the bandage by passing the end around the limb once and tucking it in.

Safety pin
These pins can secure all types of roller bandage. Fold the end of the bandage under, then tuck your finger between the bandage and the victim's skin to prevent injury as you insert the pin (right). Make sure that, once fastened, the pin lies flat (far right).

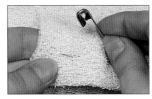

INSERTING PIN

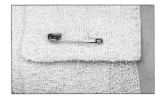

BANDAGE SECURED WITH PIN

CHOOSING THE CORRECT SIZE OF BANDAGE

Before applying a roller bandage, check that it is tightly rolled and of a suitable width for the injured area. Different parts of the body need particular widths of bandage – small areas such as fingers require narrow bandages, while large areas such as limbs need wide ones. It is better for a roller bandage to be too wide than too narrow. The bandages shown on the right are the recommended sizes for an adult. Smaller sizes may be needed for a child.

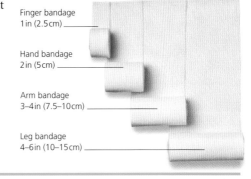

Finger bandage
1 in (2.5 cm)

Hand bandage
2 in (5 cm)

Arm bandage
3–4 in (7.5–10 cm)

Leg bandage
4–6 in (10–15 cm)

APPLYING A ROLLER BANDAGE

Follow these general rules when you are applying a roller bandage:

● Keep the rolled part of the bandage (the "head") uppermost as you work (the unrolled part is called the "tail").

● Position yourself toward the front of the victim, on the injured side.

● While you are working, make sure that the injured part is supported in the position in which it will remain after bandaging.

❶ CAUTION

Once you have applied the bandage, check the circulation in the limb beyond it (p.51). This is especially important if you are applying an elasticized or tensor bandage because these mold to the shape of the limb and may become tighter if the limb swells.

1 Place the tail of the bandage below the injury. Working from the inside of the limb outward, make two straight turns with the bandage to anchor the tail in place.

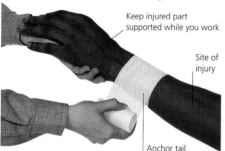

Keep injured part supported while you work

Site of injury

Anchor tail

2 Make a series of spiraling turns with the bandage. Wind it from the inside to the outside of the upper surface of the limb, and work up the limb. Make sure that each new turn covers between one-half and two-thirds of the previous turn of bandaging.

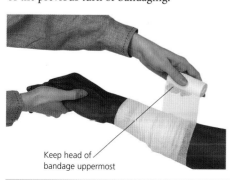

Keep head of bandage uppermost

3 Finish with one straight turn, and secure the end of the bandage (opposite). If the bandage is too short, apply another one in the same way so that the injured area is covered.

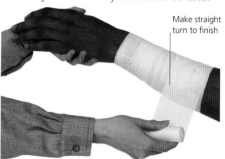

Make straight turn to finish

4 As soon as you have finished, check the circulation beyond the bandage (p.51). If necessary, unroll the bandage until the blood supply returns, and reapply it more loosely.

Press and release nail to check circulation

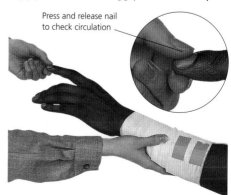

ELBOW AND KNEE BANDAGES

Roller bandages can be used on elbows and knees to hold dressings in place or support soft tissue injuries such as strains or sprains. To ensure that there is effective support, flex the joint slightly, then apply the bandage in a figure eight rather than the standard spiraling turns (p.53). Work from the inside to the outside of the upper surface of the joint. Extend the bandaging far enough on either side of it to exert an even pressure.

1 Support the injured limb, in a comfortable position for the victim, with the joint partially flexed if possible.

2 Place the tail of the bandage on the inner side of the joint. Pass the bandage over and around to the outside of the joint. Make one-and-a-half turns, so that the end of the bandage is fixed and the joint is covered.

> **⚠ WARNING**
>
> Do not apply the bandage so tightly that the circulation to the limb is impaired.

5 Continue to bandage diagonally above and below the joint in a figure eight. Increase the bandaged area by covering about two-thirds of the previous turn each time.

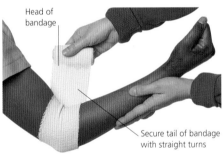

Head of bandage

Secure tail of bandage with straight turns

3 Pass the bandage to the inner side of the limb, just above the joint. Make a turn around the limb, covering the upper half of the bandage from the first turn.

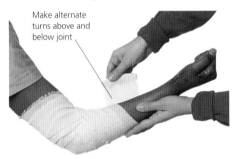

Make alternate turns above and below joint

6 To finish bandaging the joint, make two straight turns around the limb, then secure the end of the bandage (p.52).

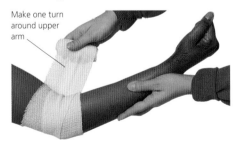

Make one turn around upper arm

4 Pass the bandage from the inner side of the upper limb to just below the joint. Make one diagonal turn below the joint to cover the lower half of the bandaging from the first straight turn.

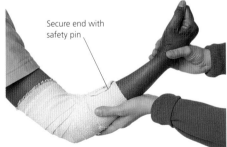

Secure end with safety pin

7 Check the circulation beyond the bandage as soon as you have finished, then every 10 minutes (p.51). If the bandage is too tight, unroll it until the blood supply returns and reapply it more loosely.

HAND AND FOOT BANDAGES

A roller bandage may be applied to hold dressings in place on a hand or foot, or to support a wrist or ankle in soft tissue injuries. A support bandage should extend well beyond the injury site to provide pressure over the whole of the injured area. The method shown below for bandaging a hand can also be used on a foot; in this case, begin bandaging at the base of the big toe and leave the heel unbandaged.

1 Place the tail of the bandage on the inner side of the wrist, by the base of the thumb. Make two straight turns around the wrist.

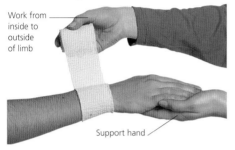

Work from inside to outside of limb

Support hand

2 Working from the inner side of the wrist, pass the bandage diagonally across the back of the hand to the nail of the little finger.

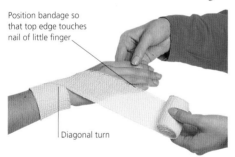

Position bandage so that top edge touches nail of little finger

Diagonal turn

3 Take the bandage under and across the fingers so that the upper edge touches the base of the nail on the index finger. Leave the thumb free.

Bandage passes around index finger

4 Leaving the thumb free, pass the bandage diagonally across the back of the hand to the outer side of the wrist. Wrap it diagonally around the wrist and over the hand again.

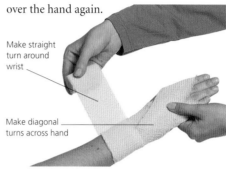

Make straight turn around wrist

Make diagonal turns across hand

5 Repeat the sequence of diagonal turns. Extend the bandaging by covering about two-thirds of the bandage from the previous turn each time. When the hand is covered, finish with two straight turns around the wrist.

6 Secure the end (p.52). As soon as you have finished, check the circulation beyond the bandage (p.51), then recheck every 10 minutes. If necessary, unroll the bandage until the blood supply returns and reapply it more loosely.

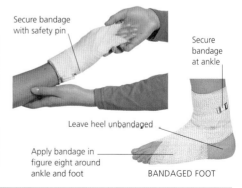

Secure bandage with safety pin

Secure bandage at ankle

Leave heel unbandaged

Apply bandage in figure eight around ankle and foot

BANDAGED FOOT

TUBULAR BANDAGE

These bandages are rolls of seamless, tubular fabric. There are two types: elasticized bandages, used to support joints such as the elbow or ankle; and tubular gauze, designed to cover a finger or toe. The gauze is used with a special applicator, supplied with the bandage. It is suitable for holding dressings

> **⚠ CAUTION**
>
> Do not encircle the finger completely with tape because this may impair circulation.

in place, but cannot exert enough pressure to control bleeding. The steps below illustrate how to apply tubular gauze to a finger.

1 Cut a piece of tubular gauze about two-and-a-half times the length of the injured finger. Slide the whole length of the tubular gauze onto the applicator, then gently slide the applicator over the finger.

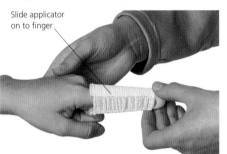

Slide applicator on to finger

2 Holding the end of the gauze on the finger, pull the applicator slightly beyond the fingertip to leave a gauze layer on the finger. Twist the applicator twice to seal the bandage over the end of the finger.

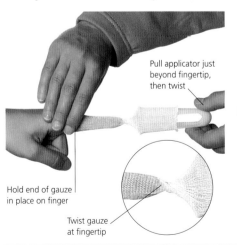

Pull applicator just beyond fingertip, then twist

Hold end of gauze in place on finger

Twist gauze at fingertip

3 While still holding the gauze at the base of the finger, gently push the applicator back over the finger to apply a second layer of gauze. Once all of it has been applied, remove the applicator from the finger.

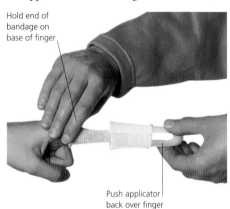

Hold end of bandage on base of finger

Push applicator back over finger

4 Secure the gauze at the base of the finger with adhesive tape. Check the circulation to the finger immediately and recheck every 10 minutes. Ask if the finger feels cold or tingly. If it does, remove the gauze and reapply it more loosely.

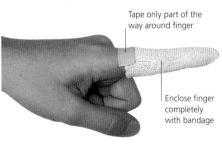

Tape only part of the way around finger

Enclose finger completely with bandage

TRIANGULAR BANDAGES

This type of bandage may be supplied in a sterile pack, as part of a first-aid kit. You can also make one by cutting or folding 10 square feet (1 square meter) of sturdy fabric (such as linen or calico) diagonally in half. It can be used in the following ways:

- Folded into a broad-fold bandage (below) to immobilize and support a limb or to secure a splint or bulky dressing.
- Folded into a narrow-fold bandage (below) to immobilize feet and ankles or hold a dressing in place.

- Used directly from a sterile pack and folded into a pad to form a sterile dressing.
- Opened to form a sling, or to hold a hand, foot, or scalp dressing in place.

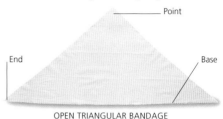

Point

End   Base

OPEN TRIANGULAR BANDAGE

MAKING A BROAD-FOLD BANDAGE

1 Open out a triangular bandage and lay it flat on a clean surface. Fold the bandage in half horizontally, so that the point of the triangle touches the center of the base.

2 Fold the triangular bandage in half again, in the same direction, so that the first folded edge touches the base. The bandage should now form a broad strip.

First folded edge aligned with base

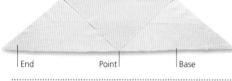

End   Point   Base

MAKING A NARROW-FOLD BANDAGE

1 Fold a triangular bandage to make a broad-fold bandage (above).

2 Fold the bandage horizontally in half again. It should form a long, narrow, thick strip of material.

STORING A TRIANGULAR BANDAGE

Keep triangular bandages in their packs so that they remain sterile until you need them. Alternatively, fold them in the way shown below so that they are ready for use or can simply be shaken open.

1 Start by folding the triangle into a narrow-fold bandage (above). Bring the two ends of the bandage into the center.

2 Continue folding the ends into the center until the bandage is a convenient size for storing. Keep the bandage in a dry place.

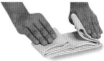

SQUARE KNOTS

When securing a triangular bandage, always use a square knot. It is secure and will not slip; it is easy to untie; and it lies flat, so it is more comfortable. Avoid tying the knot around or directly over the injury itself, since this may cause discomfort.

TYING A SQUARE KNOT

1 Pass the left end (dark) over and under the right end (light).

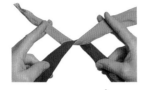

3 Pass the right end (dark) over and under the left end (light).

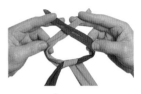

2 Lift both ends of the bandage above the rest of the material.

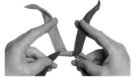

4 Pull the ends to tighten the knot, then tuck them under the bandage.

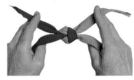

UNTYING A SQUARE KNOT

1 Pull one end and one piece of bandage firmly so that it straightens.

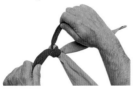

2 Hold the knot and pull the straightened end through it.

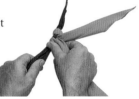

HAND AND FOOT COVER

An open triangular bandage can be used to hold a dressing in place on a hand or foot, but it will not provide enough pressure to control bleeding. The method for covering a hand (below) can also be used for a foot, with the bandage ends tied at the ankle.

1 Lay the bandage flat and fold the base to form a hem. Place the hand on the bandage, fingers toward the point. Fold the point over the hand.

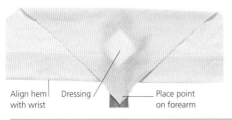

Align hem with wrist   Dressing   Place point on forearm

2 Pass the ends around the wrist in opposite directions and tie them in a square knot. Pull the point gently to tighten the bandage. Fold the point up over the knot and tuck it in.

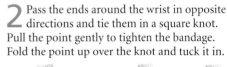

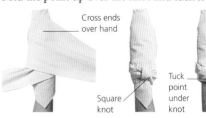

Cross ends over hand

Tuck point under knot

Square knot

SCALP BANDAGE

A triangular bandage may be used to hold a dressing in position on top of a victim's head. It cannot, however, provide enough pressure to control bleeding; to hold a dressing in position on a bleeding wound, use a roller bandage (pp.52–53). Before applying a scalp bandage, ask the injured person to sit down, if possible, because this will make it easier for you to reach all parts of his head.

1 Fold a hem along the base of the bandage. Place the bandage on the injured person's head with the hem underneath and the center of the base just above his eyebrows.

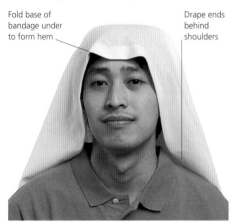

Fold base of bandage under to form hem

Drape ends behind shoulders

3 Bring the crossed ends to the front of the head. Tie the ends in a square knot (opposite) at the center of the forehead, positioning it over the hem of the bandage. Tuck the free part of each end under the knot.

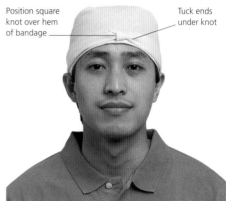

Position square knot over hem of bandage

Tuck ends under knot

2 Wrap the ends of the bandage securely around the head, tucking the hem just above his ears. Cross the two ends at the nape of the neck, over the point of the bandage.

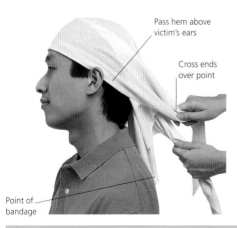

Pass hem above victim's ears

Cross ends over point

Point of bandage

4 Steady the victim's head with one hand and draw the point down to tighten the bandage. Then fold the point up over the ends and pin it at the crown of his head. If you do not have a pin, tuck the point over the ends.

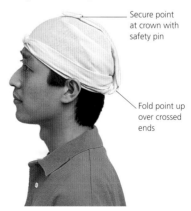

Secure point at crown with safety pin

Fold point up over crossed ends

ARM SLING

An arm sling holds the forearm in a horizontal or slightly raised position. It provides support for an injured upper arm, wrist, or forearm, or a simple rib fracture (p.164) and is used for a victim whose elbow can be bent. An elevation sling (opposite) is used to keep the forearm and hand raised in a higher position.

1 Ensure that the injured arm is supported with its hand slightly raised. Fold the base of the bandage under to form a hem. Place the bandage with the base parallel to the victim's body and level with her little finger nail. Pass the upper end under the injured arm and pull it around the neck to the opposite shoulder.

Pass end over shoulder and around back of neck

Hold point beyond elbow

2 Fold the lower end of the bandage up over the forearm and bring it to meet the upper end at the shoulder.

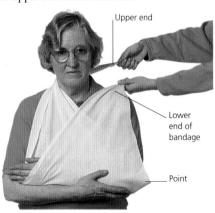

Upper end

Lower end of bandage

Point

3 Tie a square knot (p.58) on the injured side, at the hollow above the collarbone. Tuck both free ends of the bandage under the knot to pad it.

Tie knot just above collarbone

Ensure sling supports forearm and hand up to little finger

4 Fold the point forward at the victim's elbow. Tuck any loose fabric around the elbow, and secure the point to the front with a safety pin. If you do not have a pin, twist the point until the fabric fits the elbow snugly; tuck it into the sling at the back of the arm.

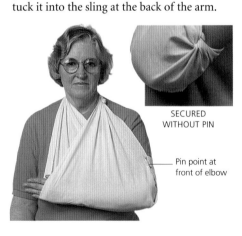

SECURED WITHOUT PIN

Pin point at front of elbow

5 As soon as you have finished, check the circulation in the fingers (p.51). Recheck every 10 minutes. If necessary, loosen and reapply the bandages and sling.

ELEVATION SLING

This form of sling supports the forearm and hand in a raised position, with the fingertips touching the shoulder. In this way, an elevation sling helps control bleeding from wounds in the forearm or hand, to minimize swelling in burn injuries, and to support the chest in complicated rib fractures (p.164).

1 Ask the victim to support his injured arm across his chest, with the fingers resting on the opposite shoulder.

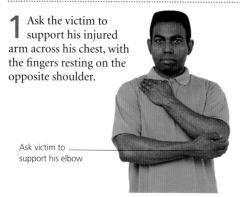

Ask victim to support his elbow

2 Place the bandage over his body, with one end over the uninjured shoulder. Hold the point just beyond his elbow.

Hold point beyond elbow of injured side

Base of bandage

3 Ask the victim to let go of his injured arm. Tuck the base of the bandage under his hand, forearm, and elbow.

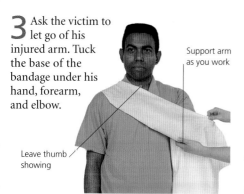

Support arm as you work

Leave thumb showing

4 Bring the lower end of the bandage up diagonally across his back, to meet the other end at his shoulder.

Bring ends together

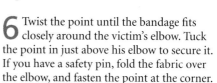

Pass lower end of bandage up across back

5 Tie the ends in a square knot (p.58) at the hollow above the collarbone. Tuck the ends under the knot to pad it.

6 Twist the point until the bandage fits closely around the victim's elbow. Tuck the point in just above his elbow to secure it. If you have a safety pin, fold the fabric over the elbow, and fasten the point at the corner.

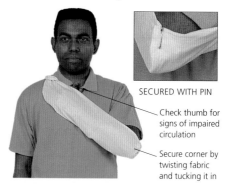

SECURED WITH PIN

Check thumb for signs of impaired circulation

Secure corner by twisting fabric and tucking it in

7 Regularly check the circulation in the thumb (p.51). If necessary, loosen and reapply the bandages and sling.

IMPROVISED SLINGS

If you need to support a victim's injured arm but do not have a triangular bandage, you can improvise a sling by using a square of any strong cloth (p.57). You can also improvise by using an item of the victim's clothing (below).

> **⚠ WARNING**
>
> If you suspect that the forearm is broken, use a cloth sling or a jacket corner to provide support. Do not use any other improvised sling: it will not provide enough support.

JACKET CORNER

Undo the victim's jacket. Fold the lower edge on the injured side up over her arm. Secure the corner of the hem to the jacket breast with a large safety pin. Tuck and pin the excess material closely around the elbow.

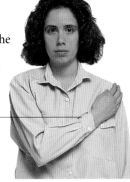

Pin excess material around elbow

Leave fingers exposed to check circulation

BUTTON-UP JACKET

Undo one button of a jacket or coat (or waistcoat). Place the hand of the injured arm inside the garment at the gap formed by the unfastened button. Advise the person to rest her wrist on the button just beneath the gap.

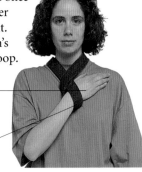

Unfasten button at center of chest

Support wrist on lower button

LONG-SLEEVED SHIRT

Lay the injured arm across the victim's chest. Pin the cuff of the sleeve to the opposite side of the front of the shirt. To improvise an elevation sling (previous page), pin the sleeve at the victim's opposite shoulder, to keep her arm raised.

Use a safety pin that is sturdy enough to take weight of arm

BELT OR THIN GARMENT

Use a belt, a tie, or a pair of suspenders or panty hose to make a "collar-and-cuff" support. Fasten the item to form a loop. Place it over the victim's head, then twist once to form a smaller loop at the front. Place the victim's hand into the loop.

Place hand in loop, where it cannot slip out

Check that cuff is not impeding circulation to hand

VICTIM HANDLING

As a general rule, when giving first aid you should leave victims in the position in which you found them until medical help arrives. You should only move a victim if he is in imminent danger, and even then only if it is safe for you to approach and you have the training and equipment to carry out the move.

This page and the next offer advice on assessing the risk of moving a victim, and give safety guidelines to help you plan any necessary moves. The subsequent pages

! WARNING

Do not move a victim unless there is an emergency situation (below) that demands that you take action.

illustrate good practice in helping victims who can walk and in carrying out moves. Note, however, that this information is no substitute for comprehensive training.

Information is given on some of the equipment for moving victims that is used by emergency services.

ASSESSING THE RISK OF MOVING A VICTIM

Before you consider moving a victim, you need to decide whether or not the person is in immediate danger and needs to be moved (below). If you do think that it is necessary to move him, you need to find out what help and equipment is available and assess how difficult it might be to carry out the procedure. Consider the following:
- Is the task really necessary? Usually, the victim can be assessed and treated in the position in which you find him.
- If a move is necessary, can the victim move himself? Ask the victim if he feels able to move; in addition, make your own assessment of his condition, using your common sense.

- What is the victim's weight and size?
- What are his injuries, and will a move make his condition worse?
- Who is available to help with the move? Are you and any helpers properly trained and physically fit?
- Will you need to use protective equipment to enter the area, and do you have such equipment available?
- Is there any equipment available to assist with moving the victim? Do you have all the items that you need?
- Is there enough space around the victim to carry out the move?
- What sort of ground will you be crossing with the victim?

SPECIAL CASE

EMERGENCY SITUATIONS
There are four emergency situations in which a victim should be moved quickly out of danger. Do this only if you will not be putting your own life at risk and you have the correct training and equipment. If you do not have these resources, you must call the emergency services instead of attempting to rescue the victim yourself.

The emergency situations are as follows:
- When a victim is in water and in imminent danger of drowning (p.28).

- When a victim is in an area on fire or an area that is filling with smoke (pp.24–25).
- When a victim is in danger from a bomb or from gunfire.
- When a victim is in or near a collapsing building or other structure.

The speed of your response depends on the level of danger, but even in the situations listed above there may be time for you to plan how to move the victim safely and correctly (p.64).

VICTIM HANDLING (continued)

ASSISTING A VICTIM SAFELY

If you need to assist or move a victim, you need to be aware of the risks that using an incorrect technique might entail. There is the possibility that you might aggravate the victim's condition, and you or any helpers could also suffer injury. You should always take time to plan the operation carefully in order to minimize these risks.

SAFETY GUIDELINES

Take the following steps to ensure safety:
● Select a method relevant to the situation, the victim's condition, and the help and equipment that is available.

● Use a team and appoint one person to coordinate the move. Make sure that the team understands the sequence of actions.
● Prepare any equipment available and make sure that the team and equipment is in position before proceeding.
● Always use the correct technique to avoid injuring the victim, yourself, or helpers.
● Try to ensure the safety and comfort of the victim, yourself, and any helpers throughout the move.
● Always explain to the victim what is happening, and encourage the victim to cooperate as much as possible.

GOOD PRACTICE IN MOVING AND HANDLING

The method that you use to help a victim will depend on the situation, the victim's condition, and whether or not you have any helpers or equipment available. Always plan a move carefully and make sure that the victim and any helpers are prepared for the move. The following sequence of actions when assisting or moving a victim will help ensure the safety and comfort of everyone involved:
● Position yourself as close as possible to the victim's body.

● Adopt a stable base, with your feet shoulder-width apart, so that you remain well-balanced.
● Maintain good posture at all times during the procedure.
● Move smoothly. Use the strongest muscles in your legs and arms to provide the power for the move.

ASSISTING THE EMERGENCY SERVICES

As a first aider, you may be asked to assist the emergency services to move a victim using specialized equipment. Always adopt the elements of good practice outlined above. However, as part of the emergency services team, you should always follow instructions given by the team.

When a victim is being rescued by helicopter, there are a number of ground safety rules to prevent injury to yourself, the victim, or any bystanders. Your main task is to control bystanders. Make sure that people are at least 55 yds (50 m) away, and that all cigarettes are extinguished. Always follow the directions of emergency personnel on scene. Never approach a helicopter unless you are told to do so by the flight crew.

ASSISTING A WALKING VICTIM

If a victim is conscious and able to walk, and you need to remove him from danger, you may be able to help him yourself. You can use the method described below to steady the victim.

If there is a transfer belt available, or if the victim has a walking aid, you can use these items to give extra stability.

 See also CONTROLLING A FALL p.66

SUPPORTING A VICTIM

1 Stand at the victim's injured or weaker side. Take hold of the hand nearest you using the palm-to-palm thumb grip: place your palm under the victim's palm, and close your fingers and thumb around her thumb. Hold the victim's arm out straight, slightly in front of her body.

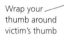

Wrap your thumb around victim's thumb

2 Pass your other arm around the victim's waist. Grasp her belt, waistband, or other clothing at her waist to support her.

3 Make sure that the victim is ready to move. Take small steps, and walk at the victim's pace. Reassure her throughout.

4 If at any stage the victim starts to fall, follow the steps for controlling a fall (p.66).

USING A TRANSFER BELT

1 Fasten the transfer belt around the victim's waist, ensuring that the shaped area of the belt fits centrally at the back.

Adjust belt so that it is comfortably tight

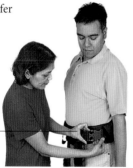

4 Place your other arm around the victim's waist, and grasp one handle of the transfer belt. Make sure that you can easily let go of the belt should the victim fall.

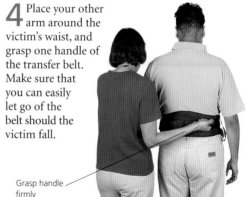

Grasp handle firmly

2 Stand by the victim's weaker side, facing the direction of movement.

3 With one hand, hold the victim's hand nearest you using the palm-to-palm thumb grip (above).

5 If the victim starts to fall, let go of the transfer belt and follow the steps for controlling a fall (p.66).

CONTROLLING A FALL

If you can see that a victim is about to collapse, perhaps because she is fainting, do not try to hold her up; instead, you need to control her fall in order to minimize the risk of injury. You should adopt the following procedure, which allows the victim to slide gently to the floor without injuring either herself or you.

1 Release your hold slightly, and move behind the victim as quickly as possible. Put your arms around the victim, but do not hold on to her.

Use your arms to direct victim's fall

2 Place your feet shoulder-width apart, so that you have a stable base, with one foot in front of the other and knees slightly bent. Allow the victim's weight to fall back against your body, but do not attempt to support her.

Keep one foot in front of the other

3 Maintaining an upright posture, allow the victim to slide down your body to a sitting position on the floor. Guide the victim to the ground

Let victim rest against your legs

4 Kneel down on the ground next to or behind the victim, and adjust her position as much as is necessary to make her comfortable.

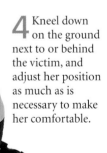

Support and reassure victim

MOVING FROM CHAIR TO FLOOR

If a seated victim is feeling faint or unwell, encourage her to sit or lie down on the floor because this may help her recover. It is much more difficult to move a victim who has already become unconscious. In this situation, you will need two other people to help you move the victim out of her seat and lay her down on the floor.

IF THE VICTIM IS CONSCIOUS

1 Advise the victim to slide off the chair slightly sideways, so that she is kneeling on one knee.

2 From kneeling, the victim should move into a half-sitting position and then sit or lie down as appropriate.

IF THE VICTIM IS UNCONSCIOUS

1 Place a slide sheet (p.69) beneath the victim's legs and feet.

2 You should kneel at the side of the chair and support the victim's head throughout the maneuver. Ask two helpers to position themselves on either side of the victim, facing her.

4 Direct the helpers to grasp the victim's clothing at the back of the hips with their outside hands and to grasp under the victim's knees with their inside hands.

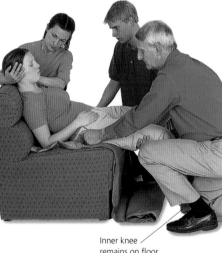

Keep hands on both side of victim's head to support it

Adjust slide sheet if necessary

Inner knee remains on floor

3 The two helpers should get into a half-kneeling position, with their inner knees on the floor and outer legs bent at a right angle with the foot on the floor.

5 Under your direction, while you continue to support the head, the helpers should slide the victim onto the sheet by transferring their body weight back onto their heels. They should then ease the victim into a sitting position on the floor.

6 Move the chair away, then lower the victim onto the slide sheet and into a lying position.

MOVING A COLLAPSED VICTIM

If a victim has collapsed, you may need to turn her over to place her in the recovery position or begin resuscitation. Do not move her from the place where you found her, however, unless she is in a position that may put her or others in danger (such as blocking an exit) or you need to give her life-saving treatment. If you need to move the victim, try to enlist several helpers. Adopt the procedures below to transfer the victim to a blanket, carry sheet, or slide sheet. A carry sheet or a blanket is used to lift a victim. A slide sheet is used to pull a victim along the floor.

PLACING VICTIM ON A CARRY SHEET/BLANKET

1 Roll the sheet or blanket lengthwise to half its usual width.

2 Space your helpers evenly on both side of the victim's body, and ask the helpers to roll the victim onto her side.

3 Place the rolled side of the sheet or blanket against the victim's back with the roll uppermost and the unrolled part on the opposite side to her body.

4 Lower the victim back over the roll and onto her other side.

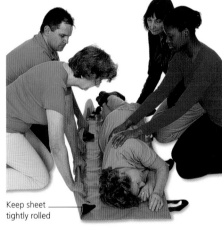

Keep sheet tightly rolled

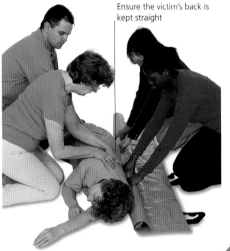

Ensure the victim's back is kept straight

5 Unroll enough of the blanket or sheet to lay the victim flat, then lower her onto it in the required position. If you are moving the victim (opposite), you should all take hold of the sheet together and then move the victim.

> **⚠ WARNING**
>
> Try not to move a victim if you suspect that she has a spinal injury. If you need to move her out of danger, use the "log-roll" technique (p.167).

MOVING EQUIPMENT

There are various items designed for moving victims. The two items described below – the slide sheet and the carry sheet – can be used by nonprofessional handlers such as first aiders or caregivers. You will need training in the use of these items. In addition, you should follow the safety guidelines given by the manufacturer.

SLIDE SHEET

This is a large reinforced nylon sheet with a low-friction underside. A slide sheet enables handlers to carry out a variety of moving procedures. These include helping to turn a victim over, moving a collapsed victim from a chair to the floor (p.67), sliding a victim along the floor, and repositioning a victim in bed.

CARRY SHEET

This sheet has a number of strong fabric handles along the sides for lifting and carrying a victim in any position. The handles allow the weight of the victim to be distributed between a team of handlers (six or eight people). Some types of carry sheet have pockets down the sides to allow poles to be inserted. Metal supports that run across the width of the carry sheet may be attached to the poles; these give the victim additional support.

When the carry sheet is used, handlers should maintain an upright posture, with a straight back and feet shoulder-width apart to provide a stable base.

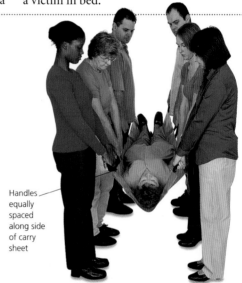

Handles equally spaced along side of carry sheet

CARRY CHAIR

This item is designed for moving a victim in a seated position, particularly through confined spaces or up and down steps. The basic carry chair has two wheels. More sophisticated chairs are available with "roll-over" wheels. This design allows the chair to be wheeled easily over rough ground and moved up and down stairs.

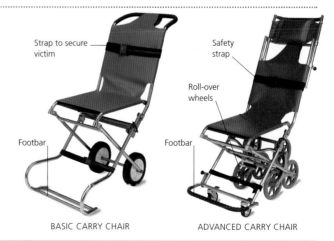

Strap to secure victim

Footbar

BASIC CARRY CHAIR

Safety strap

Roll-over wheels

Footbar

ADVANCED CARRY CHAIR

STRETCHERS AND BOARDS

These items are commonly used by the emergency services. They are designed for carrying victims to ambulances, to shelter, or out of danger. A variety of equipment is available, from basic canvas sheets with poles to specialized stretchers for particular rescue situations and boards for victims with spinal injuries. You should test stretchers regularly for wear and tear and make sure that they can support a victim's weight.

ORTHOPEDIC STRETCHER

This device, also called a "scoop" stretcher, is used to lift a victim onto an ambulance stretcher in the position in which he is found, with minimal movement of the body. This stretcher is not designed to carry victims far. It splits in half lengthwise and the halves are slid under the victim, then rejoined. Once the victim is on the stretcher, the halves are separated and removed. It should be used only by trained medical personnel.

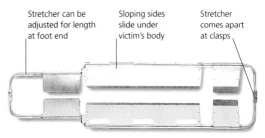

Stretcher can be adjusted for length at foot end

Sloping sides slide under victim's body

Stretcher comes apart at clasps

SPINAL BOARD

This full-body immobilization board is for moving a victim when a spinal injury is suspected. The victim is rolled or slid onto it and then lifted onto an ambulance stretcher. Make sure that the victim is securely strapped to the board. The victim remains on the board during transport to and arrival at the hospital.

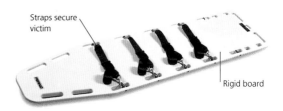

Straps secure victim

Rigid board

AMBULANCE STRETCHER

This stretcher is commonly used only by trained personnel. The collapsible stretcher is usually carried in an ambulance and can be secured in the back of a moving vehicle. It is fully adjustble, from a flat to a chairlike position, to suit the patient. The height of the stretcher is also adjustable to facilitate transfers from the stretcher to a hospital bed.

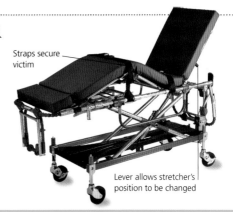

Straps secure victim

Lever allows stretcher's position to be changed

3

T<small>O STAY ALIVE</small> we need an adequate supply of oxygen to enter the lungs and be transferred to all cells in the body through the bloodstream. If a person is deprived of oxygen, the brain begins to fail. The person will lose consciousness, the heartbeat and breathing will cease, and death results.

RESUSCITATION

To restore oxygen to the brain, the airway must be open so that oxygen can enter the body; breathing must be restored to enable oxygen to enter the bloodstream via the lungs; and blood must circulate to all tissues and organs.

Therefore, the priority in treating any collapsed victim is to establish an open airway and maintain breathing and circulation. Because there are certain important differences in the treatment for children and infants, this chapter gives separate step-by-step instructions for adults, children, and infants. Techniques for treating an adult, child, or infant who is choking are also given in this chapter.

✚ FIRST-AID PRIORITIES

- Maintain an open airway, check breathing, and resuscitate.
- If victim is choking, relieve airway obstruction if possible.

CONTENTS

Breathing and circulation............72

Life-saving priorities..................73

Adult resuscitation chart............75

Unconscious adult......................76

Child resuscitation chart............86

Unconscious child
(1–7 years)............................87

Infant resuscitation chart...........94

Unconscious infant
(under 1 year)......................95

Choking summary charts...........99

Choking adult........................100

Choking child
(1–7 years)...........................101

Choking infant
(under 1 year)......................102

LIEE-SAVING PROCEDURES

BREATHING AND CIRCULATION

Oxygen is essential to support life. Without it, cells in the body die – those in the brain survive only a few minutes without oxygen. Oxygen is taken in when we inhale (*see* THE RESPIRATORY SYSTEM, p.104), and it is then circulated to all the body tissues via the circulatory system (p.118). It is vital to maintain breathing and circulation in order to sustain life.

BREATHING

The process of breathing enables air, which contains oxygen, to be taken into the air sacs (alveoli) in the lungs. Here, the oxygen is transferred across blood vessel walls into the blood, where it combines with the hemoglobin in the blood cells. The waste product of breathing, carbon dioxide, is released and exhaled in the breath.

CIRCULATION

When oxygen has been transferred to the blood cells, it has to be circulated to all the body tissues (via blood vessels). The "pump" that maintains this circulation is the heart. Oxygen-rich blood is carried from the lungs to the heart through the pulmonary veins. The heart pumps the oxygen-rich blood to the rest of the body in blood vessels called arteries. Other blood vessels called veins bring deoxygenated blood back from the tissues to the heart (p.118). The heart pumps this blood, via the pulmonary arteries, to the lungs, where it is oxygenated and carbon dioxide is removed.

▶ **See also** HOW BREATHING WORKS p.105
● THE HEART AND BLOOD VESSELS p.118
● THE RESPIRATORY SYSTEM p.104

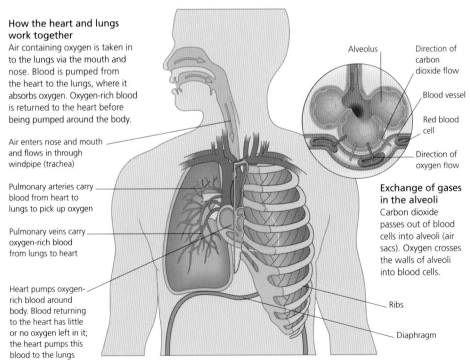

How the heart and lungs work together
Air containing oxygen is taken in to the lungs via the mouth and nose. Blood is pumped from the heart to the lungs, where it absorbs oxygen. Oxygen-rich blood is returned to the heart before being pumped around the body.

Air enters nose and mouth and flows in through windpipe (trachea)

Pulmonary arteries carry blood from heart to lungs to pick up oxygen

Pulmonary veins carry oxygen-rich blood from lungs to heart

Heart pumps oxygen-rich blood around body. Blood returning to the heart has little or no oxygen left in it; the heart pumps this blood to the lungs

Alveolus

Direction of carbon dioxide flow

Blood vessel

Red blood cell

Direction of oxygen flow

Exchange of gases in the alveoli
Carbon dioxide passes out of blood cells into alveoli (air sacs). Oxygen crosses the walls of alveoli into blood cells.

Ribs

Diaphragm

LIFE-SAVING PRIORITIES

The procedures set out in this chapter can assist a victim's breathing and circulation until emergency aid arrives.

With a pulseless victim, your priorities are to maintain an open airway, breathe for the victim (to get oxygen into the body), and maintain blood circulation (to get oxygen-rich blood to the tissues). In addition, a machine called a defibrillator (pp.82–83) can deliver a controlled electric shock to restore a normal heartbeat. The following factors increase the chances of survival if all elements are complete:

- Help is called quickly.
- Blood circulation is maintained by rescue breathing and chest compressions (together known as cardiopulmonary resuscitation or CPR).
- In an adult victim with no signs of circulation, a defibrillator is used promptly.
- The victim reaches a hospital quickly for specialized treatment and advanced care.

Chain of survival
Four elements increase the chances of a pulseless victim surviving. If any one of the elements in this chain is missing, the chances are reduced.

Early help	Early CPR	Early defibrillation	Early advanced care
Dial 9•1•1 or call EMS so that a defibrillator and expert help can be brought to the victim.	Chest compressions and rescue breaths are used to "buy time" until expert help arrives.	A controlled electric shock from a defibrillator is given. This jolts the heart into a normal rhythm.	Specialized treatment by paramedics and at the hospital stabilizes the victim's condition.

IMPORTANCE OF AN OPEN AIRWAY

An unconscious victim's airway may become narrowed or blocked. This is due to muscular control being lost, allowing the tongue to fall back and block the airway. When this happens, the victim's breathing becomes difficult and noisy or breathing may become completely impossible.

Lifting the chin and tilting the head back lifts the tongue from the entrance to the air passage, allowing the victim to breathe.

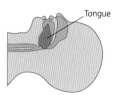 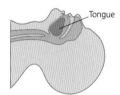

Blocked airway
In an unconscious victim, the tongue falls back, blocking the throat and airway.

Open airway
In the head tilt, chin lift position, the tongue is lifted from the back of the throat: the airway is clear.

BREATHING FOR A VICTIM

The air we exhale contains about 16 percent oxygen (5 percent less than in the air we inhale) in addition to a small amount of carbon dioxide. Exhaled breath therefore contains enough oxygen to supply another person with oxygen – and keep him alive – when it is forced into the victim's lungs during rescue breathing.

By giving rescue breaths, you can force air into the victim's air passages. This air reaches the air sacs (alveoli) in the lungs, and oxygen is then transferred to the tiny blood vessels within the lungs.

When you remove your mouth from the victim's mouth, the chest falls and air containing waste products is exhaled.

LIFE-SAVING PRIORITIES (continued)

MAINTAINING CIRCULATION

If the heart stops beating, blood does not circulate through the body. As a result, vital organs, most importantly the brain, become starved of oxygen. Brain cells are unable to survive for more than a few minutes without a supply of oxygen.

Some circulation can be maintained artificially by chest compressions. These compressions act as a mechanical aid to the heart to get blood flowing around the body. Pushing down vertically on the lower half of the breastbone squeezes the heart against the backbone, expelling blood from the heart's chambers and forcing it into the tissues. As pressure is released, the chest rises, and replacement blood is "sucked" in to refill the heart; this blood is then forced out of the heart by the next compression.

To ensure that the blood is adequately supplied with oxygen, chest compressions must be combined with rescue breathing.

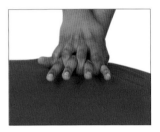

Giving chest compressions
Pushing down on the chest, using the correct technique, can maintain blood circulation.

RESTORING HEART RHYTHM

A defibrillator, or automated external defibrillator (AED), can be used to attempt to reverse an abnormal heart rhythm. Early defibrillation is an important element in the chain of survival; the earlier it is used after a cardiac arrest (when the heart has stopped beating and there is no circulation), the greater the chance of the victim surviving.

Before using a defibrillator you must be trained in its use and be able to carry out cardiopulmonary resuscitation (CPR), which is the combination of chest compressions with rescue breathing.

Defibrillators can be found in many public places, such as railway stations and shopping centers.

WHEN TO CALL 9·1·1 OR EMS

If you have a helper, send him to call 9·1·1 or EMS as soon as you know that the victim is not breathing. If you are on your own, your course of action depends on the age of the victim and the likely cause of the unconsciousness.

CHILD OR INFANT VICTIM
Unconsciousness in an infant or child under 8 years is most likely to be due to a breathing problem. For this reason, you should give rescue breaths and chest compressions for 1 minute before leaving the child to call 9·1·1 or EMS.

ADULT VICTIM
If an adult victim's pulselessness is due to a heart problem, or you do not know what has happened, call 9·1·1 or EMS immediately after noting that breathing is absent. Early medical help, including the use of a defibrillator, is vital.

However, if the pulselessness is due to injury, drowning, or choking, and no help is available, give chest compressions and rescue breaths for 1 minute, then call 9·1·1 or EMS. In these cases, pulselessness is more likely to be due to a breathing problem than a heart condition.

ADULT RESUSCITATION CHART

The sequence below summarizes the main actions you need to take when dealing with an adult, or child aged 8 or over, who is unconscious. The chart assumes that you have already checked for any danger to yourself or the victim. The pages that follow give you full details on how to carry out each step in the resuscitation sequence.

CHECK RESPONSIVENESS
- Try to get a response by asking questions and gently shaking his shoulders (p.76).
- Is there a response?

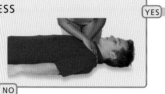

YES → Leave the victim in the position found, and summon help if needed.

NO

OPEN THE AIRWAY; CHECK FOR BREATHING
- Tilt the head back to open the airway (p.77), removing any obvious obstruction. Check for breathing (p.77).
- Is he breathing?

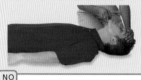

YES → Check for life-threatening injuries. Place the victim in the recovery position (pp.84–85), and summon help.

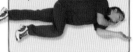

NO

Send a helper to **CALL 9•1•1 OR EMS**

RESCUE BREATHING
- Give two effective rescue breaths (pp.78–79).

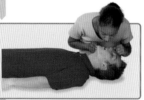

⚠ WARNING

If you are alone, call 9•1•1 or EMS as soon as you know the victim is not breathing – unless the pulselessness is due to injury, choking, or drowning. In these cases, give chest compressions and rescue breaths for 1 minute before calling 9•1•1 or EMS (see WHEN TO CALL 9•1•1 OR EMS, opposite).

ASSESS FOR CIRCULATION
- Check for signs of circulation for not more than 10 seconds (p.80).
- Are there signs of circulation?

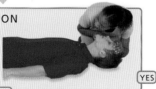

YES → Continue giving rescue breaths. Check for signs of circulation after every minute (about 10 breaths). If the victim starts breathing but remains unconscious, place him in the recovery position (pp.84–85).

NO

BEGIN CPR
- Alternate 15 chest compressions with two rescue breaths (p.80–81).
- Repeat as necessary.

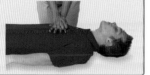

UNCONSCIOUS ADULT

The following pages give instructions for all the techniques that may be needed in the resuscitation of an unconscious adult.

Always approach and treat the victim from the side, kneeling down next to his head or chest. You will then be in the correct position for carrying out all the possible stages of resuscitation: opening the victim's airway; checking breathing and circulation; and giving rescue breaths and chest compressions (together called cardiopulmonary resuscitation or CPR).

At each stage in the process, you will have decisions to make – for example, is the victim breathing? The steps given here tell you what to do next in each situation.

The first priority is to open the victim's airway so that he can breathe or you can give effective rescue breaths. If breathing and circulation return at any stage, place the victim in the recovery position. If he is not breathing and there are no signs of circulation, the correct use of a defibrillator will increase the chance of survival.

HOW TO CHECK RESPONSE

On discovering a collapsed person, you should first establish whether he is conscious or unconscious. Do this by gently shaking his shoulders. Ask "What has happened?" or give a command: "Open your eyes." Speak loudly and clearly.

> **❶ CAUTION**
> Always assume that there is a neck injury and shake the shoulders very gently.

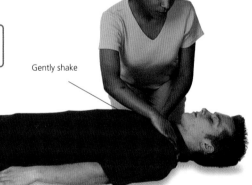

Gently shake

IF THERE IS A RESPONSE

1 If there is no further danger, leave the person in the position in which he was found and summon help if needed.

2 Treat any condition found and monitor vital signs – level of response, pulse, and breathing (pp.42–43).

3 Continue monitoring the victim either until help arrives or he recovers.

IF THERE IS NO RESPONSE

1 Shout for help. If possible, leave the victim in the position in which he was found and open the airway.

2 If this is not possible, turn him onto his back and open the airway.

▶ **Go to** HOW TO OPEN THE AIRWAY opposite

HOW TO OPEN THE AIRWAY

1 Kneel by the person's head. Place one hand on his forehead. Gently tilt his head back. As you do this, the mouth will fall open.

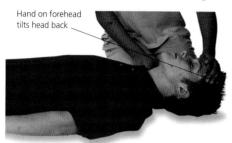

Hand on forehead tilts head back

3 Place the fingertips of your other hand under the point of the victim's chin and lift the chin.

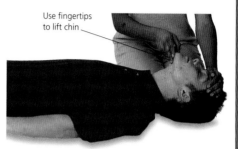

Use fingertips to lift chin

2 Pick out any obvious obstructions, such as dislodged dentures or broken teeth, from the victim's mouth. Do not do a finger sweep. Leave well-fitting dentures in place.

4 Check to see if the victim is now breathing.

(▶) **Go to** HOW TO CHECK BREATHING below

HOW TO CHECK BREATHING

Keeping the airway open, look, listen, and feel for breathing: look for chest movement, listen for sounds of breathing, and feel for breath on your cheek. Do this for no more than 10 seconds before deciding that breathing is absent.

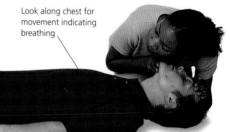

Look along chest for movement indicating breathing

IF THE VICTIM IS BREATHING

1 Check the victim for any life-threatening injuries, such as severe bleeding, and treat as necessary.

2 Place the victim in the recovery position. Monitor vital signs – level of response, pulse, and breathing (pp.42–43).

(▶) **Go to** HOW TO PLACE IN RECOVERY POSITION pp.84–85

IF THE VICTIM IS NOT BREATHING

1 CALL 9·1·1 OR EMS. Send a helper if available. If alone, see WHEN TO DIAL 9·1·1 OR CALL EMS, p.74.

2 Give two effective rescue breaths and then check for signs of circulation.

(▶) **Go to** HOW TO GIVE RESCUE BREATHS pp.78–79

UNCONSCIOUS ADULT (continued)

HOW TO GIVE RESCUE BREATHS

1 Make sure that the victim's airway is still open, by keeping one hand on his forehead and two fingers of the other hand under the tip of his chin.

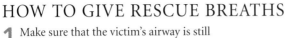

Keep chin lifted so that airway is open

2 Move the hand that was on the forehead down to the nose. Pinch the soft part of the nose with the finger and thumb. Open the victim's mouth.

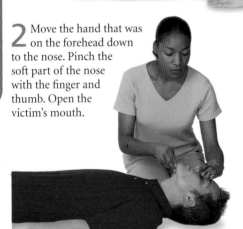

3 If you have a face shield or pocket mask (below), place it over the victim's mouth. Take a deep breath to fill your lungs with air and place your lips around the victim's mouth, making sure you have a good seal.

Continue to pinch the nose while taking a breath

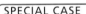

SPECIAL CASE

USING A FACE SHIELD OR POCKET MASK

First aiders may receive training in the use of these aids for hygienic purposes. Face shields are plastic barriers with a reinforced hole to fit over the victim's mouth. The mask is more substantial and has a valve.

If you are trained to use one of these aids, carry it with you at all times and use it if you need to resuscitate a victim. If you do not have a mask or shield with you, do not hesitate to give rescue breaths.

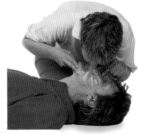

USING A FACE SHIELD

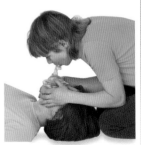

USING A POCKET MASK

4 Blow steadily into the victim's mouth until the chest rises. This usually takes about 2 seconds.

5 Maintaining head tilt and chin lift, take your mouth off the victim's mouth and see if his chest falls. If the chest rises visibly as you blow and falls fully when you lift your mouth away, you have given an effective breath. Give two effective breaths, then check for signs of circulation.

▶ **Go to** HOW TO CHECK FOR CIRCULATION p.80

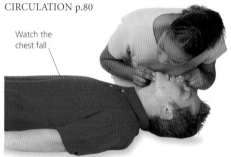

Watch the chest fall

IF YOU CANNOT ACHIEVE EFFECTIVE BREATHS

- Recheck the head tilt and chin lift.
- Recheck the victim's mouth. Remove any obvious obstructions, but do not do a finger sweep of the mouth.
- Make no more than five attempts to achieve two effective breaths.

If you still cannot achieve two effective breaths, check the victim for signs of circulation.

▶ **Go to** HOW TO CHECK FOR CIRCULATION p.80

⚠ WARNING

If you know that the victim has choked, and you cannot achieve effective breaths, you must immediately begin giving chest compressions and rescue breaths to try to relieve the obstruction quickly (*see* HOW TO GIVE CPR, pp.80–81).

SPECIAL CASE

MOUTH-TO-NOSE RESCUE BREATHING

In situations such as rescue from water, or where injuries to the mouth make it impossible to achieve a good seal, you may choose to use the mouth-to-nose method for giving rescue breaths. With the victim's mouth closed, form a tight seal with your lips around the nose and blow steadily into the victim's nose. Then allow the mouth to fall open to let the air escape.

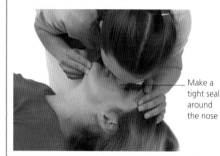

Make a tight seal around the nose

SPECIAL CASE

MOUTH-TO-STOMA RESCUE BREATHING

A victim who has had the voice box surgically removed breathes through a stoma (opening) in the front of the neck rather than the mouth and nose. Always check for a stoma before giving rescue breaths. If you find a stoma, close off the mouth and nose with your thumb and fingers and then breathe into the stoma.

Close off victim's mouth and nose with your thumb and fingers

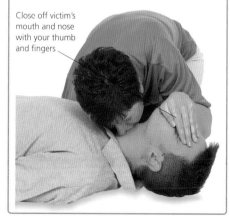

UNCONSCIOUS ADULT (continued)

HOW TO CHECK FOR CIRCULATION

Still kneeling beside the victim's head, look, listen, and feel for signs of circulation, such as breathing, coughing, or movement. Carry out this check for no more than 10 seconds.

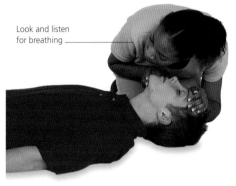

Look and listen for breathing

IF SIGNS OF CIRCULATION ARE ABSENT

Begin giving chest compressions with rescue breaths (cardiopulmonary resuscitation – CPR) immediately.

▶ Go to HOW TO GIVE CPR below

IF YOU ARE SURE YOU HAVE DETECTED SIGNS OF CIRCULATION

1 Continue rescue breathing. After every 10 breaths (about 1 minute), recheck for signs of circulation. If the victim starts to breathe but remains unconscious, turn him into the recovery position (pp.84–85).

2 Monitor vital signs – level of response, pulse, and breathing (pp.42–43). Be prepared to turn him onto his back again to restart rescue breathing (pp.78–79).

HOW TO GIVE CPR

1 Compressions are administered to the center of the chest. The following steps are the most accurate method for locating the best spot for compressions. Kneel beside the victim. With the index and middle fingers of your lower hand, locate the lowermost rib on that side. Slide your fingertips along the rib to where the lowermost ribs meet at the breastbone. Place your middle finger at this point and your index finger beside it on the lower breastbone.

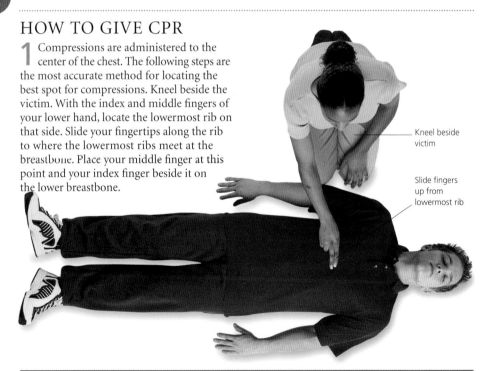

Kneel beside victim

Slide fingers up from lowermost rib

2 Place the heel of your other hand on the breastbone, and slide it down until it reaches your index finger. This is the point at which you should apply pressure.

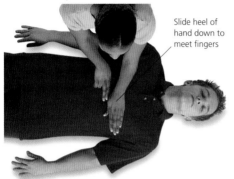

Slide heel of hand down to meet fingers

3 Place the heel of your first hand on top of the other hand, and interlock your fingers.

Keep fingers clear of chest

4 Leaning well over the victim, with your arms straight, press down vertically on the breastbone and depress the chest by about 1½–2 in (4–5 cm). Release the pressure without removing your hands from his chest.

5 Compress the chest 15 times at a rate of 100 compressions per minute. The time taken for compression and release should be about the same.

6 Tilt the head, lift the chin, and give two rescue breaths (pp.78–79).

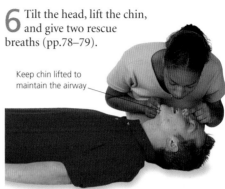

Keep chin lifted to maintain the airway

7 Continue this cycle of alternating 15 chest compressions with two rescue breaths. Continue CPR until: emergency help arrives and takes over; the victim makes a movement or takes a spontaneous breath; or you become so exhausted that you cannot carry on.

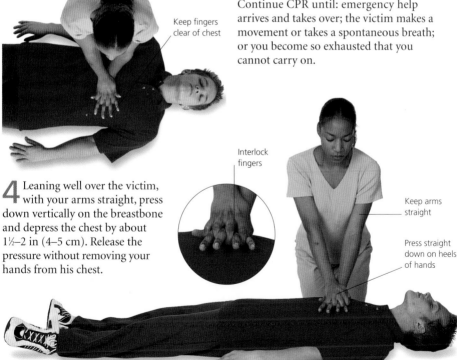

Interlock fingers

Keep arms straight

Press straight down on heels of hands

UNCONSCIOUS ADULT (continued)

HOW TO USE A DEFIBRILLATOR

When the heart stops and there are no signs of circulation, a cardiac arrest has occurred. The most common cause is an abnormal rhythm of the heart known as ventricular fibrillation. This abnormal rhythm can occur when insufficient oxygen reaches the heart or when the heart is damaged as a result of a heart attack. A machine called an automated external defibrillator (AED), or defibrillator, can be used to correct the heart rhythm. Defibrillators are available in many public places, including shopping centers and airports. The defibrillator analyzes the victim's heart rhythm and tells you what action to take at each stage. However, you must be trained in its use and be able to carry out CPR (pp.80–81).

In most cases where a defibrillator is called for, you will have already started the life-saving sequence. When the defibrillator arrives, stop what you are doing and start using the defibrillator.

---

❶ CAUTION

● Make sure that no one is touching the victim because this will interfere with the defibrillator readings.

● Do not turn off the defibrillator or remove the pads at any point, even if the victim appears to have recovered.

1 Switch on the defibrillator and check that the electrode leads are plugged in. Remove or cut through clothing covering the chest and quickly wipe away any sweat. Shave chest hair if it is excessive because it will prevent the pads from sticking to the skin.

2 Remove the backing paper from the electrode pads and attach them to the victim's chest in the position indicated on the pads.

3 The defibrillator will start analyzing the heart rhythm; make sure that no one is touching the victim. Follow the spoken and/or visual prompts (opposite). These will advise you when a shock is indicated, when to check for signs of circulation (p.80), and when to give chest compressions and rescue breaths (*see* HOW TO GIVE CPR, p.80–81).

4 Continue to follow the prompts from the defibrillator until the emergency services arrive and advanced care is available. If at any time the victim starts breathing, place him in the recovery position (pp.84–85). Leave the defibrillator attached.

Make sure helper does not touch victim while machine is analyzing

Defibrillator

Place electrode pads on each side of heart

SEQUENCE OF DEFIBRILLATOR INSTRUCTIONS

The defibrillator will give a series of visual and verbal prompts as soon as it is switched on. Some older machines may tell you to check the pulse. In this case, you must in fact check for circulation. Do not waste time trying to find the pulse. Continue to follow the prompts given by the defibrillator until advanced care is available.

- Switch defibrillator on and make sure leads are connected.
- Attach pads to victim's chest.

Defibrillator gets ready to analyze the victim's heart. It may state "Stand clear, analyzing now" or just "Analyzing." Make sure no one is touching the victim or the defibrillator will be unable to analyze. Is shock advised?

YES

Defibrillator advises that a shock is needed. The machine charges up; an alarm sounds when the machine is ready.

Defibrillator instructs you to deliver the shock.
- Make sure everyone is clear of the victim.
- Push the shock button.
Defibrillator delivers the shock and then reanalyzes the heart rhythm. You may be prompted to give up to three shocks.

Defibrillator instructs you to check for circulation (older machines may state "check pulse" – always check circulation).
- Check for signs of circulation (p.80) for no more than 10 seconds. Is there circulation?

YES

- Check airway and breathing (p.77).

NO

- Start CPR (pp.80–81) as instructed. Continue for 1 minute (until machine prompts you to stop).

The defibrillator reanalyzes heart rhythm.

NO

Defibrillator advises that no shock is needed.

Defibrillator instructs you to check for circulation (older machines may state "check pulse" – always check circulation).
- Look for signs of circulation (p.80) for no more than 10 seconds. Is there circulation?

YES

- Check airway and breathing (p.77).

NO

- Start CPR (pp.80–81) Continue for 1 minute (until machine prompts you to stop).

The defibrillator reanalyzes heart rhythm.

UNCONSCIOUS ADULT (continued)

HOW TO PLACE IN RECOVERY POSITION

1 Kneel beside the injured person. Remove glasses and any very bulky objects, such as cell phones and large bunches of keys, from the pockets. Do not search the pockets for small items.

2 Make sure that both of the legs are straight.

3 Place the arm that is nearest you at a right angle to the body, with the elbow bent and the palm facing upward.

---

❶ WARNING

If you suspect that the victim may have sustained a spinal injury, maintain an open airway with the victim in the position in which he was found or by using the jaw thrust method (p.167).

---

❶ CAUTION

If the victim is found lying on his side or front, not all of these steps will be necessary to place him in the recovery position.

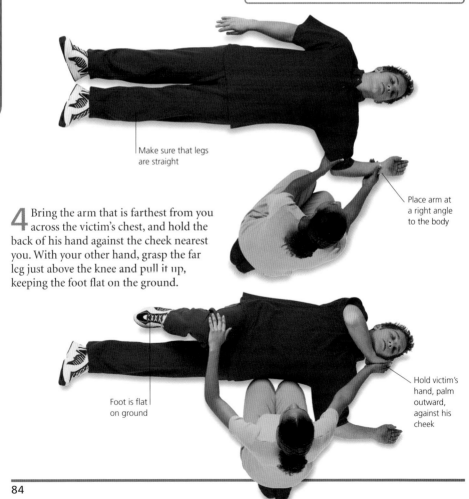

Make sure that legs are straight

Place arm at a right angle to the body

4 Bring the arm that is farthest from you across the victim's chest, and hold the back of his hand against the cheek nearest you. With your other hand, grasp the far leg just above the knee and pull it up, keeping the foot flat on the ground.

Foot is flat on ground

Hold victim's hand, palm outward, against his cheek

5 Keeping the victim's hand pressed against his cheek, pull on the far leg and roll the victim toward you and onto his side.

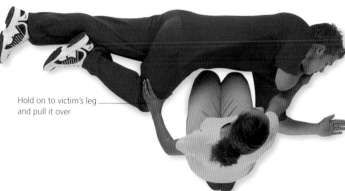

Hold on to victim's leg and pull it over

6 Adjust the upper leg so that both the hip and the knee are bent at right angles.

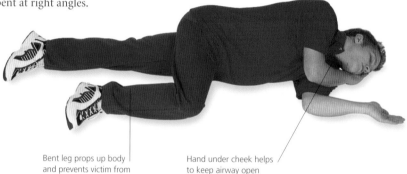

Bent leg props up body and prevents victim from rolling forward

Hand under cheek helps to keep airway open

7 Tilt the victim's head back so that the airway remains open. If necessary, adjust the hand under the cheek to make sure that the head remains tilted and the airway stays open.

8 If it has not already been done, DIAL 9·1·1 OR CALL EMS. Monitor and record vital signs – level of response, pulse, and breathing (pp.42–43).

9 If the victim has to be left in the recovery position for longer than 30 minutes, roll him onto his back, and then turn him onto the opposite side – unless other injuries prevent you from doing this.

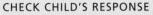

CHILD RESUSCITATION CHART

The resuscitation method used depends on the child's age and size. In children aged 1–7, respiratory failure (absence of breathing) is the main reason for the heart to stop. Ask a helper to call 9·1·1 or EMS while you treat the child, but if you are alone, resuscitate for 1 minute before calling for help.

For a child aged 8 or over, use the adult resuscitation sequence (pp.75–85).

CHECK CHILD'S RESPONSE
- Try to get a response by asking questions and gently tapping the child's shoulder.
- Is there a response?

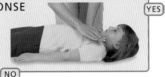

YES → Leave the child in the position found and summon help if needed.

NO

OPEN THE AIRWAY; CHECK FOR BREATHING
- Tilt the head back to open the airway (p.88), removing any obvious obstruction. Check for breathing (p.88).
- Is the child breathing?

YES → Check for life-threatening injuries. Place the child in the recovery position (pp.92–93) and summon help.

NO

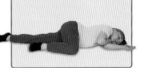

Send a helper to **DIAL 9·1·1 OR CALL EMS**

BREATHE FOR CHILD
- Give two effective rescue breaths (p.89).

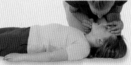

❶ WARNING
If you are alone, carry out rescue breathing and chest compressions for 1 minute before leaving the child to call 9·1·1 or EMS (see WHEN TO DIAL 9·1·1 OR CALL EMS, p.74).

ASSESS FOR CIRCULATION
- Check for circulation for no more than 10 seconds (p.90).
- Are there signs of circulation?

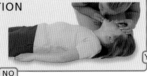

YES → Continue rescue breathing. After every 20 breaths (about 1 minute) recheck for signs of circulation. If the child starts to breathe but remains unconscious, place her in the recovery position (pp.92–93).

NO

COMMENCE CPR
- Alternate five chest compressions with one rescue breath (pp.90–91).
- Repeat as necessary.

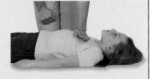

UNCONSCIOUS CHILD (1–7 years)

The following pages give full instructions for resuscitating a child aged 1–7 who is found collapsed. For a child aged 8 or over, use the adult resuscitation procedure (pp.75–85).

Always approach and treat the child from the side, kneeling down next to the head or chest. You will then be in the correct position for doing all the possible stages of resuscitation: opening the airway, checking the breathing and circulation, and giving rescue breaths and chest compressions (together known as cardiopulmonary resuscitation or CPR).

At each stage you will have decisions to make. The steps given here will guide you through each technique, then advise you on what to do next. Your first priority is to ensure that the airway is open and clear so that the child can breathe or you can give effective rescue breaths if needed. If normal breathing and circulation resume, place the child in the recovery position (pp.92–93).

Call 9·1·1 or EMS immediately if a child who has a known heart disease collapses suddenly because early access to advanced care may be life-saving.

HOW TO CHECK FOR RESPONSE

On discovering a collapsed child, you should first establish whether she is conscious or unconscious. Do this by speaking loudly and clearly to the child. Ask "What has happened?" or give a command: "Open your eyes." Place one hand on her shoulder, and gently tap her.

Gently tap shoulder

IF THERE IS A RESPONSE

1 If there is no further danger, leave the child in the position in which she was found and summon help if needed.

2 Treat any condition found and regularly monitor vital signs – level of response, pulse, and breathing (pp.42–43)

3 Continue this until either help arrives or the child recovers.

IF THERE IS NO RESPONSE

1 Shout for help. If possible, leave the child in the position in which she was found, then open the airway.

2 If this is not possible, turn the child onto her back and open the airway.

(▶) Go to HOW TO OPEN THE AIRWAY, p.88.

UNCONSCIOUS CHILD (continued)

HOW TO OPEN THE AIRWAY

1 Kneel by the child's head. Place one hand on her forehead. Gently tilt her head back. As you do this, the mouth will fall open.

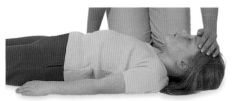

2 Pick out any obvious obstructions from the mouth. Do not do a finger sweep.

Use fingertips only to remove obstruction

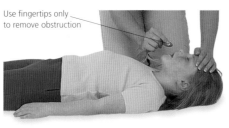

3 Place the fingertips of your other hand under the point of the child's chin and gently lift the chin.

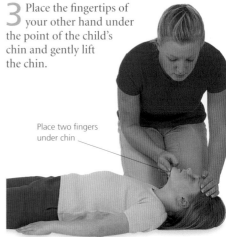

Place two fingers under chin

4 Check to see if the child is now breathing.

▶ Go to HOW TO CHECK BREATHING below

HOW TO CHECK BREATHING

Keep the airway open and look, listen, and feel for breathing – look for chest movement, listen for sounds of breathing, and feel for breath on your cheek. Do this for no more than 10 seconds.

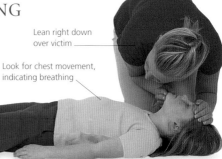

Lean right down over victim

Look for chest movement, indicating breathing

IF THE CHILD IS BREATHING

1 Check for life-threatening injuries such as severe bleeding. Treat as necessary.

2 Place the child in the recovery position. Regularly monitor her vital signs – level of response, pulse, and breathing (pp.42–43).

▶ Go to HOW TO PLACE IN RECOVERY POSITION pp.92–93

IF THE CHILD IS NOT BREATHING

1 Ask a helper to DIAL 9·1·1 OR CALL EMS.

2 Give two effective rescue breaths (right) and then check for signs of circulation.

▶ Go to HOW TO GIVE RESCUE BREATHS opposite

HOW TO GIVE RESCUE BREATHS

1 Ensure the airway is still open by keeping one hand on the child's forehead and two fingers of the other hand under her chin.

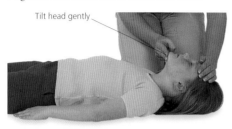

Tilt head gently

2 Pinch the soft part of the child's nose with the finger and thumb of the hand that was on the forehead. Make sure that her nostrils are closed to prevent air from escaping. Open her mouth.

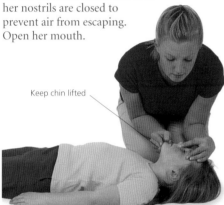

Keep chin lifted

3 Take a deep breath to fill your lungs with air. Place your lips around the child's mouth, making sure that you form an airtight seal.

Make sure that nostrils are tightly closed

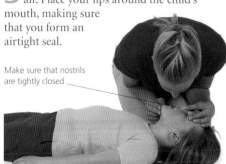

4 Blow steadily into the child's mouth until the chest rises.

5 Maintaining head tilt and chin lift, take your mouth off the child's mouth and see if her chest falls. If the chest rises visibly as you blow and falls fully when you lift your mouth, you have given an effective breath. Give two effective breaths, then check for signs of circulation.

▶ **Go to** HOW TO CHECK FOR CIRCULATION p.90

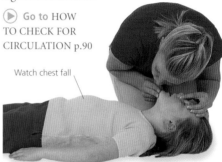

Watch chest fall

IF YOU CANNOT ACHIEVE EFFECTIVE BREATHS

- Recheck the head tilt and chin lift.
- Recheck the child's mouth. Remove any obvious obstructions, but do not do a finger sweep of the mouth.
- Make no more than five attempts to achieve two effective breaths.

If you still cannot achieve two effective breaths, check the child for signs of circulation.

▶ **Go to** HOW TO CHECK FOR CIRCULATION p.90

---

❶ WARNING

If you know that the child has choked, and you cannot achieve effective breaths, you must immediately begin giving chest compressions to try to relieve the obstruction quickly (see HOW TO GIVE CPR, p.90).

UNCONSCIOUS CHILD (continued)

HOW TO CHECK FOR CIRCULATION

Still kneeling beside the child's head, look, listen, and feel for signs of circulation, such as breathing, coughing, or movement. Check for these signs of circulation for no more than 10 seconds.

Look and listen for breathing

IF THERE ARE NO SIGNS OF CIRCULATION

Begin chest compressions and rescue breaths (cardiopulmonary resuscitation – CPR) immediately. Continue for 1 minute, then DIAL 9•1•1 OR CALL EMS.

▶ Go to HOW TO GIVE CPR below

IF YOU ARE SURE YOU HAVE DETECTED SIGNS OF CIRCULATION

1 Continue rescue breathing for 1 minute. Then DIAL 9•1•1 OR CALL EMS. After every 20 breaths (about 1 minute), check for signs of circulation. If the child starts to breathe but remains unconscious, place her in the recovery position (pp.92–93).

2 Monitor and record vital signs – level of response, pulse, and breathing (pp.42–43). Be prepared to turn the child on to her back again to restart rescue breathing (p.89).

HOW TO GIVE CPR

1 Compressions are administered to the center of the chest. The following steps are the most accurate method for locating the best spot for compressions. Use the fingertips of your lower hand to locate her lowermost rib on that side. Slide your fingertips along the rib to where the lowermost ribs meet at the breastbone. Place your middle finger at this point and your index finger beside it on the lower breastbone.

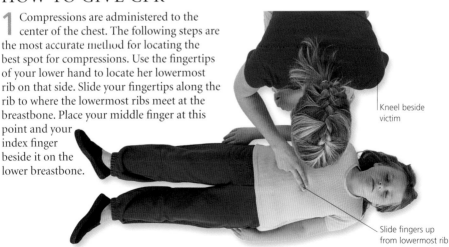

Kneel beside victim

Slide fingers up from lowermost rib

2 Place the heel of your other hand on the breastbone and slide it down until it reaches your index finger. This is the point at which you will apply pressure.

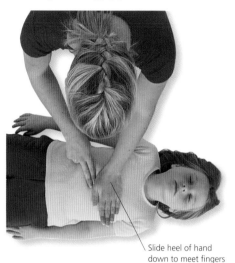

Slide heel of hand down to meet fingers

3 Use the heel of one hand only to apply pressure – keep your fingers raised so that you do not apply pressure to the child's ribs.

Keep fingers clear of chest

4 Leaning well over the child, with your arm straight, press down vertically on the breastbone and depress the chest by 1–1½ in (2½–4 cm). Release the pressure without removing your hand.

5 Compress the chest five times, at a rate of 100 compressions per minute. Compression and release should take the same amount of time.

6 Tilt the head, lift the chin, and give one rescue breath (p.89).

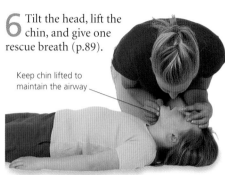

Keep chin lifted to maintain the airway

7 Continue this cycle of alternating five chest compressions with one rescue breath. Continue CPR until emergency help arrives and takes over; the child makes a movement or takes a spontaneous breath; or you become so exhausted that you cannot continue.

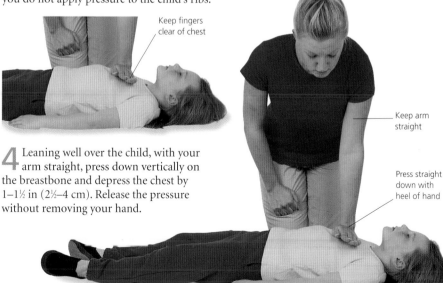

Keep arm straight

Press straight down with heel of hand

UNCONSCIOUS CHILD (continued)

HOW TO PLACE IN RECOVERY POSITION

1 Kneel beside the child. Remove glasses and any very bulky objects from the pockets, but do not search for small items.

> **⚠ WARNING**
>
> If you suspect a spinal injury, maintain the airway with the child in the position in which she was found or by using the jaw thrust method (p.167).

2 Make sure that both of the child's legs are straight. Place the arm that is nearest you at a right angle to the child's body, with the elbow bent and the palm facing upward.

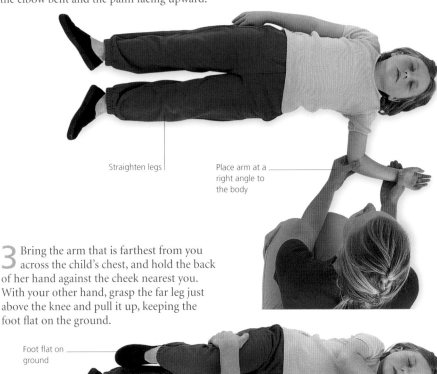

Straighten legs

Place arm at a right angle to the body

3 Bring the arm that is farthest from you across the child's chest, and hold the back of her hand against the cheek nearest you. With your other hand, grasp the far leg just above the knee and pull it up, keeping the foot flat on the ground.

Foot flat on ground

Hold child's hand, palm outward, against her cheek

> **⚠ CAUTION**
>
> If the child is found lying on her side or front, not all of these steps will be necessary to place her in the recovery position.

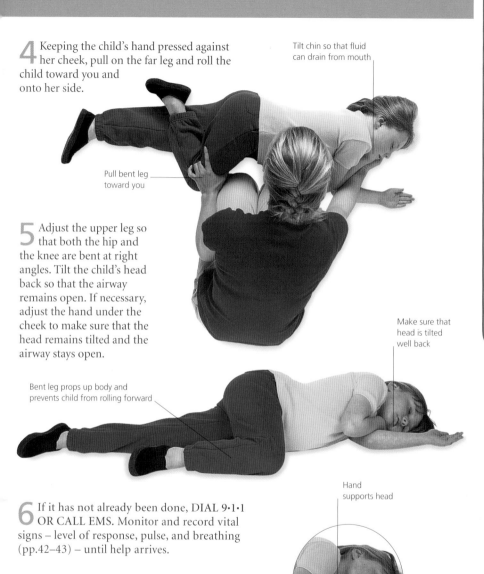

4 Keeping the child's hand pressed against her cheek, pull on the far leg and roll the child toward you and onto her side.

Tilt chin so that fluid can drain from mouth

Pull bent leg toward you

5 Adjust the upper leg so that both the hip and the knee are bent at right angles. Tilt the child's head back so that the airway remains open. If necessary, adjust the hand under the cheek to make sure that the head remains tilted and the airway stays open.

Make sure that head is tilted well back

Bent leg props up body and prevents child from rolling forward

Hand supports head

6 If it has not already been done, DIAL 9·1·1 OR CALL EMS. Monitor and record vital signs – level of response, pulse, and breathing (pp.42–43) – until help arrives.

7 If the child has to be left in the recovery position for longer than 30 minutes, you should roll her onto her back, then turn her onto the opposite side – unless other injuries prevent you from doing this.

INFANT RESUSCITATION CHART

In infants under 1 year, a problem with breathing is the most probable reason for the heart to stop. As soon as you have established that the infant is not breathing, ask a helper to call 9•1•1 or EMS while you treat the infant.

CHECK INFANT'S RESPONSE

- Gently tap or flick the sole of the infant's foot. Never shake an infant.
- Is there a response?

YES → Take the infant with you to summon help if needed.

NO ↓

OPEN THE AIRWAY; CHECK FOR BREATHING

- Place one hand on the infant's forehead and very gently tilt the head back. Remove any obvious obstruction. Lift the chin. Check for breathing (p.96).
- Is the infant breathing?

YES → Check for life-threatening injuries. Hold the infant in the recovery position (p.98) and summon help.

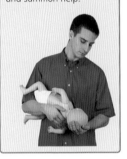

NO ↓

Send a helper to **DIAL 9•1•1 OR CALL EMS.**

↓

BREATHE FOR THE INFANT

- Give two effective rescue breaths (pp.96–97).

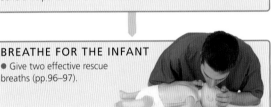

⊙ WARNING

If you are alone, carry out rescue breathing and chest compressions for 1 minute before taking the infant with you to call 9•1•1 or EMS (see WHEN TO DIAL 9•1•1 OR CALL EMS, p.74).

↓

ASSESS FOR CIRCULATION

- Check for signs of circulation for no more than 10 seconds (p.97).
- Are there signs of circulation?

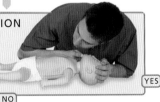

YES → Continue rescue breathing. After every 20 breaths (about 1 minute), recheck for signs of circulation. If the infant starts to breathe but remains unconscious, hold him in the recovery position (p.98).

NO ↓

COMMENCE CPR

- Alternate five chest compressions with one rescue breath (p.98).
- Repeat as necessary.

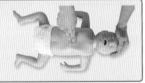

UNCONSCIOUS INFANT (under 1 year)

The following pages give full instructions for resuscitating an infant under 1 year who is found in an apparently lifeless condition. For an older infant, you should use the child resuscitation procedure (pp.86–93).

Always treat the infant from the side. You will then be in the correct position for doing all the possible stages of resuscitation: opening the airway; checking breathing and circulation; and giving rescue breaths and chest compressions (together known as cardiopulmonary resuscitation or CPR).

The steps given here guide you through each technique, then advise you on what to do next. Your first priority is to ensure that the airway is open and clear. If breathing and circulation resume, hold the infant in the recovery position (p.98). Dial 9·1·1 or call EMS immediately if an infant has known heart disease.

HOW TO CHECK FOR RESPONSE

Gently tap or flick the sole of the infant's foot and call his name to see if he responds. Never shake an infant.

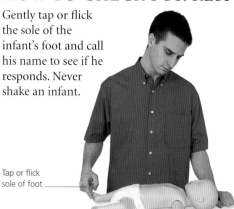

Tap or flick sole of foot

IF THERE IS A RESPONSE

Take the infant with you to summon help if needed. Monitor vital signs – level of response, pulse, and breathing (pp.42–43) – until help arrives.

IF THERE IS NO RESPONSE

Shout for help, then open the airway.

(▶) Go to HOW TO OPEN THE AIRWAY below

HOW TO OPEN THE AIRWAY

1 Place one hand on the infant's forehead and very gently tilt the head back.

2 Pick out any obvious obstructions from the mouth. Do not do a finger sweep.

Use your fingertips to remove obstructions

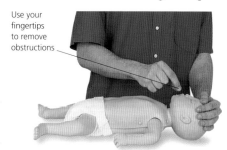

3 Place one fingertip of the other hand under the point of the chin. Gently lift the chin. Do not push on the soft tissues under the chin as this may block the airway.

Use one finger to tilt chin gently

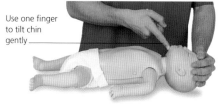

4 Check to see if the infant is now breathing.

(▶) Go to HOW TO CHECK BREATHING p.96

UNCONSCIOUS INFANT (continued)

HOW TO CHECK BREATHING

Keep the airway open and look, listen, and feel for breathing – look for chest movement, listen for sounds of breathing, and feel for breath on your cheek. Do this for no more than 10 seconds.

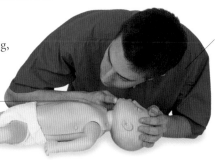

Lean right down over infant

Look for chest movement, which indicates breathing

IF THE INFANT IS BREATHING

1 Check the infant for life-threatening injuries, such as severe bleeding, and treat if necessary.

2 Hold the infant in the recovery position. Regularly monitor vital signs – level of response, pulse, and breathing (pp.42–43).

▶ Go to HOW TO HOLD IN RECOVERY POSITION p.98

IF THE INFANT IS NOT BREATHING

1 Ask a helper to DIAL 9•1•1 OR CALL EMS.

2 Give two effective rescue breaths and then check for signs of circulation.

▶ Go to HOW TO GIVE RESCUE BREATHS below

HOW TO GIVE RESCUE BREATHS

1 Make sure that the airway is still open by keeping one hand on the infant's forehead and one fingertip of the other hand under the tip of his chin.

2 Take a breath. Place your lips around the infant's mouth and nose to form an airtight seal. If you cannot make a seal around the mouth and nose, close the infant's mouth and make a seal around the nose only.

3 Blow steadily into the infant's lungs until the chest rises.

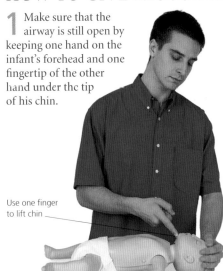

Use one finger to lift chin

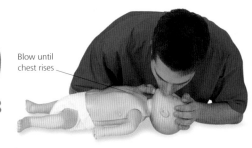

Blow until chest rises

4 Maintaining head tilt and chin lift, take your mouth off the infant's face and see if the chest falls. If the chest rises visibly as you blow and falls fully when you lift your mouth away, you have given an effective breath.

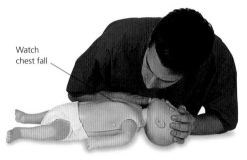

Watch chest fall

5 Give another effective rescue breath and then check for circulation.

▶ Go to HOW TO CHECK FOR CIRCULATION below.

IF YOU CANNOT ACHIEVE EFFECTIVE BREATHS

- Recheck the head tilt and chin lift.
- Recheck the infant's mouth. Remove any obvious obstructions, but do not do a finger sweep of the mouth.
- Check that you have a firm seal around the mouth and nose.
- Make no more than five attempts to achieve two effective breaths. If you still cannot achieve two effective breaths, check the infant for signs of circulation.

▶ Go to HOW TO CHECK FOR CIRCULATION below.

> **❶ WARNING**
>
> If you know that the infant has choked, and you cannot achieve effective breaths, you must immediately begin giving chest compressions to try to relieve the obstruction quickly (see HOW TO GIVE CPR, p.98).

HOW TO CHECK FOR CIRCULATION

Look, listen, and feel for signs of circulation, such as breathing, coughing, or movement. Check for these signs of circulation for no more than 10 seconds.

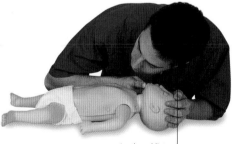

Look and listen for breathing

IF THERE ARE NO SIGNS OF CIRCULATION

Begin chest compressions and rescue breaths (cardiopulmonary resuscitation – CPR) immediately. Continue for 1 minute, then DIAL 9·1·1 OR CALL EMS.

▶ Go to HOW TO GIVE CPR p.98

IF YOU ARE SURE YOU HAVE DETECTED SIGNS OF CIRCULATION

1 Continue rescue breaths for 1 minute, then DIAL 9·1·1 OR CALL EMS.
After every 20 breaths (about 1 minute), check for signs of circulation.

2 If the infant begins to breathe but remains unconscious, hold him in the recovery position.

▶ Go to HOW TO HOLD IN RECOVERY POSITION p.98

UNCONSCIOUS INFANT (continued)

HOW TO GIVE CPR

1 Place the infant on his back on a flat surface, at about waist height in front of you, or on the floor. Place the fingertips of your lower hand along an imaginary line joining the infant's nipples. Take care not to press on the tip of the breastbone or the abdomen.

3 Compress the chest five times, at a rate of 100 times per minute. Compression and release should take the same amount of time.

4 After five compressions, maintain head tilt and chin lift, and give one rescue breath through the mouth and nose (pp.96–97).

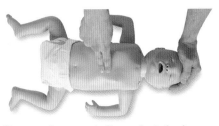

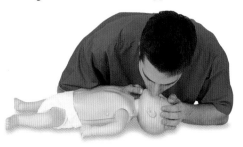

2 Press down vertically on the infant's breastbone and depress the chest by –1 in (1–2.5 cm). Release the pressure without losing the contact between your fingers and the breastbone.

5 Continue this cycle of alternating five chest compressions with one rescue breath. Continue CPR until emergency help arrives and takes over; the infant makes a movement or takes a spontaneous breath; or you become so exhausted that you cannot continue.

Press down firmly and rhythmically

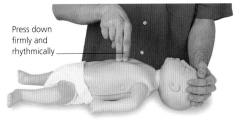

HOW TO HOLD IN RECOVERY POSITION

1 Cradle the infant in your arms with his head tilted downward. This position prevents him from choking on his tongue or from inhaling vomit.

2 Monitor and record vital signs – level of response, pulse, and breathing (pp.42–43) – until help arrives.

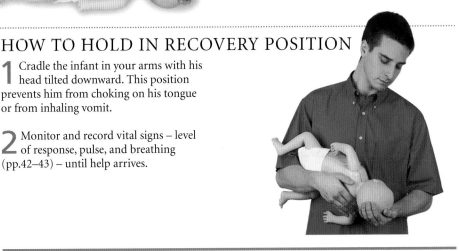

CHOKING SUMMARY CHARTS

The following pages explain how to treat a choking adult, child, or infant. The charts below summarize how to treat choking in a conscious victim. In an adult or a child, always encourage coughing first, and start the procedures described when the victim shows signs of weakening.

> **⚠ WARNING**
>
> If at any stage the victim becomes unconscious, open the airway, check breathing and, if necessary, begin rescue breaths. If you cannot achieve effective breaths, you must immediately begin giving chest compressions to try to relieve the obstruction quickly (p.80, p.90, p.98).

PROCEDURE FOR ADULT *see* p.100

DETERMINE WHETHER THE PERSON IS CHOKING ● Ask the person "Are you choking?" ● If the person can speak or cough, do not interfere.	If the person cannot speak or cough, hold the person from behind and **GIVE UP TO FIVE ABDOMINAL THRUSTS**	**CONTINUE GIVING ABDOMINAL THRUSTS** If unconscious, lay the victim down and perform CPR until the blockage clears.

PROCEDURE FOR CHILD (1–7 years) *see* p.101

DETERMINE WHETHER THE CHILD IS CHOKING ● Ask the child "Are you choking?" ● If the child can speak or cough, do not interfere	If the child cannot speak or cough **PREPARE TO GIVE ABDOMINAL THRUSTS** ● Stand or kneel behind the child. ● Make a fist with one hand and place it against her abdomen.	**GIVE ABDOMINAL THRUSTS** ● Grasp your fist with your other hand and press into her abdomen with a quick upward thrust.	Repeat abdominal thrusts as necessary. If the child becomes unconscious, lay her down and perform CPR. **DIAL 9•1•1 OR CALL EMS** Continue until help arrives.

PROCEDURE FOR INFANT (under 1 year) *see* p.102

GIVE UP TO FIVE BACK SLAPS ● Check the mouth and remove any obvious obstruction.	If the obstruction is still present **GIVE UP TO FIVE CHEST THRUSTS** ● Check the mouth; remove any obvious obstruction.	If the obstruction does not clear after three cycles of back slaps and chest thrusts **DIAL 9•1•1 OR CALL EMS** Continue until help arrives.

CHOKING ADULT

A foreign object that is stuck at the back of the throat may block the throat or cause a muscular spasm. If blockage of the airway is partial, the person should be able to clear it; if it is complete he will be unable to speak, breathe, or cough, and will lose consciousness. Be prepared to begin rescue breaths and chest compressions. The throat muscles may relax, leaving the airway sufficiently open for rescue breathing.

RECOGNITION

With partial obstruction:
- Coughing and distress.
- Difficulty speaking.

With complete obstruction:
- Inability to speak, breathe, or cough, and eventual loss of consciousness.

▶ **See also** UNCONSCIOUS ADULT pp.75–86

✚ YOUR AIMS

- To remove the obstruction.
- To dial 9•1•1 or call EMS.

❗ WARNING

If at any stage the person becomes unconscious, open the airway, check breathing, and give rescue breaths (pp.77–79). If you cannot achieve effective breaths, immediately begin giving chest compressions to try to relieve the obstruction quickly (*see* HOW TO GIVE CPR, pp.80–81).

1 Determine if the person is choking. Ask her "Are you choking?" If the person is able to speak or cough, there is no need to interfere. If the person cannot speak or cough, then you should prepare to administer abdominal thrusts.

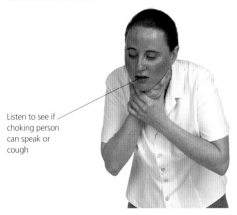

Listen to see if choking person can speak or cough

2 Give abdominal thrusts. Stand behind the person and put both arms around the upper part of the abdomen. Make sure that she is still bending far forward. Clench your fist and place it (thumb inward) between the navel and the bottom of the breastbone. Grasp your fist with your other hand. Pull sharply inward and upward up to five times.

Stand behind person

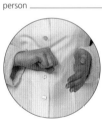

Make a fist with one hand, and position it with thumb side against the abdomen

3 Check her mouth. If the obstruction is still not cleared, repeat steps 2 and 3 up to three times, checking the mouth after each step.

4 If the obstruction still has not cleared, DIAL 9•1•1 OR CALL EMS. Continue until help arrives or the person becomes unconscious.

CHOKING CHILD (1–7 years)

Young children are particularly prone to choking. A child may choke on food, or may put small objects into his mouth and cause a blockage of the airway.

If a child is choking, you need to act quickly. If he loses consciousness, be prepared to begin rescue breaths and chest compressions. The throat muscles may relax, leaving the airway sufficiently open for rescue breathing.

RECOGNITION

With partial obstruction:
- Coughing and distress.
- Difficulty speaking.

With complete obstruction:
- Inability to speak, breathe, or cough, and eventual loss of consciousness.

 See also UNCONSCIOUS CHILD pp.87–93

＋ YOUR AIMS

- To remove the obstruction.
- To dial 9•1•1 or call EMS.

1 If the child is breathing, encourage him to cough; this may clear the obstruction. If she cannot speak or cough, proceed to step 2.

2 Wrap your arms around the child's abdomen just above the hips. Make a fist with one hand and place the thumb side of your fist against the middle of her abdomen, just above her navel.

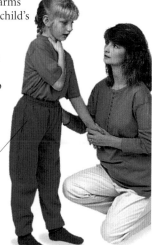

Get her to cough up the obstruction if she can.

Make sure that child is bending far forward

3 Try abdominal thrusts. Put your arms around the child's upper abdomen. Make sure that he is bending well forward. Place your fist between the navel and the bottom of the breastbone, and grasp it with your other hand. Pull sharply inward and upward up to five times. Stop if the obstruction clears. Check his mouth.

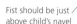

Fist should be just above child's navel

4 If the obstruction is still not cleared, repeat steps 2–3 up to three times.

5 If the obstruction still has not cleared, DIAL 9•1•1 OR CALL EMS. Continue until help arrives or the child becomes unconscious.

❶ WARNING

If at any stage the child becomes unconscious, open the airway, check breathing, and give rescue breaths (pp.88–89). If you cannot achieve effective breaths, immediately begin giving chest compressions to try to relieve the obstruction quickly (*see* HOW TO GIVE CPR, pp.90–91).

CHOKING INFANT (under 1 year)

An infant may readily choke on food or on very small objects in the mouth. The infant will rapidly become distressed, and you need to act quickly to clear any obstruction.

If the infant becomes unconscious, be prepared to give rescue breaths and chest compressions. In an unconscious infant, the throat muscles may relax, leaving the airway sufficiently open for rescue breathing. If rescue breaths fail, chest compressions may clear the obstruction.

RECOGNITION

With partial obstruction:
● Coughing and distress.
● Difficulty crying or making any other noise.

With complete obstruction:
● Inability to breathe or cough, and eventual loss of consciousness.

▶ **See also** UNCONSCIOUS INFANT pp.95–98

➕ YOUR AIMS

● To remove the obstruction.
● To arrange urgent transport to a hospital if necessary.

❶ WARNING

If at any stage the infant becomes unconscious, open the airway, check breathing, and give rescue breaths (p.96). If you cannot achieve effective breaths, immediately begin chest compressions to try to relieve the obstruction quickly (*see* HOW TO GIVE CPR, p.98).

1 If the infant is distressed, shows signs of becoming weak, or stops breathing or coughing, lay him face down along your forearm, with his head low, and support his back and head. Give up to five back slaps.

Make sure that head is below level of chest

2 Check the infant's mouth; remove any obvious obstructions with your fingertips. Do not do a finger sweep of the mouth.

3 If this fails to clear the obstruction, turn the infant onto his back and give up to five chest thrusts. Using two fingers, push inward against the infant's breastbone, at the level of the nipple line.

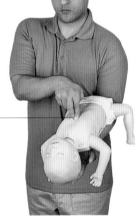

Push on breastbone with your fingertips, one finger's breadth below nipple line

4 Perform five chest thrusts, at a rate of one every 3 seconds. The aim is to relieve the obstruction with each chest thrust rather than necessarily doing all five. Check the mouth.

5 If the obstruction is not cleared, repeat steps 1–4 three times. If the obstruction still has not cleared, take the infant with you to DIAL 9·1·1 OR CALL EMS. Continue until help arrives or the infant becomes unconscious.

4

OXYGEN IS ESSENTIAL TO LIFE. Every time we inhale, air containing oxygen enters the lungs. This oxygen is then transferred to the blood, to be transported around the body. Breathing and the exchange of oxygen and carbon dioxide (a waste product from body tissues) are described as "respiration," and the structures that enable us to breathe make up the respiratory system.

WHAT CAN GO WRONG
Respiration can be impaired in various ways. The airways may be blocked; the exchange of oxygen and carbon dioxide in the lungs may be affected by inhalation of smoke or fumes; the function of the lungs may be impaired by chest injury; or the breathing mechanism may be affected by conditions such as asthma. Problems with respiration can be life threatening and require urgent first aid.

CONTENTS

The respiratory system..............104

Hypoxia....................................106

Airway obstruction...................107

Hanging and strangulation.......108

Drowning................................109

Inhalation of fumes.................110

Penetrating chest wound.........112

Hyperventilation.....................114

Asthma...................................115

Croup....................................116

RESPIRATORY PROBLEMS

✚ FIRST-AID PRIORITIES

- ● Assess the victim's condition.
- ● Identify and remove the cause of the problem and provide fresh air.
- ● Comfort and reassure the victim.
- ● Maintain an open airway, check breathing, and be prepared to resuscitate if necessary.
- ● Obtain medical aid if necessary. Dial 9•1•1 or call EMS if you suspect a serious illness or injury.

THE RESPIRATORY SYSTEM

This system comprises the mouth, nose, windpipe (trachea), lungs, and pulmonary blood vessels. Respiration involves the process of breathing and the exchange of gases (oxygen and carbon dioxide) in the lungs and in cells throughout the body.

We inhale air in order to take oxygen into the lungs, and we exhale to expel the waste gas carbon dioxide, a by-product of respiration.

When we inhale, air is drawn through the nose and mouth into the airway and the lungs. In the lungs, oxygen is taken from air sacs (alveoli) into the pulmonary capillaries. At the same time, carbon dioxide is released from the capillaries into the alveoli. This gas is then expelled as we exhale.

An average man's lungs can hold approximately 10 pints (6 liters) of air; a woman's lungs can hold about 7 pints (4 liters).

Structure of the respiratory system

The lungs form the central part of the respiratory system. Together with the circulatory system, they perform the vital function of gas exchange in order to distribute oxygen around the body and remove carbon dioxide.

Lungs are two spongy organs that occupy a large part of chest cavity

Pleural membrane has two layers, separated by a lubricating fluid, which surround and protect each of the lungs

Epiglottis

Larynx

Windpipe (trachea) extends from larynx to two main bronchi

Main bronchi branch from base of windpipe (trachea) into each lung and divide into smaller airways (bronchioles)

Bronchioles are small air passages that branch from bronchi and eventually open into alveoli (air sacs) within lungs

Rib

Intercostal muscles span spaces between ribs

Capillary

Alveolus

Alveoli cross section
A network of tiny blood vessels (capillaries) surrounds each alveolus (air sac). The thin walls of both structures allow oxygen to diffuse into the blood and carbon dioxide to leave it.

Diaphragm is a sheet of muscle that separates chest and abdominal cavities

How breathing works

The breathing process consists of the actions of inhaling (inspiration) and exhaling (expiration), followed by a pause. Pressure differences between the lungs and the air outside the body determine whether air is drawn in or expelled. When the air pressure in the lungs is lower than outside, air is drawn in; when pressure is higher, air is expelled. The pressure within the lungs is altered by the movements of the two main sets of muscles involved in breathing: the intercostal muscles and the diaphragm.

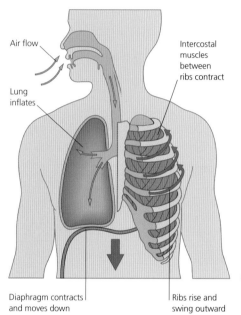

Air flow

Intercostal muscles between ribs contract

Lung inflates

Diaphragm contracts and moves down

Ribs rise and swing outward

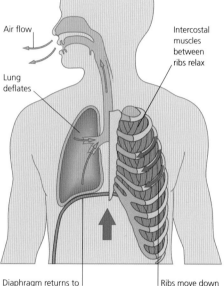

Air flow

Intercostal muscles between ribs relax

Lung deflates

Diaphragm returns to domed position

Ribs move down and inward

Inhaling
The intercostal muscles (the muscles between the ribs) and the diaphragm contract, causing the chest cavity to expand, and the lungs expand to fill the space. As a result, the pressure inside the lungs is reduced, and air is drawn into the lungs.

Exhaling
The intercostal muscles relax, and the rib cage returns to its resting position, while the diaphragm relaxes and resumes its domed shape. As a result, the chest cavity becomes smaller, and pressure inside the lungs increases. Air flows out of the lungs to be exhaled.

How breathing is controlled

Breathing is regulated by a set of nerve cells in the brain called the respiratory center. This center responds to changes in the level of carbon dioxide in the blood. When the level rises, the respiratory center responds by stimulating the intercostal muscles and the diaphragm to contract, and a breath occurs. Our breathing rate can be altered consciously under normal conditions. It also changes in response to abnormal levels of carbon dioxide, or to low levels of oxygen, or with stress, exercise, injury, or illness.

HYPOXIA

This condition arises when insufficient oxygen reaches body tissues from the blood. There are a number of causes (below), ranging from suffocation or poisoning to impaired lung or brain function. The condition is accompanied by a variety of symptoms, depending on the degree of hypoxia. If not treated quickly, hypoxia is potentially fatal because a sufficient level of oxygen is vital for the normal function of all the body organs and tissues.

In a healthy person, the amount of oxygen in the air is more than adequate for the body tissues to function normally. However, in a person who is ill or injured, a reduction in oxygen reaching the tissues results in deterioration of body function.

Mild hypoxia reduces a person's ability to think clearly, but the body responds to this by increasing the rate and depth of breathing (previous page). However, if the oxygen supply to the brain cells is cut off for as little as 3–4 minutes, the brain cells will begin to die. All the conditions covered in this chapter can result in hypoxia.

RECOGNITION

In moderate and severe hypoxia, there may be:
- Rapid breathing.
- Breathing that is distressed or gasping.
- Difficulty speaking.
- Gray–blue skin (cyanosis). At first, this will affect the extremities such as the lips, nailbeds, and earlobes, but, as the hypoxia worsens, cyanosis will affect the whole body.
- Anxiety.
- Restlessness.
- Headache.
- Nausea and possibly vomiting.
- Cessation of breathing if the hypoxia is not quickly reversed.

▶ See also ANAPHYLACTIC SHOCK p.123
● ASTHMA p. 115 ● BURNS TO THE AIRWAY p.197 ● CROUP p.116 ● DROWNING p.109
● HANGING AND STRANGULATION p.108
● INHALATION OF FUMES p.110
● PENETRATING CHEST WOUND p.112
● STROKE p.183

CONDITIONS CAUSING LOW BLOOD OXYGEN (HYPOXIA)

Condition	Causes
Insufficient oxygen in inspired air	Suffocation by smoke or gas ● Changes in atmospheric pressure, for example at high altitude or in a depressurized aircraft
Airway obstruction	Blocking or swelling of the airway ● Hanging or strangulation ● Something covering the mouth and nose ● Asthma ● Choking ● Anaphylaxis
Conditions affecting the chest wall	Crushing, for example by a fall of earth or sand or pressure from a crowd ● Chest wall injury with multiple rib fractures or constricting burns
Impaired lung function	Lung injury ● Collapsed lung ● Lung infections, such as pneumonia
Damage to the brain or nerves that control respiration	A head injury or stroke that damages the breathing center in the brain ● Some forms of poisoning ● Paralysis of nerves controlling the muscles of breathing, as in spinal cord injury
Impaired oxygen uptake by the tissues	Carbon monoxide or cyanide poisoning ● Shock

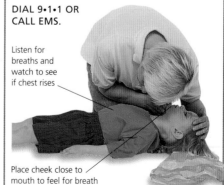

AIRWAY OBSTRUCTION

The airway may be obstructed internally, for example, by an object that is stuck at the back of the throat, or externally. The main causes of obstruction are:

- Inhalation of a foreign object such as food or false teeth – choking.
- Blockage by the tongue when a victim is unconscious.
- Blockage from blood or vomit.
- Internal swelling of the throat occurring with burns, scalds, stings, or anaphylaxis.
- Injuries to the face or jaw.
- Asthma.
- External pressure on the neck, as in hanging or strangulation (p.108).

Dry peanuts, which can swell up when in contact with body fluids, pose a particular danger in young children because they can obstruct one of the bronchi.

Airway obstruction requires prompt action from the first aider; be prepared to give rescue breaths and chest compressions if the victim stops breathing (*see* LIFE-SAVING PROCEDURES, pp.71–102).

RECOGNITION

- Features of hypoxia (opposite) such as gray–blue tinge to the lips, earlobes, and nailbeds (cyanosis).
- Difficulty speaking and breathing.
- Noisy breathing.
- Red, puffy face.
- Signs of distress from the victim, who may point to the throat or grasp the neck.
- Flaring of the nostrils.
- A persistent dry cough.

The information on this page is appropriate for all causes of airway obstruction, but if you need detailed instructions for specific situations, refer to the relevant pages.

See also ASTHMA p. 115 ● BURNS TO THE AIRWAY p.197 ● CHOKING ADULT p.100 ● CHOKING INFANT p.102 ● CHOKING CHILD p.101 ● DROWNING p.109 ● HANGING AND STRANGULATION p.108 ● INHALATION OF FUMES p.110

YOUR AIMS

- To remove the obstruction.
- To restore normal breathing.
- To seek medical aid.

❶ WARNING

If the victim is unconscious, open the airway and check for breathing; be prepared to give rescue breaths and chest compressions if necessary (*see* LIFE-SAVING PROCEDURES, pp.71–102).

DIAL 9•1•1 OR CALL EMS.

1 Remove the obstruction if it is external or visible in the mouth.

2 If the victim is conscious and breathing normally, reassure her, but keep her under observation. Monitor and record vital signs – level of response, pulse, and breathing (pp.42–43). Be prepared to give rescue breaths and chest compressions if necessary (*see* LIFE-SAVING PROCEDURES, pp.71–102).

3 Even if the victim appears to have made a complete recovery, call a doctor or take or send the victim to a hospital.

Listen for breaths and watch to see if chest rises

Place cheek close to mouth to feel for breath

HANGING AND STRANGULATION

If pressure is exerted on the outside of the neck, the airway is squeezed and the flow of air to the lungs is cut off. The main causes of such pressure are:

- Hanging – suspension of the body by a noose around the neck.
- Strangulation – constriction or squeezing around the neck or throat.

Sometimes, hanging or strangulation may occur accidentally – for example, by ties or clothing becoming caught in machinery. Hanging may cause a broken neck; for this reason, a victim in this situation must be handled extremely carefully.

See also LIFE-SAVING PROCEDURES pp.71–102 • SPINAL INJURY pp.165–167

RECOGNITION
- A constricting article around the neck.
- Marks around the victim's neck.
- Rapid, difficult breathing; impaired consciousness; gray-blue skin (cyanosis).
- Congestion of the face, with prominent veins and, possibly, tiny red spots on the face or on the whites of the eyes.

YOUR AIMS
- To restore adequate breathing.
- To arrange urgent transport to a hospital.

CAUTION
- Do not move the victim unnecessarily, in case of spinal injury.
- Do not destroy or interfere with any material that has been constricting the neck, such as knotted rope; police may need it as evidence.

1 Quickly remove any constriction from around the victim's neck. Support the body while you do so if it is still hanging. Be aware that the body may be very heavy.

Hold rope clear, but not tight

Cut away from victim

2 Lay the victim on the ground. Open the airway and check breathing. If she is not breathing, be prepared to give rescue breaths and chest compressions if necessary (*see* LIFE-SAVING PROCEDURES, pp.71–102). If she is breathing, place her in the recovery position.

Make sure that airway is open

Tuck hand under cheek

3 DIAL 9·1·1 OR CALL EMS even if she appears to recover fully.

DROWNING

Death by drowning occurs when air cannot get into the lungs, usually because a small amount of water has entered the lungs. This may also cause a spasm of the throat.

When a drowning person is rescued, water may gush from the mouth. This water is from the stomach and should be left to drain of its own accord. Do not attempt to force water from the stomach because the victim may vomit and then inhale it.

A victim from a drowning incident should always receive medical attention even if he seems to recover at the time. Any water entering the lungs causes them to become irritated, and the air passages may begin to swell several hours later – a condition known as secondary drowning.

The victim may also need to be treated for hypothermia (pp.206–208).

> See also HYPOTHERMIA pp.206–208
> ● LIFE-SAVING PROCEDURES pp.71–102
> ● WATER RESCUE p.28

✚ YOUR AIMS

● To restore adequate breathing.
● To keep the victim warm.
● To arrange urgent transport to a hospital.

1 If you are rescuing the victim from the water to safety, keep her head lower than the rest of the body to reduce the risk of her inhaling water (p.28).

2 Lay the victim down on her back on a rug or coat. Open the airway and check breathing; be prepared to give rescue breaths and chest compressions if necessary (*see* LIFE-SAVING PROCEDURES, pp.71–102). If the victim is breathing, place her in the recovery position (pp.84–85).

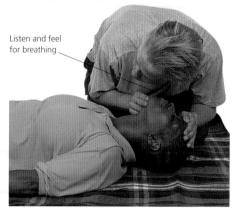

Listen and feel for breathing

3 Treat the victim for hypothermia; remove wet clothing if possible and cover her with dry blankets. If the victim regains full consciousness, give her a warm drink.

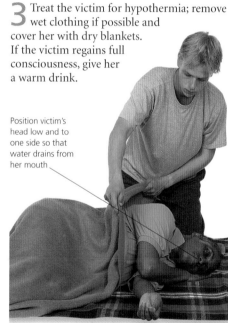

Position victim's head low and to one side so that water drains from her mouth

4 DIAL 9·1·1 OR CALL EMS even if she appears to recover fully.

❶ WARNING

Water in the lungs and the effects of cold can increase resistance to rescue breaths and chest compressions: you may have to do both at a slower rate than normal.

INHALATION OF GASES

The inhalation of smoke, gases (such as carbon monoxide), or toxic vapors can be lethal. A victim who has inhaled gases is likely to have low levels of oxygen in his body tissues (see HYPOXIA, p.106) and therefore needs urgent medical attention. Do not attempt to carry out a rescue if it is likely to put your own life at risk; gases that have built up in a confined space may quickly overcome anyone who is not wearing protective equipment.

SMOKE INHALATION
Any person who has been enclosed in a confined space during a fire should be assumed to have inhaled smoke. Smoke from burning plastics, foam padding, and synthetic wall coverings is likely to contain poisonous gases. Victims should also be examined for other injuries due to the fire.

INHALATION OF CARBON MONOXIDE
Carbon monoxide is a poisonous gas that is produced by burning. It acts directly on red blood cells, preventing them from carrying oxygen to the body tissues. If the gas is inhaled in large quantities – for example, from smoke or vehicle exhaust fumes in a confined space – it can very quickly prove fatal. However, lengthy exposure to even a small amount of carbon monoxide – for example, due to a leakage of gases from a defective heater or flue – may also result in severe, or possibly fatal, poisoning.

Carbon monoxide has no taste or smell, so take care if you suspect a leak.

> ▶ See also BURNS TO THE AIRWAYS, p.197
> ● FIRES p.24 ● HYPOXIA p.106 ● LIFE-SAVING
> PROCEDURES pp.71–102

EFFECTS OF GAS INHALATION

Gas	Source	Effects
Carbon monoxide	Exhaust fumes of motor vehicles ● Smoke from most fires ● Back-drafts from blocked chimney flues ● Emissions from defective gas heaters	*Prolonged exposure to low levels:* Headache ● Confusion ● Aggression ● Nausea and vomiting ● Incontinence *Brief exposure to high levels:* Gray–blue skin coloration with a faint red tinge ● Rapid, difficult breathing ● Impaired consciousness, leading to unconsciousness
Smoke	Fires: smoke is a bigger killer than fire itself. Smoke is low in oxygen (which is used up by the burning of the fire) and may contain toxic gases from burning materials	Rapid, noisy, difficult breathing ● Coughing and wheezing ● Burning in the nose or mouth ● Soot around the mouth and nose ● Unconsciousness
Carbon dioxide	Tends to accumulate and become dangerously concentrated in deep enclosed spaces, such as coal pits, wells, and underground tanks	Breathlessness ● Headache ● Confusion ● Unconsciousness
Solvents and fuels	Glues ● Cleaning fluids ● Lighter fuels ● Camping gas and propane-fuelled stoves. Solvent abusers may use a plastic bag to concentrate the vapor (especially with glues)	Headache and vomiting ● Impaired consciousness ● Airway obstruction from using a plastic bag or from choking on vomit may result in death ● Cardiac arrest is potential cause of death, and this may occur following inhalation of the very cold gases that are released from pressurized containers

1 DIAL 9·1·1 OR CALL EMS. Ask for both fire and ambulance services. If the victim's clothing is still burning, try to extinguish the flames (p.25).

Support the victim

2 If it is necessary to escape from the source of the gases, move the victim into fresh air (*see* VICTIM HANDLING, pp.63–64).

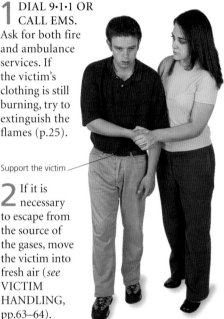

3 Support the victim and encourage him to breathe normally. Treat any obvious burns (pp.192–197) or other injuries.

Encourage the victim to sit upright to aid breathing

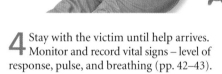

4 Stay with the victim until help arrives. Monitor and record vital signs – level of response, pulse, and breathing (pp. 42–43).

Listen for breathing

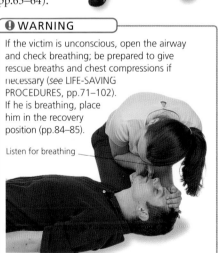

Monitor his pulse

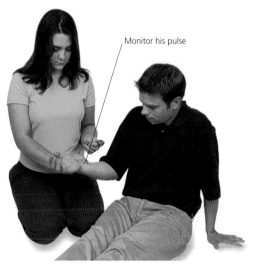

PENETRATING CHEST WOUND

The heart and lungs, and the major blood vessels around them, lie within the chest (thorax), protected by the breastbone and the 12 pairs of ribs that make up the ribcage. The rib cage extends far enough downward to protect organs such as the liver and spleen in the upper part of the abdomen.

If a sharp object penetrates the chest wall, there may be severe internal damage within the chest and the upper abdomen. The lungs are particularly susceptible to injury, either by being damaged themselves or from wounds that perforate the two-layered membrane (pleura) surrounding and protecting each lung. Air can then enter between the membranes and exert pressure on the lung, and the lung may collapse – a condition called pneumothorax.

Pressure around the affected lung may build up to such an extent that it also affects the uninjured lung. As a result, the victim becomes increasingly breathless. This buildup of pressure may prevent the heart from refilling with blood properly, impairing the

circulation and causing shock – a condition known as a tension pneumothorax. Sometimes, blood collects in the pleural cavity and puts pressure on the lungs.

▶ **See also** HYPOXIA, p.106 ● LIFE-SAVING PROCEDURES p.71–102 ● SHOCK pp.120–121

RECOGNITION

● Difficult and painful breathing, possibly rapid, shallow, and uneven.
● Victim feels an acute sense of alarm.
● Features of hypoxia (p.106), including gray–blue skin coloration (cyanosis).

There may also be:
● Coughed-up frothy, red blood.
● A crackling feeling of the skin around the site of the wound, caused by air collecting in the tissues.
● Blood bubbling out of the wound.
● Sound of air being sucked into the chest as the victim inhales.
● Veins in the neck becoming prominent.

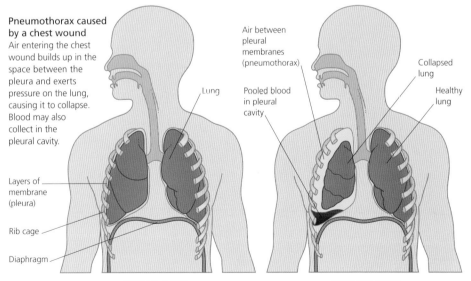

Pneumothorax caused by a chest wound
Air entering the chest wound builds up in the space between the pleura and exerts pressure on the lung, causing it to collapse. Blood may also collect in the pleural cavity.

Lung

Layers of membrane (pleura)

Rib cage

Diaphragm

NORMAL LUNGS

Air between pleural membranes (pneumothorax)

Collapsed lung

Pooled blood in pleural cavity

Healthy lung

PNEUMOTHORAX

1 Put on disposable gloves if available. Encourage the victim to lean toward the injured side and use the palm of his hand to cover the wound.

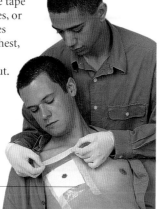

Completely cover the wound to stop air from being drawn into the chest cavity

2 Place a sterile dressing or nonfluffy clean pad over the wound and surrounding area. Cover with a plastic bag, foil, or plastic wrap. Secure firmly with adhesive tape on three edges, or with bandages around the chest, so that the dressing is taut.

Leave fourth side untaped to allow air under pressure during expiration to escape

3 DIAL 9·1·1 OR CALL EMS. While waiting for help, continue to support the victim in the same position as long as he remains conscious.

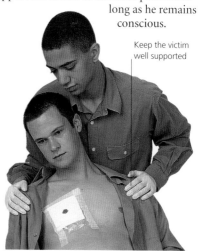

Keep the victim well supported

4 Monitor and record vital signs (pp.42–43) until medical help arrives. If condition worsens, remove dressing immediately.

⚠ WARNING

If the victim becomes unconscious, open the airway and check breathing; be prepared to give rescue breaths and chest compressions, if necessary (see LIFE-SAVING PROCEDURES, pp.71–102). If breathing, place him in the recovery position (pp.84–85), lying on his injured side to help the healthy lung work effectively.

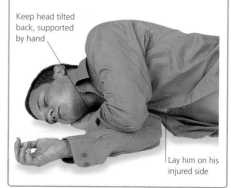

Keep head tilted back, supported by hand

Lay him on his injured side

HYPERVENTILATION

Excessive breathing (hyperventilation) is commonly a manifestation of acute anxiety and may accompany a panic attack. It may occur in susceptible individuals who have recently experienced an emotional or psychological shock.

Hyperventilation causes an abnormal loss of carbon dioxide from the blood, leading to chemical changes within the blood. These changes lead to symptoms such as unnaturally fast breathing, dizziness, and trembling and tingling in the hands. As breathing returns to normal, these symptoms will gradually subside.

RECOGNITION

● Unnaturally fast, deep breathing.

There may also be:
● Attention-seeking behavior.
● Dizziness or faintness.
● Trembling or marked tingling in the hands.
● Cramps in the hands and feet.

▶ See also PANIC ATTACK p.242

✚ YOUR AIMS

● To remove the person from the cause of distress.
● To reassure the person and calm her down.

1 When speaking to the person, be firm but kind and reassuring.

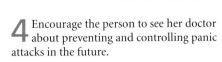

3 If she is not able to regain control of her breathing, ask her to rebreathe her own exhaled air from a paper bag. Tell her to breathe in and out slowly, using the bag, about 10 times and then breathe without the bag for 15 seconds. She should continue to alternate this cycle of breathing with and without the bag until the need to breathe rapidly has passed.

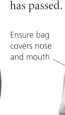

Ensure bag covers nose and mouth

2 If possible, lead the person away to a quiet place where she may be able to regain control of her breathing more easily and quickly. If this is not possible, ask any bystanders to leave.

4 Encourage the person to see her doctor about preventing and controlling panic attacks in the future.

ASTHMA

In an asthma attack, the muscles of the air passages in the lungs go into spasm and the linings of the airways swell. As a result, the airways become narrowed, which makes breathing difficult.

Sometimes there is a recognized trigger for an attack, such as an allergy, a cold, a particular drug, or cigarette smoke. At other times, there is no obvious trigger. Many sufferers have sudden attacks at night.

People with asthma usually deal with their own attacks, using a "reliever" inhaler at the first sign of an attack. Most reliever inhalers have blue caps. A plastic diffuser, or "spacer," can be fitted to an inhaler to help the victim breathe in the medication more effectively. Preventer inhalers usually have brown or white caps and are used regularly

RECOGNITION

- Difficulty breathing, with a very prolonged exhaling phase.

There may also be:
- Wheezing as the victim exhales.
- Difficulty speaking and whispering.
- Features of hypoxia (p.106), such as a gray–blue tinge to the lips, earlobes, and nailbeds (cyanosis).
- Distress and anxiety.
- Cough.
- In a severe attack, exhaustion. Rarely, the victim loses consciousness and stops breathing.

by people with asthma to help prevent attacks. However, preventer inhalers are not an effective treatment for asthma attacks and should not be used in this situation.

YOUR AIMS

- To ease breathing.
- To obtain medical help if necessary.

1 Keep calm and reassure the person. Get her to take a puff of her reliever inhaler. It should relieve the asthma attack within a few minutes. Ask her to breathe slowly and deeply.

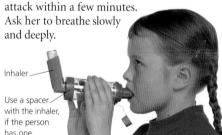

Inhaler

Use a spacer with the inhaler, if the person has one

2 Let her adopt the position that she finds most comfortable – often sitting down. Do not make her lie down.

3 A mild asthma attack should ease within 3 minutes. If it does not, ask her to take another dose from the same inhaler.

ⓘ CAUTION

If this is the first attack, or if the attack is severe and any one of the following occurs:
- the inhaler has no effect after 5 minutes,
- the person is getting worse,
- breathlessness makes talking difficult,
- she is becoming exhausted,

DIAL 9•1•1 OR CALL EMS.

Help her use her inhaler every 5–10 minutes. Monitor and record her breathing and pulse every 10 minutes (pp.42–43).

ⓘ WARNING

If the person loses consciousness, open the airway and check breathing; be prepared to give rescue breaths and chest compressions if necessary (see LIFE-SAVING TECHNIQUES, pp.71–102).

DIAL 9•1•1 OR CALL EMS

If the person is breathing, place her in the recovery position (pp.84–85). Monitor her vital signs – level of response, pulse, and breathing (pp.42–43) – until help arrives.

CROUP

An attack of severe breathing difficulty in very young children is known as croup. It is caused by inflammation in the windpipe and larynx. Croup can be alarming but usually passes without lasting harm. Attacks of croup usually occur at night and may recur before the child settles.

EPIGLOTTITIS RISK

If an attack of croup persists or is severe, and is accompanied by fever, call 9·1·1 or EMS. There is a small risk that the child is suffering from a rare, crouplike condition called epiglottitis, in which the epiglottis (p.104), a small, flaplike structure in the throat, becomes infected and swollen and may block the airway completely. The child then needs urgent medical attention.

> ### RECOGNITION
>
> ● Distressed breathing in a young child.
>
> *There may also be:*
>
> ● A short, barking cough.
>
> ● A crowing or whistling noise, especially on breathing in (stridor).
>
> ● Blue–gray skin (cyanosis).
>
> ● In severe cases, the child using muscles around the nose, neck, and upper arms in trying to breathe.
>
> *Suspect epiglottitis if:*
>
> ● A child is sitting bolt upright and is in respiratory distress.
>
> ● The child has a high temperature.

> ### ✚ YOUR AIMS
>
> ● To comfort and support the child.
> ● To obtain medical help if necessary.

1 Sit the child up on your knee, supporting her back. Calmly reassure the child. Try not to panic because this will only alarm her and is likely to make the attack worse.

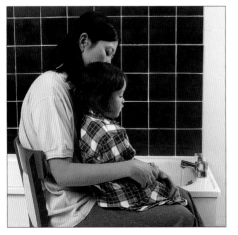

2 Create a steamy atmosphere: either take the child into the bathroom and run the hot water, or boil some water in the kitchen. Encourage her to sit and breathe in the steam; this should ease her breathing. Keep the child clear of running hot water or steam. Also try taking the child outside to breath cool air.

3 Call a doctor or, if croup is severe, DIAL 9·1·1 OR CALL EMS.

4 When the child is put back to bed, create a humid atmosphere in her bedroom – for example, by hanging a wet towel over a radiator in the room. The humidity may prevent an attack from recurring.

> ### ❶ CAUTION
>
> Do not put your fingers down the child's throat. This can cause the throat muscles to go into spasm and block the airway.

5

CONTENTS

The heart and blood vessels......118

Shock..120

Internal bleeding......................122

Anaphylactic shock..................123

Angina pectoris........................124

Acute heart failure...................124

Heart attack.............................125

Fainting....................................126

THE HEART AND the network of blood vessels are collectively known as the circulatory (cardiovascular) system. This system keeps the body supplied with blood, which carries oxygen and nutrients to all body tissues.

The circulatory system may be disrupted in two main ways: severe bleeding and fluid loss may cause the volume of blood to fall, depriving the organs of oxygen; or age or disease may cause the system to break down. The techniques described in this section show how a first aider can help maintain an adequate blood supply to a victim's heart and brain. In minor incidents, first aid should ensure the casualty's recovery. In serious cases, such as a heart attack, your action may be vital in preserving life until help arrives.

✚ FIRST-AID PRIORITIES

- Assess the victim's condition.
- Comfort and reassure the victim.
- Position the victim to improve the blood supply to the vital organs.
- Loosen tight clothing to ease breathing and improve circulation.
- Maintain an open airway, check breathing, and be prepared to resuscitate if necessary.
- Obtain medical aid if necessary. Call 9•1•1 or EMS if you suspect a serious illness or injury.

THE HEART AND BLOOD VESSELS

The circulatory system consists of the heart and the blood vessels. These structures supply the body with a constant flow of blood, which brings oxygen and nutrients to the tissues and carries waste products away.

Blood is pumped around the body by rhythmic contractions (beats) of the heart muscle. The blood runs through a network of vessels, divided into three types: arteries, veins, and capillaries. The force that is exerted by the blood flow through the main arteries is called blood pressure. It varies with the strength and phase of the heartbeat, the elasticity of the arterial walls, and the volume and thickness of the blood.

How blood circulates
Oxygen-rich (oxygenated) blood passes from the lungs to the heart, then travels to body tissues via the arteries. Blood that has given up its oxygen (deoxygenated blood) returns to the heart through the veins.

Brachial artery

Aorta carries oxygenated blood to body tissues

Vena cava carries deoxygenated blood from body tissues to heart

Radial artery

Femoral artery

Carotid artery

Jugular vein

Brachial vein

Pulmonary arteries carry deoxygenated blood to lungs

Pulmonary veins carry oxygenated blood from lungs to heart

Heart pumps blood around body

Radial vein

Femoral vein

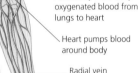

Small artery (arteriole)

Capillary

Small vein (venule)

Capillary networks
Networks of fine blood vessels (capillaries) link arteries and veins within body tissues. Oxygen and nutrients pass from the blood into the tissues; waste products pass from the tissues into the blood, through capillaries.

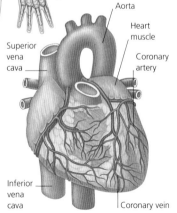

Aorta

Heart muscle

Superior vena cava

Coronary artery

Inferior vena cava

Coronary vein

The heart
This muscular organ pumps blood around the body and then to the lungs to pick up oxygen. Coronary blood vessels supply the heart muscle with oxygen and nutrients.

```
KEY
```
▮ Vessels carrying oxygenated blood
▮ Vessels carrying deoxygenated blood

How the heart functions

The heart pumps blood by muscular contractions called heartbeats, which are controlled by electrical impulses generated in the heart. Each beat has three phases: diastole, when blood enters the heart; atrial systole, when blood is squeezed out of the atria (collecting chambers); and ventricular systole, when blood leaves the heart.

In diastole, the heart relaxes. Oxygen-rich (oxygenated) blood from the lungs flows via the pulmonary veins into the left atrium. Blood that has given up its oxygen to body tissues (deoxygenated blood) flows from the venae cavae (large veins) to the right atrium.

In atrial systole, the two atria contract and the valves between the atria and the ventricles (pumping chambers) open so that blood flows into the ventricles.

During ventricular systole, the ventricles contract. The thick-walled left ventricle forces blood into the aorta (main artery), which carries it to the rest of the body. The right ventricle pumps blood into the pulmonary artery, which carries it to the lungs to collect more oxygen.

Blood flow through the heart

The heart's right side pumps deoxygenated blood from the body to the lungs. The left side pumps oxygenated blood to the whole of the body.

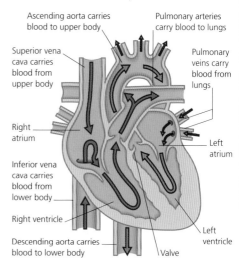

Ascending aorta carries blood to upper body

Pulmonary arteries carry blood to lungs

Superior vena cava carries blood from upper body

Pulmonary veins carry blood from lungs

Right atrium

Left atrium

Inferior vena cava carries blood from lower body

Right ventricle

Descending aorta carries blood to lower body

Valve

Left ventricle

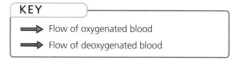

KEY

➡ Flow of oxygenated blood

➡ Flow of deoxygenated blood

Composition of blood

There are about 10 pints (6 liters), or 1 pint per 17 pounds of body weight (1 liter per 13 kilograms), of blood in the average adult body. Roughly 55 percent of the blood is clear yellow fluid (plasma). The platelets and red and white blood cells suspended in this fluid make up the other 45 percent.

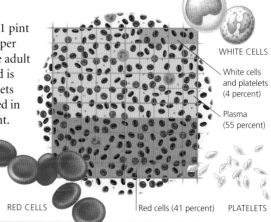

WHITE CELLS

White cells and platelets (4 percent)

Plasma (55 percent)

Red cells (41 percent)   PLATELETS

RED CELLS

The blood cells

Red blood cells contain hemoglobin, a red pigment that enables the cells to carry oxygen. White blood cells play a role in defending the body against infection. Platelets help blood clot.

SHOCK

This life-threatening condition occurs when the circulatory system (which distributes oxygen to the body tissues and removes waste products) fails and, as a result, vital organs such as the heart and brain are deprived of oxygen. It requires immediate emergency treatment to prevent permanent organ damage and death.

Shock can be made worse by fear and pain. Whenever there is a risk of shock developing, reassuring the victim and making her comfortable may be sufficient to prevent her from deteriorating.

CAUSES OF SHOCK
The most common cause of shock is severe blood loss. If this exceeds 2 pints (1.2 liters), which is about one-fifth of the normal blood volume, shock will occur. This degree of blood loss may result from wounds. It may also be caused by hidden bleeding from internal organs (p.122), blood escaping into a body cavity, or bleeding from damaged blood vessels due to a closed fracture (p.151). Loss of other body fluids can also result in shock. Conditions that can cause heavy fluid loss include diarrhea, vomiting, blockage in the intestine, and severe burns.

In addition, shock may occur when there is adequate blood volume but the heart is unable to pump the blood. This problem can be due to severe heart disease, heart

attack, or acute heart failure. Other causes of shock include overwhelming infection, lack of certain hormones, low blood sugar (hypoglycemia), hypothermia, severe allergic reaction (anaphylactic shock), drug overdose, and spinal cord injury.

▶ See also ANAPHYLACTIC SHOCK p.123
● LIFE-SAVING PROCEDURES pp.71–102
● SEVERE BLEEDING pp.130–131 ● SEVERE
BURNS AND SCALDS pp.194–195

RECOGNITION

Initially:
● A rapid pulse.
● Pale, cold, clammy skin; sweating.

As shock develops:
● Gray–blue skin (cyanosis), especially inside the lips. A fingernail or earlobe, if pressed, will not regain its colour immediately.
● Weakness and dizziness.
● Nausea, and possibly vomiting.
● Thirst.
● Rapid, shallow breathing.
● A weak, "thready" pulse. When the pulse at the wrist disappears, about half of the blood volume will have been lost.

As the brain's oxygen supply weakens:
● Restlessness and aggressiveness.
● Yawning and gasping for air.
● Unconsciousness.

Finally, the heart will stop.

EFFECTS OF BLOOD OR FLUID LOSS

Approximate volume lost	Effects on the body
1 pint (about 0.5 liter)	Little or no effect; this is the quantity normally taken in a blood-donor session
Up to 3.5 pints (2 liters)	Release of hormones such as epinephrine, quickening the pulse and inducing sweating ● Small blood vessels in nonvital areas, such as the skin, shut down to divert blood and oxygen to the vital organs ● Shock becomes evident
3.5 pints (2 liters) or more (over one third of normal volume in the average adult)	As blood or fluid loss approaches this level, the pulse at the wrist may become undetectable ● Victim will usually lose consciousness ● Breathing may cease and the heart may stop

+ YOUR AIMS

- To recognize shock.
- To treat any obvious cause of shock.
- To improve the blood supply to the brain, heart, and lungs.
- To arrange urgent transport to a hospital.

! CAUTION

- Do not let the victim eat, drink, smoke, or move unnecessarily. If she complains of thirst, moisten her lips with a little water.
- Do not leave the victim unattended, except to call for help.
- Do not try to warm the victim with a hot-water bottle or any other direct source of heat.

1 Treat any possible cause of shock that you can detect, such as severe bleeding (pp.130–131) or serious burns (p.194).

2 Lay the victim down on a blanket to insulate her from the cold ground. Constantly reassure her.

3 Raise and support her legs to improve the blood supply to the vital organs. Take care if you suspect a fracture.

Raise victim's legs so that they are higher than her heart

Keeping head low may prevent victim losing consciousness

4 Loosen tight clothing at the neck, chest, and waist to reduce constriction in these areas.

5 Keep the victim warm by covering her body and legs with coats or blankets.
DIAL 9·1·1 OR CALL EMS.

6 Monitor and record vital signs – level of response, pulse, and breathing (pp.42–43). If the person becomes unconscious, open the airway and check breathing; be prepared to give rescue breaths and chest compressions if necessary (*see* LIFE-SAVING PROCEDURES, pp.71–102).

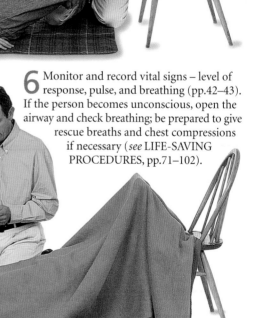

Take pulse at wrist

Protect victim from cold with coats or blankets

INTERNAL BLEEDING

Bleeding inside body cavities may follow an injury, such as a fracture or a penetrating wound, but can also occur spontaneously – for example, bleeding from a stomach ulcer. The main risk from internal bleeding is shock (pp.120–121). In addition, blood can build up around organs such as the lungs or brain and exert damaging pressure on them.

You should suspect internal bleeding if a victim develops signs of shock without obvious blood loss. Check for any bleeding from body openings (orifices) such as the ear, mouth, urethra, or anus (below).

 See also CEREBRAL COMPRESSION p.181
● CRUSH INJURY p.133

▶ Treat as for SHOCK pp.120–121

RECOGNITION

- ● Initially, pale, cold, clammy skin. If bleeding continues, skin may turn blue-gray (cyanosis).
- ● Rapid, weak pulse.
- ● Thirst.
- ● Rapid, shallow breathing.
- ● Confusion, restlessness, and irritability.
- ● Possible collapse and unconsciousness.
- ● Bleeding from body openings (orifices).
- ● In cases of violent injury, "pattern bruising" – an area of discolored skin with a shape that matches the pattern of clothes, crushing objects, or restraining objects (such as a seat belt).
- ● Pain.
- ● Information from the victim that indicates recent injury or illness; previous similar episodes of internal bleeding; or use of drugs to control a medical condition such as thrombosis (in which unwanted clots form in blood vessels).

POSSIBLE SIGNS OF INTERNAL BLEEDING

Signs of bleeding vary depending on the site of the blood loss, but the most obvious feature is a discharge of blood from a body opening (orifice). Blood loss from any orifice is significant and can lead to shock (pp.120–121). In addition, bleeding from some orifices can indicate a serious underlying injury or illness.

Site	Appearance of blood	Cause of blood loss
Mouth	Bright red, frothy, coughed-up blood	Bleeding in the lungs
	Vomited blood, red or dark reddish brown, resembling coffee grounds	Bleeding within the digestive system
Ear	Fresh, bright red blood	Injury to the inner or outer ear ● Perforated eardrum
	Thin, watery blood	Leakage of fluid from around brain due to head injury
Nose	Fresh, bright red blood	Ruptured blood vessel in the nostril
	Thin, watery blood	Leakage of fluid from around brain due to head injury
Anus	Fresh, bright red blood	Hemorrhoids ● Injury to the anus or lower intestine
	Black, tarry, offensive-smelling stool (melena)	Disease or injury to the intestine
Urethra	Urine with a red or smoky appearance and occasionally containing clots	Bleeding from the bladder, kidneys, or urethra
Vagina	Either fresh or dark blood	Menstruation ● Miscarriage ● Pregnancy or recent childbirth ● Disease of, or injury to, the vagina or uterus

ANAPHYLACTIC SHOCK

This condition is a severe allergic reaction affecting the whole body. In susceptible individuals, it may develop within seconds or minutes of contact with a trigger factor and is potentially fatal. Possible triggers include the following:

- Skin or airborne contact with particular materials.
- The injection of a specific drug.
- The sting of a certain insect.
- The ingestion of a food such as peanuts.

In an anaphylactic reaction, chemicals are released into the blood that widen (dilate) blood vessels and constrict (narrow) air passages. Blood pressure falls dramatically, and breathing is impaired. The tongue and throat can swell, increasing the risk of

hypoxia (p.106). The amount of oxygen reaching the vital organs is severely reduced.

A victim with anaphylactic shock needs emergency treatment with an injection of epinephrine (adrenaline). First-aid priorities are to ease breathing and minimize shock until specialized help arrives.

RECOGNITION

- Anxiety.
- Widespread red, blotchy skin eruption.
- Swelling of the tongue and throat.
- Puffiness around the eyes.
- Impaired breathing, ranging from a tight chest to severe difficulty; the victim may wheeze and gasp for air.
- Signs of shock (pp.120–121).

➕ YOUR AIM

- To arrange urgent transport to a hospital.

1 DIAL 9·1·1 OR CALL EMS.
Give any information you have on the cause of the victim's condition.

2 Check whether the victim is carrying the necessary medication – a syringe or an auto-injector (see below) of epinephrine (adrenaline) for self-administration. Help her use it. If the victim is unable to administer the medication, and you have been trained to use an auto-injector, give it to her yourself.

3 If the victim is conscious, help her sit up in the position that best relieves any breathing difficulty.

4 Treat the victim for shock (pp.120–121) if necessary.

SPECIAL CASE

EpiPens are one type of auto-injector

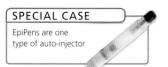

⚠ WARNING

If the victim becomes unconscious, open the airway and check breathing; be prepared to give rescue breaths and chest compressions if necessary (see LIFE-SAVING PROCEDURES, pp.71–102). If the victim is breathing, place her in the recovery position (pp.84–85).

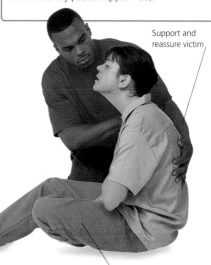

Support and reassure victim

Sitting position should help to ease victim's breathing

ANGINA PECTORIS

The term "angina pectoris" means literally "a constriction of the chest." Angina occurs when coronary arteries, which supply the heart muscle with blood, become narrowed and cannot carry sufficient blood to meet increased demands during exertion or excitement. An attack forces the victim to rest; the pain should ease soon afterward.

RECOGNITION

- Vicelike central chest pain, often spreading to the jaw and down one or both arms.
- Pain easing with rest.
- Shortness of breath.
- Weakness, which is often sudden and extreme.
- Feeling of anxiety.

YOUR AIMS

- To ease strain on the heart by ensuring that the victim rests.
- To obtain medical help if necessary.
- To help the victim with any medication.

⚠ WARNING

If the pain persists, or returns, suspect a heart attack (opposite)

DIAL 9•1•1 OR CALL EMS.

Treat by giving the victim a full-dose (300 mg) aspirin pill to chew. Constantly monitor and record vital signs – level of response, pulse, and breathing (pp.42–43).

If the victim becomes unconscious, open the airway and check breathing; be prepared to give rescue breaths and chest compressions if necessary (see LIFE-SAVING PROCEDURES, pp.71–102).

1 Help the person sit down. Make sure that she is comfortable and reassure her. This action should help her breathing.

2 If the person has medication for angina, such as pills or a pump-action or aerosol spray, let her administer it herself. If necessary, help her take it.

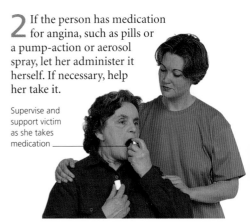

Supervise and support victim as she takes medication

3 Encourage her to rest, and keep any bystanders away. The attack should ease within a few minutes.

ACUTE HEART FAILURE

In heart failure, the heart muscle is over-strained or damaged and cannot pump sufficient blood to the body tissues. Fluid may also build up in the lungs, leading to breathing difficulties. A possible cause of heart failure is a clot in a coronary artery (coronary thrombosis). Attacks of acute heart failure occur suddenly, often at night.

RECOGNITION

- Severe breathlessness.
- Often, but not always, signs and symptoms of heart attack (opposite).

▶ **Treat as for** HEART ATTACK opposite

HEART ATTACK

A heart attack is most commonly caused by a sudden obstruction of the blood supply to part of the heart muscle – for example, because of a clot in a coronary artery (coronary thrombosis). The main risk is that the heart will stop beating.

The effects of a heart attack depend largely on how much of the heart muscle is affected; many victims recover completely. Drugs such as aspirin, and medications that dissolve the clot, are used to limit the extent of damage to the heart muscle.

See also LIFE-SAVING PROCEDURES pp.71–102

See also LIFE-SAVING PROCEDURES pp.71–102

RECOGNITION

● Persistent, vicelike central chest pain, often spreading to the jaw and down one or both arms. Unlike angina pectoris (opposite), the pain does not ease when the victim rests.

● Breathlessness, and discomfort occurring high in the abdomen, which may feel like severe indigestion.

● Collapse, often without any warning.

● Sudden faintness or dizziness.

● A sense of impending doom.

● "Ashen" skin, and blueness at the lips.

● A rapid, weak, or irregular pulse.

● Profuse sweating.

● Extreme gasping for air ("air hunger").

YOUR AIMS

● To encourage the victim to rest.

● To arrange urgent transport of the victim to a hospital.

❶ WARNING

If the victim becomes unconscious, open the airway and check breathing; be prepared to give rescue breaths and chest compressions if needed (*see* LIFE-SAVING PROCEDURES, pp.71–102).

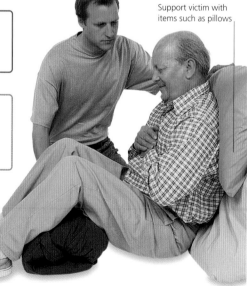

Support victim with items such as pillows

1 Make the victim as comfortable as possible to ease the strain on his heart. A half-sitting position, with the victim's head and shoulders well supported and his knees bent, is often best.

2 DIAL 9·1·1 OR CALL EMS. State that you suspect a heart attack. If the victim asks you to do so, call his own doctor as well.

3 If the victim is fully conscious, give him a full-dose (300mg) aspirin pill and advise him to chew it slowly.

4 If the victim has medicine for angina, such as pills or a pump-action or aerosol spray, help him take it. Encourage the victim to rest.

5 Constantly monitor and record vital signs – level of response, pulse, and breathing (pp.42–43) – until help arrives.

FAINTING

A faint is a brief loss of consciousness caused by a temporary reduction of the blood flow to the brain. Fainting may be a reaction to pain, exhaustion, lack of food, or emotional stress. It is also common after long periods of physical inactivity, such as standing or sitting still, especially in a warm atmosphere. This inactivity causes blood to pool in the legs, reducing the amount of blood reaching the brain.

When a person faints, the pulse rate becomes very slow. However, the rate soon

RECOGNITION
- A brief loss of consciousness that causes the victim to fall to the floor.
- A slow pulse.
- Pale, cold skin and sweating.

picks up and returns to normal. A person who has fainted usually makes a rapid and complete recovery.

See also LIFE-SAVING PROCEDURES pp.71–102

YOUR AIMS
- To improve blood flow to the brain.
- To reassure the person as she recovers and make her comfortable.

1 When a person feels faint, advise her to lie down. Kneel down, raise her legs, and support her ankles on your shoulders; this helps improve the blood flow to the brain.

Support ankles on your shoulders

Raise legs to improve blood flow to brain

Watch face for signs of recovery

2 Make sure that the person has plenty of fresh air; ask someone to open a window. In addition, ask any bystanders to stand clear.

3 As she recovers, reassure her and help her sit up gradually. If she starts to feel faint again, advise her to lie down again, and raise and support her legs until she recovers fully.

WARNING

If the person does not regain consciousness quickly, open the airway and check breathing; be prepared to give rescue breaths and chest compressions if necessary (see LIFE-SAVING PROCEDURES, pp.71–102).

DIAL 9•1•1 OR CALL EMS.

6

BREAKS IN THE SKIN or the body surfaces are known as wounds. Open wounds allow blood and other fluids to be lost from the body and enable germs to enter. In a closed wound, bleeding is confined within the body tissues and is most easily recognized by bruising. Wounds can be daunting, particularly if there is a lot of bleeding, but prompt action will reduce the amount of blood lost and minimize shock.

UNDERSTANDING TREATMENT
The way in which an injury is inflicted and the force that is exerted determine the effect of the wound on the body and influence its treatment. This chapter covers recommended treatments for all types of wounds. When you treat any wound, it is important to wear gloves and follow good hygiene procedures to protect both yourself and the injured person from cross-infection (p.15).

CONTENTS

Bleeding and types of wounds..128

Severe bleeding.................... 130

Impalement............................ 132

Amputation........................... 132

Crush injury.......................... 133

Cuts and abrasions................. 134

Foreign object in a cut............ 135

Bruising................................ 136

Infected wound..................... 136

Scalp and head wounds........... 137

Eye wound............................ 138

Bleeding from the ear............. 138

Nosebleed............................ 139

Bleeding from the mouth......... 140

Knocked-out tooth.................. 140

Wound to the palm................. 141

Wound at a joint crease........... 141

Abdominal wound................... 142

Vaginal bleeding.................... 143

Bleeding varicose vein............. 144

FIRST-AID PRIORITIES

- Assess the victim's condition.
- Comfort and reassure the victim.
- Take care with hygiene; wear gloves.
- Control blood loss by applying pressure and elevating the injured part.
- Minimize shock.
- Obtain medical help, if necessary. Call 9•1•1 or EMS if you suspect a serious illness or injury.

WOUNDS AND BLEEDING

BLEEDING AND TYPES OF WOUNDS

Blood circulates in vessels called arteries, veins, and capillaries (p.118). When a blood vessel is damaged, several mechanisms are activated to control blood loss: the vessel constricts, and a series of chemical reactions occur to form a blood clot – a "plug" over the damaged area (below). If blood vessels are torn or severed, uncontrolled blood loss may occur before clotting can take place, and shock (pp.120–121) may develop.

TYPES OF BLEEDING

Bleeding (hemorrhage) is classified by the type of blood vessel that is damaged.

Arteries carry bright red, oxygen-rich blood under pressure from the heart. If an artery is damaged, bleeding may be profuse. Blood will spurt out of it in time with the heartbeat. If a main artery is severed, it may jet blood several feet high. In this case, the volume of circulating blood will fall rapidly.

Blood from veins, having given up its oxygen into the tissues, is dark red. It is under less pressure than arterial blood, but vein walls can widen greatly and the blood can "pool" inside them. If a major vein is damaged, blood may gush from it profusely.

Bleeding from capillaries occurs with any wound. At first, bleeding may be brisk, but blood loss is usually slight. A blow may rupture capillaries under the skin, causing bleeding into the tissues (bruising).

How blood clots

When a blood vessel is severed or damaged, it constricts (narrows) in order to prevent excessive amounts of blood from escaping. Injured tissue cells at the site of the wound, together with specialized blood cells called platelets, then trigger a series of chemical reactions that result in the formation of a substance called fibrin. Strands (filaments) of fibrin come together to form a mesh, which traps blood cells to make a blood clot. The clot releases a pale-colored fluid known as serum, which contains antibodies and specialized cells; this serum begins the process of repairing the damaged area.

At first, the blood clot is a jellylike mass. Later, it dries into a crust (scab) that seals and protects the site of the wound until the healing process is complete.

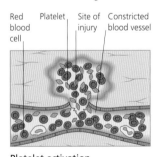

Red blood cell | Platelet | Site of injury | Constricted blood vessel

Platelet activation
In the first stage of clotting, cells in the blood called platelets come into contact with the damaged vessel wall. They become sticky and start to clump at the site of the injury.

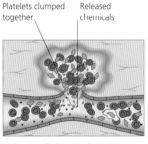

Platelets clumped together | Released chemicals

Release of chemicals
The clumped platelets and the damaged tissue release chemicals that trigger a complex chain of reactions. This process creates substances that enable clotting.

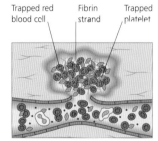

Trapped red blood cell | Fibrin strand | Trapped platelet

Fibrin formation
Threads of fibrin form a mesh at the site of the injury. The fibrin mesh traps more blood cells at the site to form a jellylike clot, usually within about 10 minutes.

Types of wounds

Wounds can be classified into a number of different types, depending on the object that produces the wound – such as a knife or a bullet – and the manner in which the wound has been inflicted.

Each of these types of wounds carries specific risks associated with surrounding tissue damage and infection.

Simple laceration

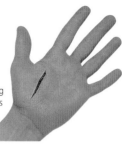

This is caused by a clean cut from a sharp-edged object such as a razor. Blood vessels are cut straight across, so bleeding may be profuse. Structures such as tendons, nerves, or arteries may be damaged.

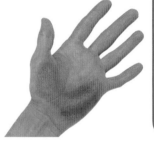

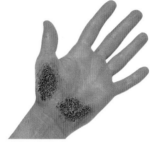

Complex laceration

Crushing or ripping forces result in tears or lacerations. These wounds may bleed less profusely than incised wounds, but there is likely to be more tissue damage. Lacerations are often contaminated with germs, so the risk of infection is high.

Abrasion (graze)

This is a superficial wound in which the topmost layers of skin are scraped off, leaving a raw, tender area. Abrasions are often caused by a sliding fall or a friction burn. They can contain embedded foreign particles that may result in infection.

Contusion (bruise)

A blunt blow or punch can rupture capillaries beneath the skin, causing blood to leak into the tissues. This process results in bruising. The skin occasionally splits. Severe contusion may indicate deeper damage, such as a fracture or an internal injury.

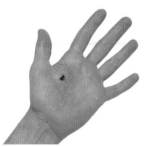

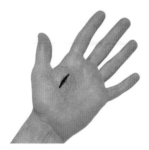

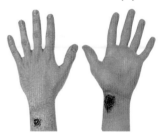

ENTRY WOUND   EXIT WOUND

Puncture wound

An injury caused by standing on a nail or being pricked by a needle will result in a puncture wound. It has a small entry site but a deep track of internal damage. Since germs and dirt can be carried far into the body, the infection risk is high.

Stab wound

This type of wound is caused by a long or bladed instrument, usually a knife, penetrating the body. Stab wounds to the trunk must always be treated seriously because of the dangers of injury to vital organs or life-threatening internal bleeding.

Gunshot wound

A bullet or other missile may drive into or through the body, causing serious internal injury and sucking in clothing and contaminants from the air. The entry wound may be small and neat; any exit wound may be large and ragged.

SEVERE BLEEDING

Severe bleeding can be dramatic and frightening. Shock is likely to develop, and the injured person may lose consciousness. If bleeding is not controlled, the heart could stop. Bleeding at the face or neck may impede the air flow to the lungs. When

treating severe bleeding, check first whether there is an object embedded in the wound; take care not to press on the object.

▶ **See also** LIFE-SAVING PROCEDURES pp.71–102 ● SHOCK pp.120–121

IF NO OBJECT IS EMBEDDED IN WOUND

+ YOUR AIMS

- To control bleeding.
- To prevent and minimize the effects of shock.
- To minimize infection.
- To arrange urgent transport to a hospital.

1 Put on disposable gloves if available. Remove or cut clothing as necessary to expose the wound (p.40).

2 Apply direct pressure over the wound with your fingers or palm, preferably over a sterile dressing or nonfluffy, clean pad (but do not waste any time by looking for a dressing). You can ask the injured person to apply direct pressure herself.

3 Raise and support the injured limb above the level of the heart to reduce blood loss. Handle the limb very gently if you suspect that there is a fracture.

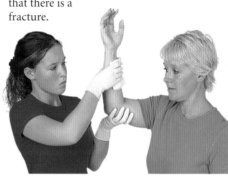

4 Help the person lie down on a blanket, if available, to protect her from the cold. If you suspect that shock may develop, raise and support her legs so that they are above the level of her heart.

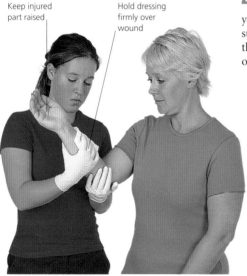

Keep injured part raised

Hold dressing firmly over wound

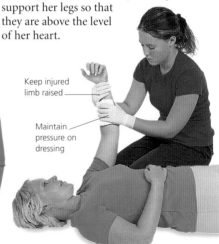

Keep injured limb raised

Maintain pressure on dressing

5 Secure the dressing with a bandage that is tight enough to maintain pressure, but not so tight that it impairs the circulation.

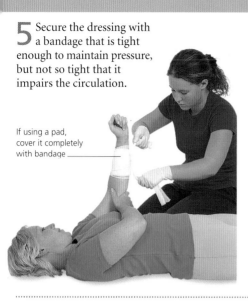

If using a pad, cover it completely with bandage ⎯⎯⎯⎯

6 If further bleeding occurs, apply a second dressing on top of the first. If blood seeps through this dressing, remove both dressings and apply a fresh one, ensuring that pressure is applied accurately to the point of bleeding.

7 Support the injured part in a raised position with a sling and/or bandaging.

8 DIAL 9·1·1 OR CALL EMS.
Monitor and record vital signs – level of response, pulse, and breathing (pp.42–43). Watch for signs of shock (pp.120–121), and check the dressings for seepage. Check the circulation beyond the bandage (p.51).

> **❶ CAUTION**
> Do not allow the injured to eat, drink, or smoke.

IF AN OBJECT IS EMBEDDED IN WOUND

> **➕ YOUR AIMS**
> ● To control bleeding without pressing the object into the wound.
> ● To prevent and minimize the effects of shock.
> ● To minimize infection.
> ● To arrange urgent transport to a hospital.

1 Put on disposable gloves if available. Press firmly on either side of the embedded object to push the edges of the wound together.

2 If the injury is to a limb, raise and support the limb above the level of the heart to reduce the blood loss.

3 Help the person lie down on a blanket, if available, to protect her from the cold. If you suspect that shock may develop, raise and support her legs so that they are above the level of her heart.

4 Build up padding on either side of the object. Carefully bandage over the object without pressing on it.

Take care not ⎯⎯⎯⎯ to press on object

5 Support the injured part in a raised position with a sling and/or bandaging to minimize swelling.

6 DIAL 9·1·1 OR CALL EMS.
Monitor and record vital signs – level of response, pulse, and breathing (pp.42–43). Watch for signs of shock (pp.120–121), and check the dressing for seepage. Check the circulation beyond the bandage (p.51).

131

IMPALEMENT

If someone has been impaled, for example by falling onto railings, you must never attempt to lift him off the object involved because you could worsen internal injuries.

Call for the emergency services immediately, giving clear details about the incident. The emergency services will bring special cutting equipment with them to free the person.

+ YOUR AIM
- To prevent further injury.

! CAUTION
Do not allow the injured to eat, drink, or smoke.

1 DIAL 9·1·1 OR CALL EMS.
Send a helper to make the call, if possible. Explain the situation clearly.

2 Support the person's body weight until the emergency services take over from you. Constantly reassure him.

AMPUTATION

A limb that has been partially or completely severed can, in many cases, be reattached by microsurgery. The operation will require a general anesthetic, so do not allow the victim to eat, drink, or smoke. It is vital to get the injured person and the amputated part to hospital as soon as possible. Shock is likely, and needs to be treated.

▶ **See also** SHOCK pp.120–121

CARE OF THE VICTIM

+ YOUR AIMS
- To minimize blood loss and shock.
- To arrange urgent transport to a hospital.

1 Put on disposable gloves if available. Control blood loss by applying pressure and raising the injured part.

2 Apply a sterile dressing, or a nonfluffy, clean pad, and secure it with a bandage. Treat for shock (pp.120–121).

3 DIAL 9·1·1 OR CALL EMS.
State that amputation is involved. Monitor and record vital signs – level of response, pulse, and breathing (pp.42–43).

CARE OF THE AMPUTATED PART

+ YOUR AIM
- To prevent deterioration of the part.

! CAUTION
- Do not wash the severed part.
- Do not allow the severed part to come into direct contact with ice.

1 Put on disposable gloves. Wrap the part in plastic wrap or a plastic bag.

2 Wrap the package in gauze or soft fabric. Place it in a container full of crushed ice.

3 Clearly mark the container with the time of injury and the person's name. Give it to the emergency service personnel yourself.

CRUSH INJURY

Traffic and building site incidents are the most common causes of crush injuries. Other possible causes include explosions, earthquakes, and train crashes.

A crush injury may include a fracture, swelling, and internal bleeding. The crushing force may also cause impaired circulation, resulting in numbness at or below the site of injury. You may not be able to detect a pulse in a crushed limb.

DANGERS OF PROLONGED CRUSHING
If a person is trapped for any length of time, two serious complications may result. First, prolonged crushing may cause

extensive damage to body tissues, especially to muscles. Once the pressure is removed, shock may develop rapidly as tissue fluid leaks into the injured area.

Second, and more dangerously, toxic substances will build up in damaged muscle tissue around a crush injury. If released suddenly into the circulation, these toxins may cause kidney failure. This process, called "crush syndrome," is extremely serious and can be fatal.

▶ **See also** FRACTURES pp.150–152
● SHOCK pp.120–121

IF CRUSHED FOR LESS THAN 15 MINUTES

➕ YOUR AIM
● To obtain specialized medical aid urgently, taking any steps possible to treat the injured.

1 Release the person quickly. Put on disposable gloves if available. Control external bleeding and cover wounds (p.130).

2 Secure and support any suspected fractures (pp.150–152). Treat for shock (pp.120–121).

3 DIAL 9·1·1 OR CALL EMS.
Give clear details of the incident. Monitor and record vital signs – level of response, pulse, and breathing (pp.42–43) – until help arrives.

IF CRUSHED FOR MORE THAN 15 MINUTES

➕ YOUR AIM
● To obtain specialized medical aid urgently.

❗ CAUTION
Do not release a person who has been crushed for more than 15 minutes.

1 DIAL 9·1·1 OR CALL EMS.
Give clear details of the incident.

2 Comfort and reassure the injured person. Monitor and record vital signs – level of response, pulse, and breathing (pp.42–43).

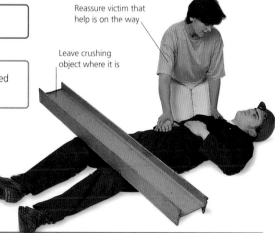

Reassure victim that help is on the way

Leave crushing object where it is

CUTS AND ABRASIONS

Bleeding from small cuts and abrasions is easily controlled by pressure and elevation. An adhesive dressing is normally all that is necessary, and the wound will heal by itself in a few days. Medical aid need only be sought in the following circumstances:

- If the bleeding does not stop.
- If there is a foreign object embedded in the cut (opposite).
- If the wound is at particular risk of infection (such as a human or animal bite, or a puncture by a dirty object).
- If an old wound shows signs of becoming infected (p.136).

TETANUS

This is a dangerous infection caused by the bacterium *Clostridium tetani*, which lives in soil as spores. If tetanus bacteria enter a wound, they may multiply in the damaged and swollen tissues and may release a poisonous substance (toxin) that spreads through the nervous system, causing muscle spasms and paralysis.

The disorder can be prevented by immunization, and people are normally given a course of tetanus immunization during childhood. However, immunization may need to be repeated in adulthood.

☐ YOUR AIM
- To minimize the risk of infection.

1 Wash your hands thoroughly, and put on disposable gloves if available.

2 If the wound is dirty, clean it by rinsing lightly under running water, or use an alcohol-free wipe. Pat the wound dry using a gauze swab and cover with sterile gauze.

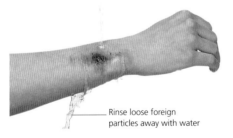

Rinse loose foreign particles away with water

❶ CAUTION

Always ask about tetanus immunization.

Seek medical advice if:
- The person has never been immunized.
- The person is uncertain about the timing and number of injections that have been given.
- It is more than 10 years since the person's last injection.

3 Elevate the injured part above the level of the heart, if possible. Avoid touching the wound directly. Support the affected limb with one hand.

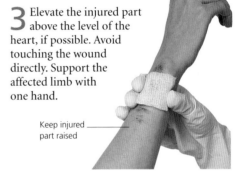

Keep injured part raised

4 Clean the surrounding area with soap and water; use clean swabs for each stroke. Pat dry. Remove the wound covering and apply an adhesive dressing. If there is a special risk of infection, advise the person to see her doctor.

Wipe away from wound, using a clean gauze swab for each stroke

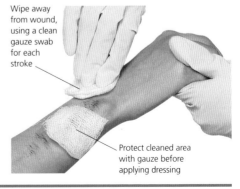

Protect cleaned area with gauze before applying dressing

FOREIGN OBJECT IN A CUT

It is important to remove foreign objects, such as small pieces of glass or grit, from wounds before beginning treatment. If such items remain in a wound, they may cause infection or delayed healing in the short term and discoloration in the long term. The best way to remove superficial pieces of glass or grit is with tweezers if you have them. Alternatively, carefully pick the pieces off the wound or rinse them off with cool water. Do not try to remove objects that are firmly embedded in the wound because you may damage the surrounding tissue and aggravate bleeding. Instead, apply dressings or bandages around them.

▶ **See also** EMBEDDED FISHHOOK p.213
● SPLINTER p.212

✚ YOUR AIMS

● To control bleeding without pressing the object into the wound.
● To minimize the risk of infection.
● To arrange transport to a hospital if necessary.

1 Put on disposable gloves if available. Control any bleeding by applying pressure on either side of the object and raising the injured part above the level of the heart.

2 Cover the wound with gauze to minimize the risk of infection.

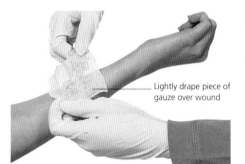

Lightly drape piece of gauze over wound

❶ CAUTION

Always ask about tetanus immunization.

Seek medical advice if:
● The person has never been immunized.
● The person is uncertain about the timing and number of injections that have been given.
● It is more than 10 years since the person's last injection.

3 Build up padding around the object until you can bandage over it without pressing down. Carefully hold the padding in place until the bandaging is complete.

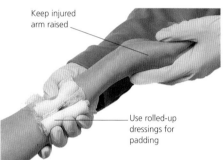

Keep injured arm raised

Use rolled-up dressings for padding

4 Arrange to take or send the injured person to a hospital if necessary.

SPECIAL CASE

LARGE OBJECTS
If the object is particularly large, and you cannot pad high enough to bandage over it without pressing on it, bandage around the object.

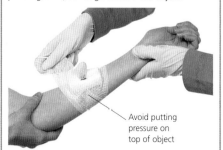

Avoid putting pressure on top of object

BRUISING

This is caused by bleeding into the skin or into tissues beneath the skin. It can either develop rapidly or emerge a few days later. Bruises that appear rapidly will benefit from first aid. Bruising can also indicate deep injury. Elderly people and those taking anticoagulant drugs can bruise very easily.

▶ See also INTERNAL BLEEDING p.122

+ YOUR AIM
- To reduce blood flow to the injury, and thus minimize swelling.

1 Raise and support the injured part in a comfortable position.

2 Apply firm pressure to the bruise using a cold compress (p.49). Keep the compress in place for at least 5 minutes.

INFECTED WOUND

Any open wound can become contaminated with microorganisms (germs). The germs may come from the source of the injury, from the air, from the breath or the fingers, or from particles of clothing embedded in a wound (as may occur in gunshot wounds). Bleeding flushes some dirt away; remaining germs may be destroyed by the white blood cells. However, if dirt or dead tissue remain in a wound, infection may spread through the body. Tetanus is also a risk.

Any wound that does not begin to heal within 48 hours is likely to be infected. A victim with a wound that is at high risk of infection may need treatment with antibiotics and/or antitetanus injections (*see* CUTS AND ABRASIONS, p.134).

RECOGNITION
- Increasing pain and soreness at the site of the wound.
- Swelling, redness, and a feeling of heat around the injury.
- Pus within, or oozing from, the wound.
- Swelling and tenderness of the glands in the neck, armpit, or groin.
- Faint red trails on the skin that lead to the glands in the neck, armpit, or groin.
- In someone who has advanced infection, signs of fever such as sweating, thirst, shivering, and lethargy.

▶ See also BLEEDING AND TYPES OF WOUND pp.128–129 ● CUTS AND ABRASIONS p.134

+ YOUR AIMS
- To prevent further infection.
- To obtain medical aid if necessary.

1 Put on disposable gloves if available. Cover the wound with a sterile dressing or a clean, nonfluffy pad and bandage in place. Do not bandage too tightly.

2 Raise and support the injured part using a sling and/or bandaging. This will help to reduce any swelling around the wound.

3 Tell the person to see his doctor. If the infection appears to be advanced (with signs of fever such as sweating, shivering, thirst, and lethargy), call a doctor or take or send the person to a hospital.

SCALP AND HEAD WOUNDS

The scalp has many small blood vessels running close to the skin surface, so any cut can result in profuse bleeding. This bleeding will often make a scalp wound appear worse than it is. In some cases, however, a scalp wound may form part of a more serious underlying injury, such as a skull fracture, or may be associated with a head or neck injury. For these reasons, you should examine someone with a scalp wound very carefully, particularly if it is possible that signs of a serious head injury are being masked by alcohol or drug intoxication. If you are in any doubt, follow the treatment for head injury (p.179). In addition, bear in mind the possibility of a neck (spinal) injury.

▶ **See also** HEAD INJURY p.179 ● SHOCK pp.120–121 ● SPINAL INJURY pp.165–167

✚ YOUR AIMS

- To control blood loss.
- To arrange transport to a hospital.

❶ WARNING

If the injured person becomes unconscious, open the airway and check breathing; be prepared to give rescue breaths and chest compressions if necessary (see LIFE-SAVING PROCEDURES, pp.71–102).

1 Put on disposable gloves if available. If there are any displaced flaps of skin at the injury site, carefully replace them over the wound. Reassure the injured person.

2 Cover the wound with a sterile dressing or a clean, nonfluffy pad. Apply firm, direct pressure on the pad. This measure will help control bleeding and reduce blood loss, minimizing the risk of shock.

3 Secure the dressing with a roller bandage. (For minor bleeding, you can keep the pad in place with a triangular bandage.)

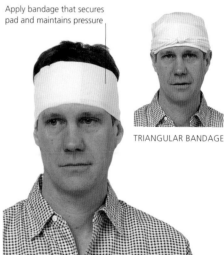

Apply bandage that secures pad and maintains pressure

TRIANGULAR BANDAGE

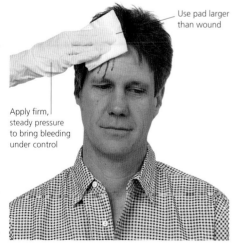

Use pad larger than wound

Apply firm, steady pressure to bring bleeding under control

4 Help the person lie down, with his head and shoulders slightly raised. Then take or send him to a hospital in the final treatment position. Regularly monitor and record vital signs – level of response, pulse, and breathing (pp.42–43).

EYE WOUND

The eye can be bruised or cut by direct blows or by sharp, chipped fragments of metal, stone, and glass.

All eye injuries are potentially serious because of the risk to the victim's vision. Even superficial abrasions to the surface (cornea) of the eye can lead to scarring or infection, with the possibility of permanent deterioration of vision.

RECOGNITION
- Intense pain and spasm of the eyelids.
- Visible wound and/or bloodshot appearance.
- Partial or total loss of vision.
- Leakage of blood or clear fluid from a wound.

See also FOREIGN OBJECT IN THE EYE p.214

YOUR AIMS
- To prevent further damage.
- To arrange transport to a hospital.

CAUTION
Do not touch or attempt to remove an embedded foreign object in the eye (p.214).

1 Help the person to lie on her back, and hold her head to keep it as still as possible. Tell her to keep both eyes still; movement of the "good" eye will cause movement of the injured one, which may damage it further.

2 Ask her to hold a sterile dressing or a clean, nonfluffy pad over the affected eye. If it will take some time to obtain medical help, secure the pad in place with a bandage.

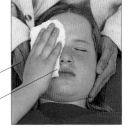

Keep head supported

Use a large, soft pad that covers eye

3 Take or send the injured person to a hospital in the treatment position.

BLEEDING FROM THE EAR

This is usually due to a burst (perforated) eardrum, caused by, for example, a foreign object pushed in the ear, a blow to the side of the head, or an explosion. Symptoms include a sharp pain, then earache, deafness, and possible dizziness. Watery blood is a serious sign: it shows that the skull is fractured and fluid is leaking from around the brain.

See also FOREIGN OBJECT IN THE EAR p.215 ● HEAD INJURY p.179

YOUR AIM
- To arrange transport to a hospital.

CAUTION
Do not tilt the person's head if you suspect a spine fracture.

1 Help the person into a half-sitting position, with his head tilted to the injured side to allow blood to drain away.

2 Put on disposable gloves if available. Hold a sterile dressing or a clean, nonfluffy pad lightly in place on the ear. Send or take the person to hospital in the treatment position.

NOSEBLEED

Bleeding from the nose most commonly occurs when tiny blood vessels inside the nostrils are ruptured, either by a blow to the nose, or as a result of sneezing, picking, or blowing the nose. Nosebleeds may also occur as a result of high blood pressure.

A nosebleed can be dangerous if the person loses a lot of blood. In addition, if bleeding follows a head injury, the blood may appear thin and watery. The latter is a very serious sign because it indicates that the skull is fractured and fluid is leaking from around the brain.

▶ See also FOREIGN OBJECT IN THE NOSE p.215 ● HEAD INJURY p.179

✚ YOUR AIMS
- To control blood loss.
- To maintain an open airway.

1 Ask the person to sit down. Advise her to tilt her head forward to allow the blood to drain from the nostrils.

2 Ask the person to breathe through her mouth (this will also have a calming effect) and to pinch the soft part of the nose. Reassure and help her if necessary.

Pinch just below hard part of nose

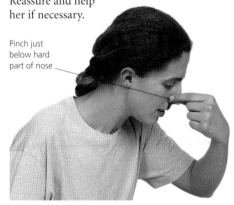

❶ CAUTION
- Do not let the head tip back; blood may run down the throat and induce vomiting.
- If bleeding stops and then restarts, tell the person to reapply pressure.
- If the nosebleed is severe, or if it lasts longer than 30 minutes in total, take or send the victim to a hospital in the treatment position.

SPECIAL CASE

CHILDREN
A young child may be worried by a nosebleed. Reassure her and give her a bowl to spit or dribble into.

Pinch child's nose

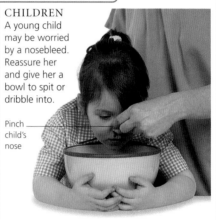

3 Tell the person to keep pinching her nose. Advise her not to speak, swallow, cough, spit, or sniff because she may disturb blood clots that have formed in the nose. Give her a clean cloth or tissue to mop up any dribbling.

4 After 10 minutes, tell the person to release the pressure. If the bleeding has not stopped, tell her to reapply the pressure for two further periods of 10 minutes.

5 Once the bleeding has stopped, and with the person still leaning forward, clean around her nose with lukewarm water.

6 Advise the person to rest quietly for a few hours. Tell her to avoid exertion and, in particular, not to blow her nose, because these actions will disturb any clots.

BLEEDING FROM THE MOUTH

Cuts to the tongue, lips, or lining of the mouth range from trivial injuries to more serious wounds. The cause is usually the person's own teeth or dental extraction.

Bleeding from the mouth may be profuse and can be alarming. In addition, there is a danger that blood may be inhaled into the lungs, causing problems with breathing.

+ YOUR AIMS

- To control bleeding.
- To safeguard the airway by preventing any inhalation of blood.

1 Ask the person to sit down, with her head forward and tilted slightly to the injured side, to allow blood to drain from her mouth.

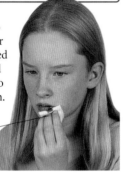

Apply pressure on wound to control bleeding

2 Put on disposable gloves if available. Place a gauze pad over the wound. Ask the person to hold the pad and press on the wound for 10 minutes.

SPECIAL CASE

BLEEDING SOCKET
To control bleeding from a tooth socket, take a gauze pad that is thick enough to stop the teeth from meeting, place it across the empty socket, and tell her to bite down on it.

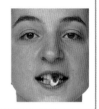

⊘ CAUTION

- If the wound is large, or if bleeding persists beyond 30 minutes or recurs, seek medical or dental advice.
- Do not wash the mouth out because this may disturb a clot.

3 If bleeding persists, replace the pad. Tell the person to let the blood dribble out; if swallowed, it may induce vomiting. Advise her to avoid drinking anything hot for 12 hours.

KNOCKED-OUT TOOTH

If a secondary (adult) tooth is knocked out, it should be replanted in its socket as soon as possible. If this is not possible, ask the person to keep the tooth inside her cheek or place the tooth in a small container of milk to prevent it from drying out.

+ YOUR AIM

- To replant the tooth as soon as possible.

⊘ CAUTION

Do not clean the tooth as you may damage the tissues, reducing the chance of reimplantation.

1 Put on disposable gloves if available. Gently push the tooth into the socket. Keep it in place by pressing a gauze pad between the bottom and top teeth.

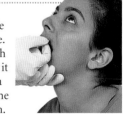

2 Ask the person to hold the tooth firmly in place. Send her to a dentist or hospital.

WOUND TO THE PALM

The palm of the hand has several large blood vessels, which is why a wound to the palm may cause profuse bleeding. There is also a risk that a deep wound to the palm may sever tendons and nerves in the hand and result in loss of feeling or movement in the fingers. If a victim has a foreign object embedded in a wound, it will be impossible for the victim to clench his fist. In such cases, you should treat the injury using the method described on p.135.

▶ See also FOREIGN OBJECT IN A CUT p.135
● SHOCK pp.120–121

+ YOUR AIMS

● To control blood loss and the effects of shock.
● To minimize the risk of infection.
● To arrange transport to a hospital.

1 Put on disposable gloves if available. Press a sterile dressing or clean pad firmly into the palm, and ask the injured person to clench his fist over it. If he finds it difficult to press hard, tell him to grasp his fist with his uninjured hand.

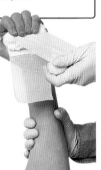

2 Bandage the fingers so that they are clenched over the pad. Tie the ends of the bandage over the top of the fingers.

Leave thumb free

Raise and support arm

3 Support the person's arm in an elevation sling (p.61) to keep it raised. Arrange to take or send him to a hospital.

WOUND AT A JOINT CREASE

Major blood vessels pass across the inside of the elbow and knee. If severed, these vessels will bleed copiously. The steps given below help to control bleeding and shock; however, they also impede the flow of blood to the lower part of the limb, so you must ensure adequate circulation to this area.

▶ See also FOREIGN OBJECT IN A CUT p.135
● SHOCK pp.120–121

+ YOUR AIMS

● To control blood loss.
● To prevent and minimize the effects of shock.
● To arrange transport to a hospital.

1 Put on disposable gloves if available. Press a sterile dressing or clean, nonfluffy pad on the injury. Bend the joint firmly to hold the pad in place and keep pressure on the wound.

2 Raise and support the limb. If possible, help the injured person to lie down with his legs raised and supported.

3 Take or send him to a hospital in the final treatment position. Every 10 minutes, check the circulation beyond the injury. If necessary, briefly release the pressure on the wound to restore normal blood flow to the lower part of the limb, then reapply pressure.

ABDOMINAL WOUND

A stab wound, gunshot, or crush injury to the abdomen may cause serious or even life-threatening wounds. Organs and major blood vessels deep inside the body may be punctured, lacerated, or ruptured. The severity of a wound may be evident from symptoms such as external bleeding and protruding abdominal contents. More commonly, there is hidden internal injury and bleeding, which may be fatal if there is any delay in emergency treatment. In addition, abdominal wounds carry a high risk of shock and infection.

▶ See also INTERNAL BLEEDING p.122
● SHOCK pp.120–121

✚ YOUR AIMS

● To minimize shock.
● To minimize the risk of infection.
● To arrange urgent transport to a hospital.

1 Put on disposable gloves if available. Help the injured person lie down on a firm surface, preferably on a blanket. Loosen any tight clothing, such as a belt or a shirt.

3 DIAL 9·1·1 OR CALL EMS. Treat the person for shock (pp.120–121). Monitor and record vital signs – level of response, pulse, and breathing (pp.42–43).

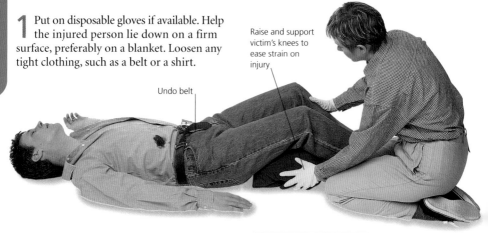

Raise and support victim's knees to ease strain on injury

Undo belt

2 Put a dressing over the wound, and secure it in place with a bandage or adhesive tape. If blood seeps through the dressing, apply another dressing or pad on top.

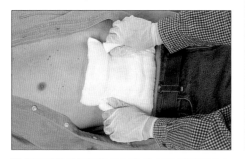

❗ WARNING

● If someone with an open wound coughs or vomits, press firmly on the dressing to prevent the contents of the abdomen from pushing through the wound and being exposed.

● Do not touch any protruding intestine. Cover the area with a clean plastic bag or plastic wrap to prevent the intestine surface from drying out. Alternatively, apply a sterile dressing.

● If the victim becomes unconscious, open the airway and check breathing; be ready to give rescue breaths and chest compressions if needed (see LIFE-SAVING PROCEDURES, pp.71–102). If he is breathing, put him in the recovery position (pp.84–85), supporting the abdomen.

VAGINAL BLEEDING

Bleeding from the vagina is most likely to be menstrual bleeding, and the woman often has abdominal cramps. However, it can also indicate a more serious condition such as miscarriage; pregnancy; recent abortion or childbirth; internal disease or infection; or injury as a result of sexual assault (below). If the bleeding is severe, shock may develop. The history of the condition is vital to diagnosis, and has some bearing on the first aid that you give. Be sensitive to the woman's feelings. She may feel embarrassed or may resent a male presence. Male first aiders should, if possible, seek the help of a female chaperone.

▶ See also MISCARRIAGE p.237 ● SHOCK pp.120–121

✛ YOUR AIMS

- To make the woman comfortable and to reassure her.
- To observe her and treat for shock.
- To arrange transport to a hospital if necessary.

❶ WARNING

If bleeding continues and is severe:
DIAL 9•1•1 OR CALL EMS.
Treat for shock (pp.120–121). Monitor and record level of response, pulse, and breathing (pp.42–43).

1 Remove the woman, if possible, to a place with some privacy. Otherwise, arrange for screening to be set up around her.

2 Find a sanitary napkin or a clean towel and give it to her to use.

3 Make the woman as comfortable as possible, in whichever position she prefers. If she chooses to sit up, prop her up with rolled-up clothing or cushions.

4 If the woman knows that her cramps are due to a menstrual period, she may take analgesics or her own medication.

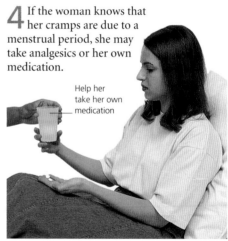

Help her take her own medication

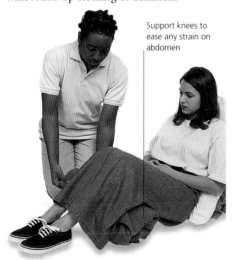

Support knees to ease any strain on abdomen

SPECIAL CASE

SEXUAL ASSAULT

If a woman has been sexually assaulted, it is vital to preserve the evidence if possible. Gently advise her to refrain from washing or using the toilet until a forensic examination has been performed by a doctor, but do not insist. If she wishes to remove clothing, keep it intact in a clean plastic bag if possible. A woman who has recently been assaulted may feel threatened by a male rescuer; a man should seek help from another woman.

BLEEDING VARICOSE VEIN

Veins contain one-way valves that keep the blood flowing toward the heart. If these valves fail, blood collects behind them and makes the veins swell. This problem, called varicose veins, usually develops in the legs.

A varicose vein has taut, thin walls and is often raised, producing typically knobbly skin over the affected area. The vein can be burst by a gentle knock, and this may result in profuse bleeding. Shock will quickly develop if bleeding is not controlled.

 See also SHOCK pp.120–121

See also SHOCK pp.120–121

+ YOUR AIMS

- To bring blood loss under control.
- To minimize shock.
- To arrange urgent transport to a hospital.

1 Put on disposable gloves if available. Help the person lie down on her back, then raise and support the injured leg as high as possible. This measure will help reduce the amount of bleeding.

2 Carefully expose the site of the bleeding. Apply firm, direct pressure on the area, using a sterile dressing, or a clean, nonfluffy pad, until the blood loss is under control.

Support leg on your shoulder during treatment

3 Remove garments such as constricting stockings because these garments may cause bleeding to continue.

4 Put a large, soft pad over the dressing; bandage it firmly enough to exert even pressure, but not so tightly that the circulation is impaired.

Bandage over dresssing

Keep leg high

5 DIAL 9·1·1 OR CALL EMS. Keep the injured leg raised and supported until help arrives. Monitor and record vital signs – level of response, pulse, and breathing (pp.42–43). Check the circulation beyond the bandage (p.51).

7

THE SKELETON is the supporting framework around which the body is constructed. It is jointed in many places, and muscles attached to the bones enable us to move. Most of our movements are controlled at will and coordinated by impulses that travel from the brain via the nerves to every muscle and joint in the body.

DIAGNOSING TYPES OF INJURY
Because it is sometimes difficult to distinguish between bone, joint, and muscle injuries, the chapter begins with an overview of how bones, muscles, and joints function and how damage occurs. First-aid treatments for most injuries, from major fractures to sprains and dislocations, are included here. Skull fracture is covered in the chapter on nervous system problems (p.176) because of the potential damage this injury can have on the brain.

+ FIRST-AID PRIORITIES

- Assess the victim's condition.
- Comfort and reassure the victim.
- Steady and support the injured part.
- Enhance the support with padding, bandages, and splints if necessary.
- Minimize shock.
- Obtain medical aid if necessary. Dial 9•1•1 or call EMS if you suspect a serious injury.

CONTENTS

The skeleton............................ 146

Bones, muscles, and joints........ 148

Fractures................................. 150

Dislocated joint........................ 153

Strains and sprains 154

Major facial fracture................ 156

Cheekbone and nose
    fractures............................. 157

Lower jaw injury....................... 157

Fractured collar bone............... 158

Shoulder injury........................ 159

Upper arm injury...................... 160

Elbow injury............................. 161

Forearm and wrist injuries 162

Hand and finger injuries.......... 163

Injury to the rib cage............... 164

Spinal injury............................ 165

Back pain................................. 168

Fractured pelvis....................... 169

Hip and thigh injuries.............. 170

Knee injury.............................. 172

Lower leg injury....................... 173

Ankle injury............................. 174

Foot and toe injuries................ 174

THE SKELETON

The body is built on a framework of bones called the skeleton. This structure supports the muscles, blood vessels, and nerves of the body. Many bones of the skeleton also protect important organs such as the brain and heart. At many points on the skeleton, bones articulate with each other by means of joints. These are supported by ligaments and moved by muscles that are attached to the bones by tendons.

The skeleton

There are 206 bones in the skeleton, providing a protective framework for the body. The skull, spine, and rib cage protect vital body structures; the pelvis supports the abdominal organs; and the bones and joints of the arms and legs enable the body to move.

Breastbone (sternum)

Twelve pairs of ribs form rib cage, which protects vital organs in chest and moves with lungs during breathing

Spine, which is formed from 33 bones (vertebrae), protects spinal cord and enables back to move

Pelvis is attached to lower part of spine and protects lower abdominal organs

Scaphoid

Wrist bones (carpals)

Hand bone (metacarpal)

Finger bone (phalanx)

BONES OF HAND

Skull protects brain and supports structures of face

Jawbone (mandible) is hinged and enables mouth to open and close

Collarbone (clavicle)

Shoulder blade (scapula)

Collarbones and shoulder blades form the shoulder girdle, to which arms are attached

Upper arm bone (humerus)

Ulna

Radius

Forearm bones

Hip joint is point at which leg bones are connected to pelvis

Thigh bone (femur)

Kneecap (patella)

Lower leg bones

Shin bone (tibia)

Splint bone (fibula)

Ankle bones (tarsals)

Foot bones (metatarsals)

Toe bones (phalanges)

Heel bone (calcaneus)

THE SPINE

The spine, or backbone, has a number of functions. It supports the head, makes the upper body flexible, helps support the body's weight, and protects the spinal cord (p.177). The spine is a column made up of 33 bones called vertebrae, which are connected by joints. Between individual vertebrae are disks of fibrous tissue, called intervertebral disks, which help to make the spine flexible and cushion it from jolts. Muscles and ligaments attached to the vertebrae stabilize the spine and control the movements of the back.

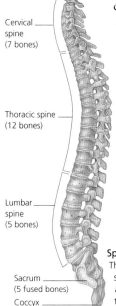

Cervical spine (7 bones)

Thoracic spine (12 bones)

Lumbar spine (5 bones)

Sacrum (5 fused bones)

Coccyx (4 fused bones)

Spinal column
The vertebrae form five groups. The cervical vertebrae support the head and neck. The thoracic vertebrae form an anchor for the ribs. The lumbar vertebrae help to support the body's weight and give stability. The sacrum supports the pelvis, and the coccyx forms the end of the spine.

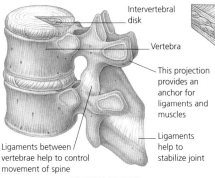

Intervertebral disk

Vertebra

This projection provides an anchor for ligaments and muscles

Ligaments help to stabilize joint

Ligaments between vertebrae help to control movement of spine

PORTION OF SPINE

Fibrous covering

Gelatinous core

SECTION OF INTERVERTEBRAL DISK

Structures that make the spine flexible
The joints connecting the vertebrae, and the discs between vertebrae, allow the spine to move. There is only limited movement between adjacent vertebrae, but together the vertebrae, discs, and ligaments allow a range of movements in the spine as a whole.

THE SKULL

This bony structure protects the brain and the top of the spinal cord. It also supports the eyes and other facial structures.

The skull is made up of several bones, most of which are fused at joints called sutures. Within the bone are air spaces (sinuses), which lighten the skull. The bones covering the brain form a dome called the cranium. Several other bones form the eye sockets, nose, cheeks, and jaws.

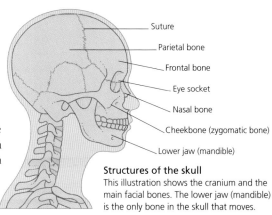

Suture

Parietal bone

Frontal bone

Eye socket

Nasal bone

Cheekbone (zygomatic bone)

Lower jaw (mandible)

Structures of the skull
This illustration shows the cranium and the main facial bones. The lower jaw (mandible) is the only bone in the skull that moves.

BONES, MUSCLES, AND JOINTS

The bones

Bone is a living tissue containing large amounts of calcium and phosphorus; these minerals make it hard, rigid, and strong. Bones can be long, short, or flat. From birth to early adulthood, bones grow by continually laying down calcium on the outside. Bones are also able to generate new tissue after an injury such as a fracture.

Age and certain diseases can weaken bones, making them brittle and susceptible to breaking or crumbling, either under stress or spontaneously. Inherited problems, or bone disorders such as rickets, cancer, and infections, can cause bones to become distorted and weakened. Damage to the bones during adolescence can shorten a bone or impair movement. In older people, a disorder called osteoporosis can cause the bones to lose density, making them brittle and prone to fractures.

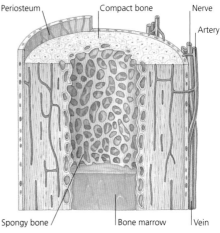

Periosteum   Compact bone   Nerve   Artery
Spongy bone   Bone marrow   Vein

Parts of a bone
Each bone is covered by a membrane (periosteum), which contains nerves and blood vessels. Under this membrane is a layer of compact, dense bone; at the core is spongy bone. In some bones, there is a cavity at the center containing soft tissue called bone marrow.

The muscles

Muscles cause parts of the body to move. Skeletal (voluntary) muscles control movement and posture. They are attached to bones by bands of strong, fibrous tissue (tendons), and many operate in groups. As one group of muscles contracts, its paired group relaxes. Smooth (involuntary) muscles operate the internal organs, such as the heart, and work constantly, even while we sleep. They are controlled by the autonomic nervous system (p.177).

Straightening the arm
The triceps muscle, at the back of the upper arm, shortens (contracts) to pull down the bones of the forearm. The biceps muscle, at the front of the arm, relaxes.

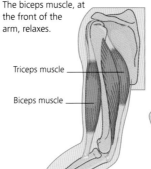

Triceps muscle

Biceps muscle

Bending the arm
The biceps muscle at the front of the arm shortens (contracts), pulling the bones of the forearm upward to bend the arm. At the same time, the triceps muscle (at the back of the arm) relaxes and lengthens.

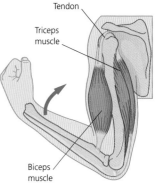

Tendon

Triceps muscle

Biceps muscle

The joints

A joint is a place at which one bone meets another. In a few joints (immovable joints), the bone edges fit firmly together or are fused. Immovable joints are found in the skull and pelvis. Most joints are movable, and there are several types (below). In these joints, the bone ends are joined by fibrous tissue called ligaments, which form a capsule around the joint. The capsule lining (synovial membrane) produces fluid to lubricate the joint; the ends of the bones are also protected by smooth cartilage. Muscles that move the joint are attached to the bones by tendons. The degree and type of movement depends on the way the ends of the bones fit together, the strength of the ligaments, and the arrangement of muscles.

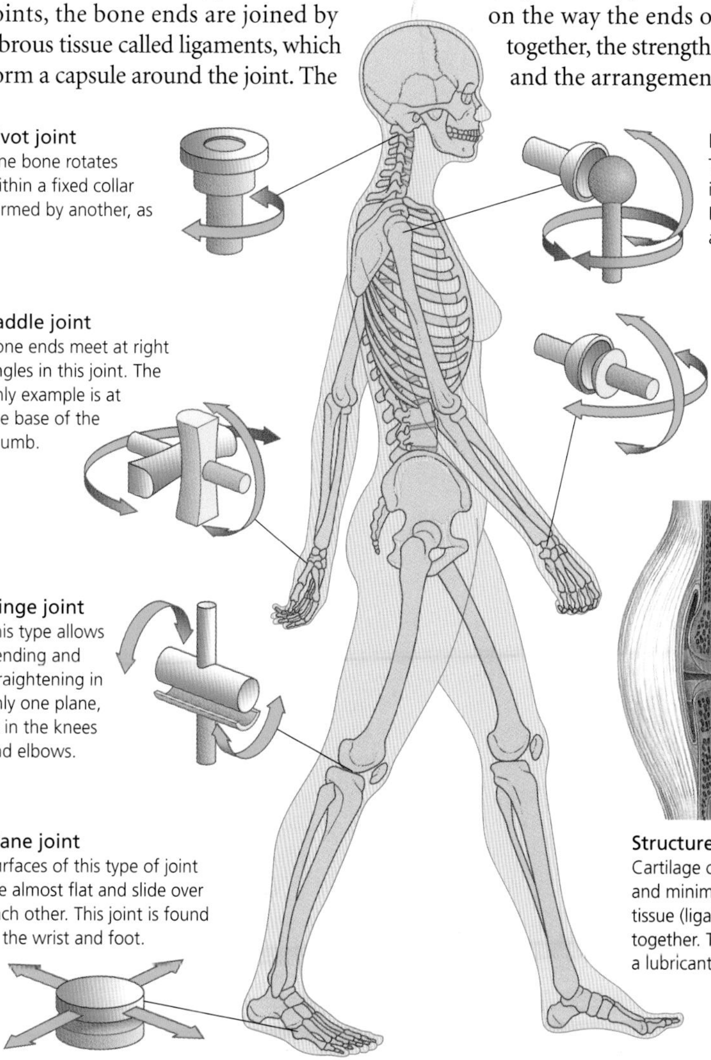

Pivot joint
One bone rotates within a fixed collar formed by another, as

Ball-and-socket joint
This allows movement in all directions. Examples are the hip and shoulder joints.

Saddle joint
Bone ends meet at right angles in this joint. The only example is at the base of the thumb.

Ellipsoidal joint
In this type of joint, movement can occur in most directions. The wrist is an example.

Bone

Synovial membrane

Ligament

Synovial fluid

Cartilage

Hinge joint
This type allows bending and straightening in only one plane, as in the knees and elbows.

Plane joint
Surfaces of this type of joint are almost flat and slide over each other. This joint is found in the wrist and foot.

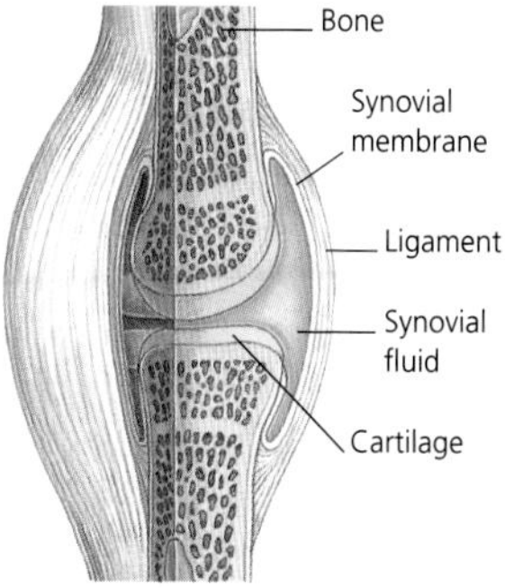

Structures of a movable joint
Cartilage covers the bone ends and minimizes friction. Bands of tissue (ligaments) hold the ends together. The joint is enclosed in a lubricant-filled capsule.

149

FRACTURES

A fracture is a break or crack in a bone. Generally, considerable force is needed to break a bone, unless it is diseased or old. However, bones that are still growing are supple and may split, bend, or crack – hence the term greenstick fracture.

Both direct and indirect force can cause bones to fracture. A bone may break at the point where a heavy blow is received – for example, when struck by a car (direct force). Fractures may also result from a twist or a wrench (indirect force).

STABLE AND UNSTABLE FRACTURES

A fracture may be stable or unstable. In a stable injury, the broken bone ends do not move, either because they are incompletely broken or they are jammed together. Such injuries are common at the wrist, shoulder, ankle, and hip. Usually, they can be gently handled without causing further damage.

In an unstable injury, the broken bone ends can easily move out of position. As a result, there is a risk that they may cause damage to blood vessels, nerves, and organs. Unstable injuries can occur if the bone is completely broken or the ligaments are torn (ruptured). Such injuries should be handled very carefully to avoid further damage.

OPEN AND CLOSED FRACTURES

In an open fracture, one of the broken bone ends may pierce the skin surface, or there may be a wound at the fracture site. An open fracture carries a high risk of becoming infected.

In a closed fracture, the skin above the fracture is intact. However, bones may be displaced (unstable) and cause damage to other internal tissues in the area. If the bone ends pierce organs or major blood vessels, there may be internal bleeding and shock (pp.120–121).

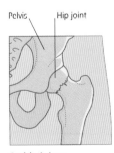

Pelvis   Hip joint   Thigh bone

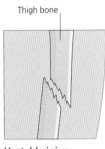

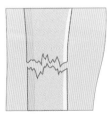

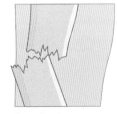

Closed fracture
The skin is not broken, although the bone ends may damage nearby tissues and blood vessels. Internal bleeding is a risk.

Open fracture
Bone is exposed at the surface where it breaks the skin. The injured person is likely to suffer bleeding and shock. Infection is a risk.

Stable injury
Although the bone is fractured, the ends of the injury remain in place. The risk of bleeding or further damage is minimal.

Unstable injury
In this type of fracture, the broken bone ends can easily be displaced by movement or muscle contraction.

► **See also** CRUSH INJURY p.133 ● INTERNAL BLEEDING p.122 ● SHOCK pp.120–121

CLOSED FRACTURE

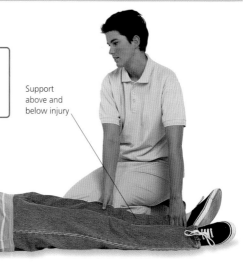

Support above and below injury

1 Advise the victim to keep still. Support the injured part with your hands, or ask a helper to do this, until it is immobilized.

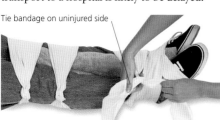

2 For firmer support, bandage the injured part to an unaffected part of the body. Make sure the bandage is tied on the uninjured side. For upper limb fractures, immobilize the arm against the trunk (pp.60–62). For lower limb fractures, bandage the injured leg to the uninjured one if transport to a hospital is likely to be delayed.

Tie bandage on uninjured side

3 Arrange to transport the injured person to a hospital as necessary. Treat for shock (pp.120–121) if necessary by raising the legs. However, do not raise the injured limb if this causes more pain.

4 Check the circulation beyond a bandage (p.51) every 10 minutes. If the circulation is impaired, loosen the bandages.

SPECIAL CASE

APPLYING TRACTION

If a fractured limb is bent or angled so that it cannot be immobilized, gentle traction may be needed to pull it straight. This action overcomes the pull of the muscles and helps reduce pain and bleeding at the fracture site.

To apply traction, pull steadily in the line of the bone until the limb is straight. Pull only in a straight line and hold until the limb is immobilized. Do not persist if traction causes intolerable pain.

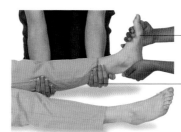

Pull injured limb if necessary

Ask a helper to support the limb

FRACTURES (continued)

OPEN FRACTURE

✚ YOUR AIMS

● To prevent blood loss, movement, and infection at the site of injury.

● To arrange transport to a hospital, with comfortable support during the trip.

SPECIAL CASE

PROTRUDING BONE
If bone is protruding, build up pads of clean, soft, nonfluffy material around the bone, until you can bandage over the pads, to protect it from any pressure.

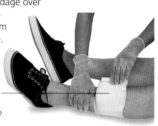

Hold padding in place with roller bandage

1 Put on disposable gloves, if available. Loosely cover the wound with a large, clean, nonfluffy pad or sterile dressing. Apply pressure to control bleeding (p.130), but do not press on a protruding bone.

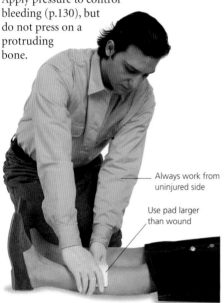

Always work from uninjured side

Use pad larger than wound

2 Carefully place clean padding over and around the dressing.

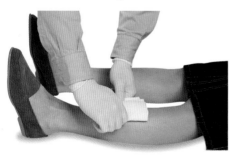

3 Secure the dressing and padding with a bandage. Bandage firmly but not so tightly that it impairs the circulation.

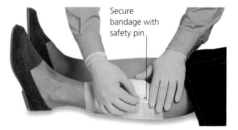

Secure bandage with safety pin

4 Immobilize the injured part as for a closed fracture (p.151), and arrange to transport the victim to a hospital.

5 Treat for shock (pp.120–121) if necessary. Monitor and record vital signs – level of response, pulse, and breathing (pp.42–43). Check the circulation beyond the bandage (p.51) every 10 minutes.

❶ CAUTION

● Do not move the person until the injured part is secured and supported, unless she is in danger.

● Do not allow the person to eat, drink, or smoke, as a general anesthetic may be needed.

● Do not press down directly on a protruding bone end.

DISLOCATED JOINT

This is a joint injury in which the bones are partially or completely pulled out of position. Dislocation can be caused by a strong force wrenching the bone into an abnormal position or by violent muscle contraction. This very painful injury most often affects the shoulder, jaw, or joints in the thumbs or fingers. Dislocations may be associated with torn ligaments (*see* SPRAINS AND STRAINS, pp.154–155), or with damage to the synovial membrane, which lines the joint capsule (p.149).

In some cases, joint dislocation can have serious consequences. If vertebrae in the spine are dislocated, the spinal cord can be damaged. Dislocation of the shoulder or hip may damage the major nerves that supply the limbs and result in paralysis. A severe dislocation of any joint may also fracture the bones involved.

In many cases, it can be difficult to distinguish a dislocation from a closed fracture (p.151). If you are in any doubt, treat the injury as a fracture.

> ● See also FRACTURES pp.150–152 ● SHOCK pp.120–121 ● STRAINS AND SPRAINS pp.154–155

RECOGNITION

There may be:
● "Sickening," severe pain, and difficulty in moving the area.
● Swelling and bruising around the joint.
● Shortening, bending, or twisting of the area.

✚ YOUR AIMS

● To prevent movement at the injury site.
● To arrange transport to a hospital, with comfortable support during the trip.

---

❶ CAUTION

● Do not try to reposition a dislocated bone into its socket because this may cause further injury.
● Do not move the person until the injured part is secured and supported, unless he is in danger.
● Do not allow the person to eat, drink, or smoke, as a general anesthetic may be needed.

---

1 Advise the person to keep still. Support the injured part, in a position of maximum comfort, before you immobilize it.

Ask person to support injured part

2 Immobilize the injured part with padding, bandages, and slings (pp.60–62). For firm support, bandage the injured part to an unaffected part of the body.

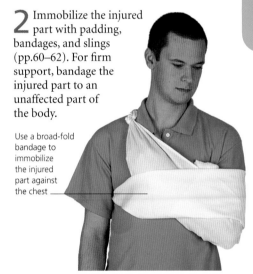

Use a broad-fold bandage to immobilize the injured part against the chest

3 Arrange transport to a hospital. Treat for shock if necessary. Monitor and record vital signs – level of response, pulse, and breathing (pp.42–43).

4 Check the circulation beyond the bandages (p.51) every 10 minutes. If the circulation is impaired, loosen the bandages.

STRAINS AND SPRAINS

The softer structures around bones and joints – the ligaments, muscles, and tendons – may be injured in several ways. Injuries to these soft tissues are commonly called strains and sprains. They occur when the tissues are overstretched and partially or completely torn (ruptured) by violent or sudden movements. For this reason strains and sprains are frequently associated with sporting activities.

MUSCLE AND TENDON INJURY

Muscles and tendons may be strained, ruptured, or bruised. A strain occurs when the muscle is overstretched and may be partially torn. This often occurs at the junction of the muscle and the tendon that joins the muscle to a bone. In a rupture, a muscle or tendon is torn completely; this may occur in the main bulk of the muscle or in the tendon. Deep bruising may be

extensive in parts of the body where there is a large bulk of muscle. Injuries in these areas are usually accompanied by bleeding into the surrounding tissues, which can lead to pain, swelling, and bruising.

Strains and sprains should be treated initially by the "RICE" procedure:
R – *Rest* the injured part.
I – Apply *Ice* or a cold compress.
C – *Compress* the injury.
E – *Elevate* the injured part.
This treatment may be sufficient to relieve the symptoms, but if you are in any doubt as to the severity of the injury, treat it as a fracture (pp.150–152).

LIGAMENT INJURY

One common form of ligament injury is a sprain. This is the tearing of a ligament at or near a joint. It is often due to a sudden or unexpected wrenching motion that pulls the bones in the joint too far apart and tears the surrounding tissues.

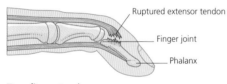

Ruptured extensor tendon

Finger joint

Phalanx

Torn finger tendon
Tendons attach muscle to bone across a joint. If a hard object strikes the end of the finger, the sudden bending may tear the extensor tendon, which passes over the top of the finger joint, from its attachment.

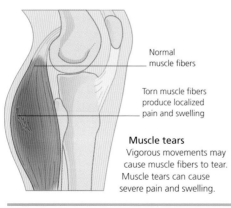

Normal muscle fibers

Torn muscle fibers produce localized pain and swelling

Muscle tears
Vigorous movements may cause muscle fibers to tear. Muscle tears can cause severe pain and swelling.

Sprained ankle
This is due to overstretching or tearing of a ligament – the fibrous cords that connect bones at a joint. In this example, one of the ligaments in the ankle is partially torn.

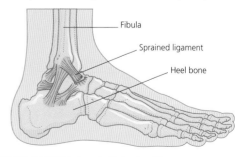

Fibula

Sprained ligament

Heel bone

- To reduce swelling and pain.
- To obtain medical aid if necessary.

1 Advise the person to sit or lie down. Support the injured part in a comfortable position.

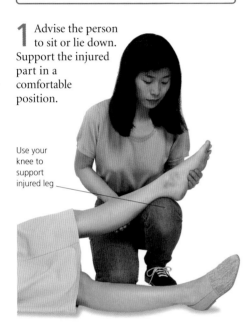

Use your knee to support injured leg

2 If the injury has just happened, cool the area by applying an ice pack or cold compress (p.49). This will help reduce swelling, bruising, and pain.

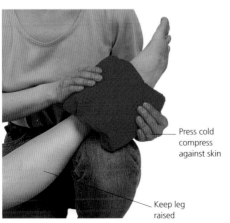

Press cold compress against skin

Keep leg raised

3 Apply gentle, even pressure (compression) to the injured part by surrounding the area with a thick layer of soft padding, such as cotton padding or plastic foam, and securing this layer of padding with a bandage. Check the circulation beyond the bandage (p.51) every 10 minutes.

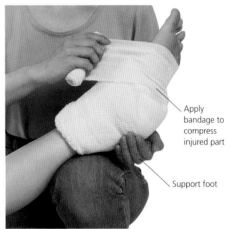

Apply bandage to compress injured part

Support foot

4 Raise (elevate) and support the injured part to reduce the flow of blood to the injury. This action will help minimize bruising in the area.

Keep limb elevated at a comfortable level

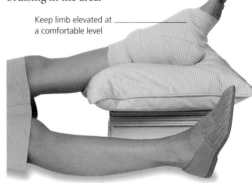

5 If the pain is severe, or the person is unable to use the injured part, take or send the person to a hospital. Otherwise, advise her to rest and to see her doctor if necessary.

MAJOR FACIAL FRACTURE

Fractures of facial bones are usually due to hard impacts. Serious facial fractures may appear horrifying. There may be distortion of the eye sockets, general swelling and bruising, and bleeding from displaced tissues or from the nose and mouth. The main danger with any facial fracture is that blood, saliva, or swollen tissue may obstruct the airway and cause breathing difficulties.

When you are examining someone with a facial injury, check for damage to the skull, brain, or neck. There is a danger that you may misinterpret the symptoms of a facial fracture as a black eye.

RECOGNITION

There may be:
- Pain around affected area; if jaw is affected, difficulty speaking, chewing, or swallowing.
- Difficulty breathing.
- Swelling and distortion of the face.
- Bruising and/or a black eye.

See also CEREBRAL COMPRESSION p.181 ● CONCUSSION p.180 ● LIFE-SAVING PROCEDURES pp.71–102 ● SHOCK pp.120–121 ● SKULL FRACTURE p.182 ● SPINAL INJURY pp.165–167

YOUR AIMS

- To keep the airway open.
- To minimize pain and swelling.
- To arrange urgent transport to a hospital.

WARNING

If the injured person is unconscious, open and clear the airway. Check breathing and be ready to give rescue breaths and chest compressions if necessary (*see* LIFE-SAVING PROCEDURES, pp.71–102).

DIAL 9•1•1 OR CALL EMS.

If the person is breathing, place him in the recovery position (pp.84–85) with his injured side downward to allow any blood or other body fluids to drain away and keep the airway clear. Keep his hand away from his face, and place soft padding under his head. Be aware of the risk of neck (spinal) injury.

CAUTION

Do not apply a bandage to the lower part of the face or lower jaw in case the injured person vomits or has difficulty breathing.

1 DIAL 9•1•1 OR CALL EMS.
If the injured person is conscious, get him to spit out any blood, displaced teeth, or dentures from his mouth.

2 Gently apply a cold compress (p.49) to the face to help reduce pain and limit potential swelling. Treat for shock (p.120–121) if necessary.

3 Regularly monitor and record vital signs – level of response, pulse, and breathing (pp.42–43) – until medical help arrives.

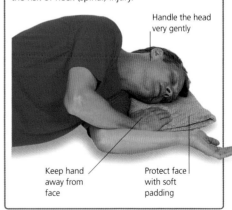

Handle the head very gently

Keep hand away from face

Protect face with soft padding

CHEEKBONE & NOSE FRACTURES

Fractures of the cheekbone and nose are usually the result of deliberate blows to the face. Swollen facial tissues are likely to cause discomfort, and the air passages in the nose may become blocked, making breathing difficult. These injuries should always be examined at a hospital.

RECOGNITION

There may be:
- Pain, swelling, and bruising.
- A wound or bleeding from the nose or mouth.

 See also NOSEBLEED p.139

YOUR AIMS
- To minimize pain and swelling.
- To arrange to transport or send the victim to a hospital.

CAUTION
If there is straw-colored fluid leaking from the nose, treat the person as for a skull fracture (p.182).

1 Gently apply a cold compress (p.49) to the injured area to help reduce pain and limit potential swelling.

2 If the victim has a nosebleed, try to stop the bleeding (p.139). Arrange to transport or send the victim to a hospital.

LOWER JAW INJURY

Jaw fractures are usually the result of direct force, such as a heavy blow to the chin. In some cases, a blow to one side of the jaw may produce indirect force, which causes a fracture on the other side. A fall on to the point of the chin can fracture the jaw on both sides. The lower jaw may also be dislocated by a blow to the face, or is sometimes dislocated by yawning.

If the face is seriously injured, with the jaw fractured in more than one place, treat as for a major facial fracture (opposite).

RECOGNITION

There may be:
- Difficulty speaking, swallowing, and moving the jaw.
- Pain and nausea when moving the jaw.
- Displaced or loose teeth and dribbling.
- Swelling and bruising inside and outside the mouth.

See also KNOCKED-OUT TOOTH p.140
- MAJOR FACIAL FRACTURE opposite.

YOUR AIMS
- To protect the airway.
- To arrange transport to a hospital.

CAUTION
Do not bandage any padding in place in case the person vomits or has difficulty breathing.

1 If the person is not seriously injured, help him sit with his head far forward to allow fluids to drain from his mouth. If loose teeth are spit out, keep them in a glass of milk to send to the hospital with him.

2 Give the person a soft pad to hold firmly against his jaw in order to support it.

3 Take or send him to a hospital, keeping his jaw supported.

FRACTURED COLLARBONE

The collarbones (clavicles) form "struts" between the shoulder blades and the top of the breastbone to help support the arms. It is rare for a collarbone to be broken by a direct blow. Usually, a fracture results from an indirect force transmitted from an impact at the shoulder or passing along the arm, for example from a fall onto an outstretched arm. Collarbone fractures often occur in young people as a result of sports activities. The broken ends of the collarbone may be displaced, causing swelling and bleeding in the surrounding tissues as well as distortion of the shoulder.

RECOGNITION

There may be:
- Pain and tenderness, increased by movement.
- Swelling and deformity of the shoulder.
- Attempts by the injured to relax muscles and relieve pain; she may support the arm at the elbow, and incline the head to the injured side.

▶ **See also** UPPER ARM INJURY p.160

YOUR AIMS
- To immobilize the injured shoulder and arm.
- To arrange transport to a hospital.

1 Help the injured person sit down. Lay the affected arm diagonally across her chest with her fingertips resting against the opposite shoulder. Ask her to support the elbow with her other hand.

3 Gently place some soft padding, such as a small towel or folded clothing, between the arm and the body to make the victim more comfortable.

4 Secure the arm to the chest with a broad-fold bandage (p.57) tied around the chest and over the sling.

Remove any restricting clothing, such as a bra strap, if it is causing discomfort

Injury makes person incline head to injured side

Ask person to support elbow

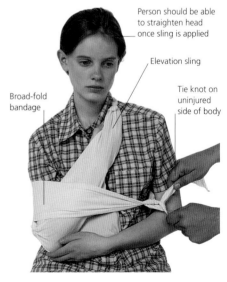

Person should be able to straighten head once sling is applied

Elevation sling

Tie knot on uninjured side of body

Broad-fold bandage

2 Support the arm on the affected side in an elevation sling (p.62).

5 Arrange to take or send the person to a hospital in a sitting position.

SHOULDER INJURY

A fall on to the shoulder or an outstretched arm, or a wrenching force, may pull the head of the arm bone (humerus) out of the joint socket. At the same time, ligaments around the shoulder joint may be torn. This painful injury is called dislocation of the shoulder. Some people have repeated dislocations and may need a strengthening operation on the affected shoulder.

A fall onto the point of the shoulder may damage the ligaments bracing the collarbone at the shoulder. Other shoulder injuries include damage to the joint capsule and to the tendons around the shoulder; these injuries tend to be common in older

RECOGNITION

There may be:

● Severe pain, increased by movement; the pain may make the injured reluctant to move.

● Attempts by the injured to relieve pain by supporting the arm and inclining the head to the injured side.

● A flat, angular look to the shoulder.

people. To treat a shoulder injury, follow the RICE procedure – *rest* the affected part, apply *ice*, *compress*, and *elevate* (p.154).

 See also DISLOCATED JOINT p.153

YOUR AIMS

● To support and immobilize the injured limb.
● To arrange transport to a hospital.

CAUTION

● Do not attempt to replace a dislocated bone into its socket.

● Do not allow the injured person to eat, drink, or smoke because a general anesthetic may be necessary at the hospital.

1 Help the injured to sit down. Gently place the arm on the affected side across her body in the most comfortable position.

2 Place a triangular bandage between the arm and the chest, in preparation for tying an arm sling (p.60).

3 Insert soft padding, such as a folded towel or clothing, between the arm and the chest, inside the bandage.

4 Finish tying the arm sling so that the arm and its padding are well supported.

Site of injury

Keep bandage clear of injury site

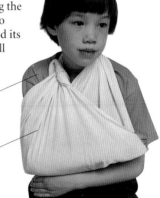

Sling is draped under the arm

Support arm while positioning padding

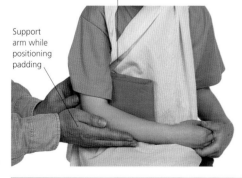

5 Secure the limb to the chest by tying a broad-fold bandage (p.57) around the chest and over the sling.

6 Arrange to take or send the person to a hospital in a sitting position.

UPPER ARM INJURY

The most serious form of upper arm injury is a fracture of the long bone in the upper arm (humerus). The bone may be fractured across the center by a direct blow. However, it is much more common, especially in elderly people, for the arm bone to break at the shoulder end, usually in a fall.

A fracture at the top of the bone is usually a stable injury (p.150), so the broken bone ends stay in place. For this reason, it may not be immediately apparent that the bone is broken, although the arm is likely to be painful. There is a possibility that the injured person will cope with the pain and leave the fracture untreated for some time.

RECOGNITION

There may be:
- Pain, increased by movement.
- Tenderness and deformity over the site of a fracture.
- Rapid swelling.
- Bruising, which may develop more slowly.

▶ **See also** FRACTURES pp.150–152

✚ YOUR AIMS

- To immobilize the arm.
- To arrange transport to a hospital.

1 Ask the injured person to sit down. Gently place the forearm horizontally across her body in the position that is most comfortable. Ask her to support her elbow if possible.

2 Place soft padding beneath the injured arm. Then tie the arm and its padding in an arm sling to support it (p.60).

3 Secure the arm by tying a broad-fold bandage (p.57) around the chest and over the sling. Try to avoid bandaging over the fracture site if possible. Arrange transport to a hospital.

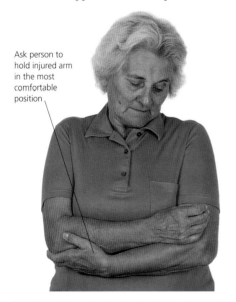

Ask person to hold injured arm in the most comfortable position

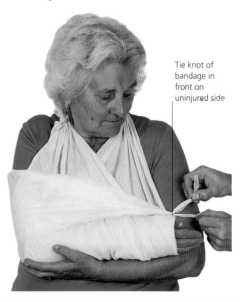

Tie knot of bandage in front on uninjured side

ELBOW INJURY

Fractures or dislocations at the elbow usually result from a fall on to the hand. Children often fracture the upper arm bone just above the elbow. This is an unstable fracture (p.150), and the bone ends may damage blood vessels. Circulation in the arm needs to be checked regularly. In any elbow injury, the elbow will be stiff and difficult to straighten. Never try to force it to bend.

RECOGNITION

There may be:

- Pain, increased by movement.
- Tenderness over the site of a fracture.
- Swelling, bruising, and deformity.
- Fixed elbow.

 See also UPPER ARM INJURY opposite

FOR AN ELBOW THAT CAN BEND

✚ YOUR AIMS

- To immobilize the arm without further injury to the joint.
- To arrange transport to a hospital.

 Treat as for UPPER ARM INJURY opposite

❶ CAUTION

Check the pulse in the affected wrist regularly (p.42). If the pulse is not present, gently straighten the elbow until the pulse returns. Support the arm in this position.

FOR AN ELBOW THAT CANNOT BEND

✚ YOUR AIMS

- To immobilize the arm without further injury to the joint.
- To arrange urgent transport to a hospital.

❶ WARNING

- Do not try to move the injured arm.
- Do not attempt to apply bandages if help is on its way.

1 Help the person lie down. Place padding, such as cushions or towels, around the elbow for comfort and support.

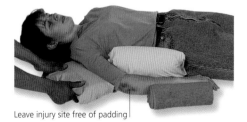

Leave injury site free of padding

2 DIAL 9·1·1 OR CALL EMS.
Check the pulse (p.42) in the injured arm until medical help arrives.

SPECIAL CASE

PREPARING FOR TRANSPORT
Put padding between the injured limb and body. Then use three folded triangular bandages to immobilize the injured limb against the trunk, at the wrist and hips (1), then above (2) and below (3) the elbow.

Tie bandages firmly on the uninjured side

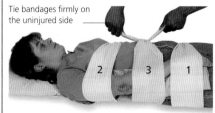

FOREARM AND WRIST INJURIES

The bones of the forearm (radius and ulna) can be fractured by an impact such as a heavy blow or a fall on to an outstretched hand. Since the bones have little fleshy covering, the broken ends may pierce the skin, producing an open fracture (p.152).

At the wrist, the most common form of fracture is a Colles' fracture, which is a break at the end of the radius. This injury often occurs in older women. In a young adult, a fall may break one of the small wrist bones (carpals).

The wrist joint is rarely dislocated but is often sprained. It can be difficult to

distinguish between a sprain and a fracture, especially if the tiny scaphoid bone (at the base of the thumb) is injured.

▶ See also DISLOCATED JOINT p.153
- FRACTURES pp.150–152

1 Ask the injured person to sit down. Gently steady and support the injured forearm by placing it across his body. Expose and treat any wound that you find, wearing disposable gloves if available.

2 Place a triangular bandage between the chest and the injured arm, as for an arm sling (p.60). Surround the forearm in soft padding, such as a small towel or a thick layer of cotton padding.

3 Fasten the arm sling around the arm and its padding using a square knot (p.58). Tie the knot at the hollow of the collarbone on the injured side.

4 If the journey to a hospital is likely to be prolonged, secure the arm to the body by tying a broad-fold bandage (p.57) over the sling. Position the bandage close to the elbow. Then arrange transport to a hospital.

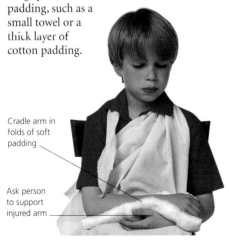

Cradle arm in folds of soft padding

Ask person to support injured arm

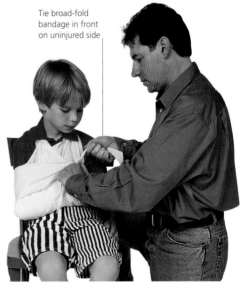

Tie broad-fold bandage in front on uninjured side

HAND AND FINGER INJURIES

The bones and joints in the hand can suffer various types of injury. Minor fractures are usually caused by direct force. The most common type – a fracture of the knuckle between the little finger and the hand – often results from a misdirected punch.

Multiple fractures, affecting many or all of the bones in the hand, are usually caused by crushing injuries. The fractures may be open, with severe bleeding and swelling, needing immediate first-aid treatment.

The joints in the fingers or thumb are sometimes dislocated or sprained as a result of a fall onto the hand (for example, while someone is skiing or ice skating).

RECOGNITION

There may be:
- Pain, increased by movement.
- Swelling, bruising, and deformity.
- In an open fracture, a wound and bleeding.

Always compare the suspected fractured hand with the normal hand because finger fractures result in deformities that may not be immediately obvious.

▶ See also CRUSH INJURY p.133
● DISLOCATED JOINT p.153 ● FRACTURES pp.150–152 ● WOUND TO THE PALM p.141

YOUR AIMS

- To immobilize and elevate the hand.
- To arrange transport to a hospital.

1 If there is any bleeding, put on disposable gloves, if available. Apply a clean, nonfluffy dressing to the wound.

2 Remove any rings before the hand begins to swell, and keep the hand raised to reduce swelling. Protect the injured area by wrapping the hand in folds of soft padding.

3 Gently support the affected arm across the body by applying an elevation sling (p.61).

4 If necessary, secure the arm to the body by tying a broad-fold bandage (p.57) around the chest and over the sling. Then arrange transport to a hospital.

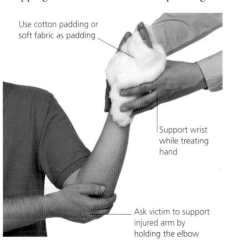

Use cotton padding or soft fabric as padding

Support wrist while treating hand

Ask victim to support injured arm by holding the elbow

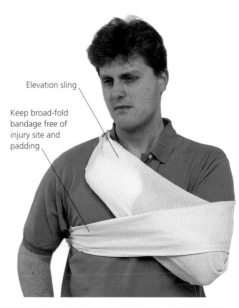

Elevation sling

Keep broad-fold bandage free of injury site and padding

INJURY TO THE RIB CAGE

One or more ribs can be fractured by direct force to the chest from a blow or a fall, or by a crush injury (p.133). If there is an open wound over the fracture, or if a fractured rib pierces a lung, the victim's breathing may be seriously impaired.

An injury to the chest can cause an area of fractured ribs to become detached from the rest of the chest wall, producing a "flail chest" injury. The detached area moves in when the victim breathes in, and out as he breathes out. This "paradoxical" breathing causes severe respiratory difficulties.

Fractures of the lower ribs may injure internal organs such as the liver and spleen and cause internal bleeding (p.122).

RECOGNITION

Depending on the severity, there may be:
- Sharp pain at the site of a fracture.
- Pain on taking a deep breath.
- Shallow breathing.
- An open wound over the fracture, through which you may hear air being "sucked" into the chest cavity.
- "Paradoxical" breathing.
- Features of internal bleeding (p.122) and shock (pp.120–121).

● **See also** ABDOMINAL WOUND p.142
● PENETRATING CHEST WOUND p.112
● SHOCK pp.120–121

YOUR AIMS
- To support the chest wall.
- To arrange transport to a hospital.

⚠ CAUTION
If you need to place the person in the recovery position (pp.84–85), lay him on his injured side. This position allows the lung on the uninjured side to work to its full capacity.

1 For fractured ribs, support the arm on the injured side in an arm sling (p.60) and take or send him to a hospital. If there is a penetrating chest wound, lean the person toward the affected side, and cover and seal the wound along three edges (p.113).

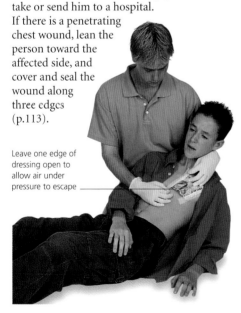

Leave one edge of dressing open to allow air under pressure to escape

2 Help him settle into the most comfortable position inclined toward the injured side. Support the arm on that side in an elevation sling (p.61). **DIAL 9·1·1 OR CALL EMS.**

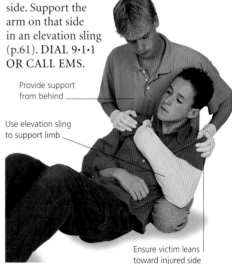

Provide support from behind

Use elevation sling to support limb

Ensure victim leans toward injured side

SPINAL INJURY

Injuries to the spine can involve one or more parts of the back and/or neck: the bones (vertebrae), the disks of tissue that separate the vertebrae, the surrounding muscles and ligaments, or the spinal cord and the nerves that branch off from it.

The most serious risk associated with spinal injury is damage to the spinal cord. Such damage can cause loss of function or sensation below the injured area. The spinal cord or nerve roots can suffer temporary damage if they are pinched by displaced or dislocated disks or by fragments of broken bone. If the cord is partly or completely severed, the damage may be permanent.

RECOGNITION

When the vertebrae are damaged, there may be:
● Pain in the neck or back at the injury site; this may be masked by other, more painful injuries.
● A step, irregularity, or twist in the normal curve of the spine.
● Tenderness in the skin over the spine.

When the spinal cord is damaged, there may be:
● Loss of control over limbs; movement may be weak or absent.
● Loss of sensation, or abnormal sensations such as burning or tingling. The injured person may say that limbs feel stiff, heavy, or clumsy.
● Loss of bladder and/or bowel control.
● Breathing difficulties.

WHEN TO SUSPECT SPINAL INJURY
The most important indicator is the mechanism of the injury. Always suspect spinal injury if abnormal forces have been exerted on the back or neck, and particularly if the injured person complains of any interference with feeling or movement.

If the incident involved violent forward or backward bending, or twisting of the spine, you must assume that the victim has sustained a spinal injury. You must take particular care to avoid unnecessary movement of the head and neck at all times to prevent further injury.

Although spinal cord injury may occur without any damage to the vertebrae, spine fracture vastly increases the risk. The areas that are most vulnerable are the bones in the neck and those in the lower back.

SOME CAUSES OF SPINAL INJURY
Any of the following circumstances should alert you to a possible spinal injury:
● Falling from a height.
● Falling awkwardly while doing gymnastics or trampolining.
● Diving into a shallow pool and hitting the bottom.
● Being thrown from a horse or motorbike.
● Sudden deceleration in a motor vehicle.
● A heavy object falling across the back.
● Injury to the head or the face.

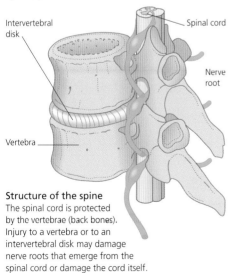

Intervertebral disk
Spinal cord
Nerve root
Vertebra

Structure of the spine
The spinal cord is protected by the vertebrae (back bones). Injury to a vertebra or to an intervertebral disk may damage nerve roots that emerge from the spinal cord or damage the cord itself.

See also HEAD INJURY p.179 ● IMPAIRED CONSCIOUSNESS p.178 ● MECHANICS OF INJURY p.31

Continued on next page

SPINAL INJURY (continued)

FOR A CONSCIOUS VICTIM

➕ YOUR AIMS

- To prevent further injury.
- To arrange urgent transport to a hospital.

❗ CAUTION

- Do not move the person from the position in which you found her unless she is in danger.
- If the person has to be moved, use the log-roll technique (opposite). An orthopedic stretcher (p.70) may be used by trained personnel.

❗ WARNING

If you suspect neck injury, ask a helper to place rolled-up blankets, towels, or items of clothing on either side of the head and neck, while you keep her head in the neutral position.

Continue to support the head and neck throughout until emergency medical services take over.

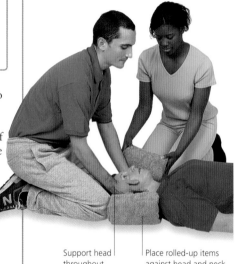

Support head throughout | Place rolled-up items against head and neck

1 Reassure the person and advise her not to move. DIAL 9·1·1 OR CALL EMS.

2 Kneel behind the head. Grasp the sides of the head firmly, with your hands over the ears. Do not completely cover her ears – she should still be able to hear you. Steady and support her head in the neutral head position, in which the head, neck, and spine are aligned. This is the least harmful head position for someone with a suspected spinal injury.

3 Continue to support the head in the neutral position until emergency medical services take over, no matter how long this may be. Get help to monitor and record vital signs – level of response, pulse, and breathing (pp.42–43).

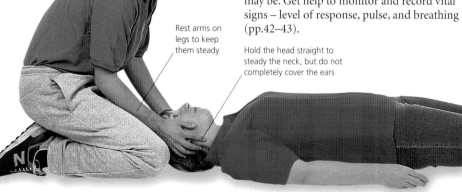

Rest arms on legs to keep them steady

Hold the head straight to steady the neck, but do not completely cover the ears

FOR AN UNCONSCIOUS VICTIM

➕ YOUR AIMS

- To maintain an open airway.
- To resuscitate the injured person if necessary.
- To prevent further spinal damage.
- To arrange urgent transport to a hospital.

1 Kneel behind the person's head. Grasp the sides of her head firmly with your hands over the ears. Steady and support her head in the neutral head position, in which the head, neck, and spine are aligned.

2 If necessary, open the airway using the jaw thrust method. Place your hands on each side of the face with your fingertips at the angles of her jaw. Gently lift the jaw to open the airway. Take care not to tilt the neck.

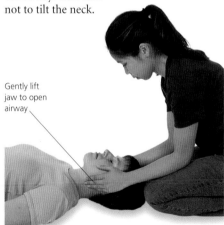

Gently lift jaw to open airway

SPECIAL CASE

LOG-ROLL TECHNIQUE

This technique should be used if you have to turn someone with a spinal injury. Ideally, you need five helpers but the move can be done with three. While you support the injured person's head and neck, ask your helpers to straighten her limbs gently. Then, ensuring that everyone works together, direct your helpers to roll the person. Keep the head, neck, trunk, and toes in a straight line at all times.

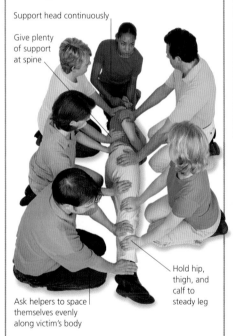

Support head continuously

Give plenty of support at spine

Hold hip, thigh, and calf to steady leg

Ask helpers to space themselves evenly along victim's body

3 Check the victim's breathing. If she is breathing, continue to support her head. Ask a helper to DIAL 9•1•1 OR CALL EMS. Only if you are alone and you need to leave the person to call for help, and if the person is unable to maintain an open airway, should you turn her into the recovery position (pp.84–85) before you leave her. Try to avoid moving the victim.

4 If the person is not breathing, and there are no signs of circulation, give rescue breaths and chest compressions (*see* LIFE-SAVING PROCEDURES, pp.71–102). If you need to turn her, use the log-roll technique (above).

5 Monitor and record vital signs – level of response, pulse, and breathing (pp.42–43) – until medical help arrives.

BACK PAIN

Pain may occur in the spine itself or in the muscles and ligaments around it. In most instances, back pain is the result of a minor problem. However, pain may be a sign of an underlying serious disorder.

CAUSES OF BACK PAIN
The most common cause of back pain is overstretching of the ligaments or muscles as the result of a fall or strenuous activity. Other common causes of back pain are "whiplash" injuries, which lead to neck pain, and pregnancy and menstruation, which often produce pain in the lower part of the back. More serious causes of back pain include a damaged disk in the spine, which may irritate or pinch the spinal cord or nerves, and kidney disease.

See also SPINAL INJURY pp.165–167

RECOGNITION
There may be:
- Dull to severe pain in the back or neck, which is usually increased by movement.
- Pain traveling down any of the limbs, possibly together with tingling and numbness.
- Spasm of the muscles, causing the neck or back to be held rigid or bent.
- Tenderness in the muscles.

Medical help will be necessary if the back pain is accompanied by muscle spasms, fever, headaches, vomiting, nausea, impaired consciousness, incontinence, or any loss of sensation or movement.

YOUR AIMS
- To relieve pain.
- To obtain medical aid if necessary.

CAUTION
If the person has severe back pain, help him lie down, and call a doctor.

1 Advise the person to lie down flat in the most comfortable position for him, either on the ground or on a firm mattress.

2 Advise him to lie as still as possible until the pain eases. Help the victim take any analgesics he has. If the symptoms persist, call his doctor or send him to a hospital.

SPECIAL CASE
NECK PAIN
You can make a temporary neck collar to relieve neck pain using folded newspaper covered by a bandage or scarf. Place the center of the collar at the front of the neck, below the chin. Pass the loose ends around her neck and tie at the front. Ensure that breathing is not impeded.

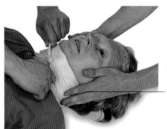

Support head while applying collar

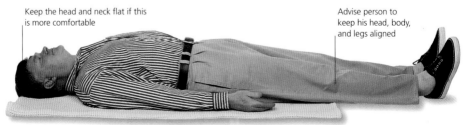

Keep the head and neck flat if this is more comfortable

Advise person to keep his head, body, and legs aligned

FRACTURED PELVIS

Injuries to the pelvis are usually caused by indirect force, such as in a car crash or by crushing. For example, the impact of a car dashboard on a knee can force the head of the thigh bone through the hip socket.

A fracture of the pelvic bones may be complicated by injury to tissues and organs inside the pelvis, such as the bladder and the urinary passages. In addition, internal bleeding associated with the fracture may be severe. This is because there are major organs and blood vessels in the pelvis. Shock often develops as a result of this bleeding, and should be treated promptly.

RECOGNITION

There may be:

- Inability to walk or even stand, although the legs appear uninjured.
- Pain and tenderness in the region of the hip, groin, or back, which increase with movement.
- Blood at the urinary outlet, especially in a man. The injured person may not be able to urinate or may find this painful.
- Signs of shock and internal bleeding.

▶ **See also** INTERNAL BLEEDING p.122
● SHOCK pp.120–121

✚ YOUR AIMS

- To minimize the risk of shock.
- To arrange urgent transport to a hospital.

❶ CAUTION

Do not bandage the legs together if this causes any more pain. In such cases, surround the injured area with soft padding such as clothing or towels.

1 Help the injured person lie down on his back. Keep his legs straight and flat or, if it is more comfortable, help him bend his knees slightly and support them with padding, such as a cushion or folded clothing.

2 Place padding between the bony points of the knees and the ankles. Immobilize the legs by bandaging them together with folded triangular bandages; secure the feet and ankles (1), then the knees (2).

3 DIAL 9·1·1 OR CALL EMS. Treat for shock (pp.120–121).

4 Monitor and record vital signs – level of response, breathing, and pulse (pp.42–43) – until help arrives.

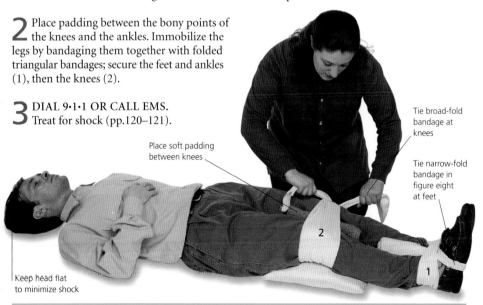

Tie broad-fold bandage at knees

Tie narrow-fold bandage in figure eight at feet

Place soft padding between knees

Keep head flat to minimize shock

HIP AND THIGH INJURIES

The most serious injury of the thigh bone (femur) is a fracture. It takes a considerable force, such as a traffic accident or a fall from a height, to fracture the shaft of the femur. This is a serious injury because the broken bone ends can pierce major blood vessels, causing heavy blood loss, and shock (pp.120–121) may result.

Fracture of the neck of the femur is common in elderly people, particularly women, whose bones become less dense and more brittle with age. This fracture is sometimes a stable injury in which the bone ends are impacted together (see FRACTURES, pp.150–152). The injured person may be able to walk with a fractured neck of femur for some period of time before the fracture is discovered. In the hip joint, the most serious, although much less common, type of injury is dislocation.

▶ **See also** DISLOCATED JOINT p.153
● FRACTURES pp.150–152 ● SHOCK pp.120–121

RECOGNITION

There may be:
● Pain at the site of the injury.
● Inability to walk.
● Signs of shock.
● Shortening of the leg and turning outward of the knee and foot, as powerful muscles move the broken bone ends over each other.

✚ YOUR AIMS

● To immobilize the lower limb.
● To arrange urgent transport to a hospital.

❶ WARNING

● Do not allow the injured person to eat, drink, or smoke, because he may need to have a general anesthetic in hospital.
● Do not raise the person's legs, even if there are signs of shock, because you may cause further internal damage.

1 Help the injured person lie down. If possible, ask a helper to gently steady and support the injured limb.

2 Gently straighten the lower leg if possible. If necessary, apply traction (p.151) at the ankle to help straighten the leg.

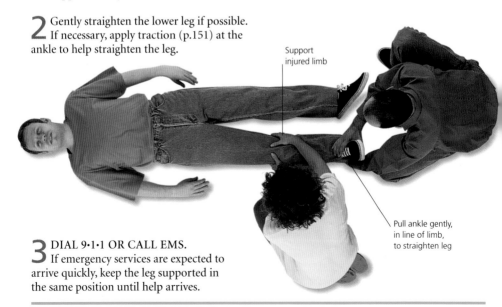

Support injured limb

Pull ankle gently, in line of limb, to straighten leg

3 DIAL 9·1·1 OR CALL EMS. If emergency services are expected to arrive quickly, keep the leg supported in the same position until help arrives.

4 If help is not expected to arrive quickly, immobilize the leg by splinting it to the uninjured one. Gently bring the sound limb alongside the injured one. Position bandages at the ankles and feet (1), then the knees (2). Add bandages above (3) and below (4) the fracture site. Insert soft padding between the legs to prevent the bony parts from rubbing against each other, then tie the bandages on the uninjured side.

5 Take any steps possible to treat the injured for shock (pp.120–121): insulate him from the cold with blankets or clothing, but do not raise his legs.

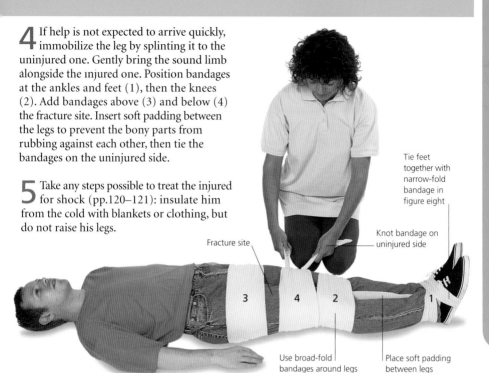

Tie feet together with narrow-fold bandage in figure eight

Knot bandage on uninjured side

Fracture site

Use broad-fold bandages around legs

Place soft padding between legs

SPECIAL CASE

PREPARING FOR TRANSPORT

If the journey to a hospital is likely to be long and rough, more sturdy support for the leg and feet will be needed. Use a specially made malleable splint or a long, solid object, such as a fence post, that will reach from the armpit to the foot.

Place the splint against the injured side. Insert padding between the legs and between the splint and the body. Tie the feet together with a narrow-fold bandage (1). Secure the splint to the body with broad-fold bandages at the chest (2), pelvis (3), knees (4), above and below the fracture site (5 and 6), and at one extra point (7). Do not bandage over the fracture.

Once the person's leg is fully immobilized, she should be moved onto the stretcher using the log-roll technique (p.167).

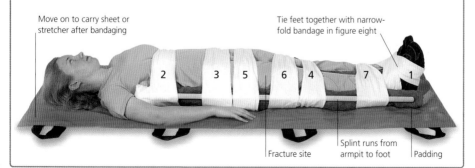

Move on to carry sheet or stretcher after bandaging

Tie feet together with narrow-fold bandage in figure eight

Fracture site

Splint runs from armpit to foot

Padding

KNEE INJURY

The knee is the hinge joint between the thighbone (femur) and shinbone (tibia). It is capable of bending, straightening, and, in the bent position, slight rotation.

The knee joint is supported by strong muscles and ligaments and protected at the front by a disk of bone called the kneecap (patella). The surfaces of the major bones are protected by disks of cartilage. These structures may be damaged by direct blows, violent twists, or sprains. Possible knee injuries include fracture of the patella, sprains, and damage to the cartilage.

A knee injury may make it impossible for the person to bend the joint, and you

See also STRAINS AND SPRAINS pp.154–155

should ensure that the she does not try to walk on the injured leg.

Bleeding or fluid in the knee joint may cause marked swelling around the knee.

RECOGNITION

There may be:
- Pain, spreading from the injury to become deep-seated in the joint.
- If the bent knee has "locked," acute pain on attempting to straighten the leg.
- Rapid swelling at the knee joint.

YOUR AIMS

- To protect the knee in the most comfortable position.
- To arrange transport to a hospital.

WARNING

- Do not attempt to straighten the knee forcibly. Displaced cartilage or internal bleeding may make it impossible to straighten the knee joint safely.
- Do not allow the person to eat, drink, or smoke, because she may need a general anesthetic at the hospital.
- Do not allow the person to walk.

1 Help the person lie down, preferably on a blanket to insulate her from the ground. Place soft padding, such as a pillow, blanket, or coat, under her injured knee to support it in the most comfortable position.

2 Wrap soft padding around the joint. Secure with bandages that extend from midthigh to the middle of the lower leg.

3 Arrange transport to a hospital. The person needs to remain in the treatment position and should therefore be transported in an ambulance.

Use roller bandage to hold padding in place

Support knee with soft padding

LOWER LEG INJURY

Injuries to the lower leg include fractures of the shinbone (tibia) and the splint bone (fibula), and tearing of the soft tissues (muscles, ligaments, and tendons).

Fractures of the tibia are usually due to a heavy blow (for example, from the bumper of a moving vehicle). Since there is little flesh over the tibia, a fracture is more likely to produce a wound. The fibula can be broken by the twisting that sprains an ankle.

> See also STRAINS AND SPRAINS
pp.154–155

RECOGNITION

There may be:
- Localized pain.
- Swelling, bruising, and deformity of the leg.
- An open wound.

YOUR AIMS
- To immobilize the leg.
- To arrange urgent transport to a hospital.

1 Help the person lie down, and carefully steady and support the injured leg. If there is an open wound, gently expose the wound and treat bleeding. Apply padding to protect the injury.

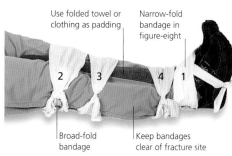

Support leg at knee and ankle

2 DIAL 9·1·1 OR CALL EMS. Support the injured leg with your hands to prevent any movement of the fracture site. Do this until help arrives.

⚠ CAUTION

If the journey to a hospital is likely to be long and rough, place soft padding on the outside of the injured leg, from the knee to the foot. Secure legs with broad-fold bandages as described above.

3 If help is delayed, support the injured leg by splinting it to the other leg. Bring the uninjured limb alongside the injured one and slide bandages under both legs. Position bandages at the feet and ankles (1), then knees (2). Add bandages above (3) and below (4) the fracture. Insert padding between the lower legs. Then tie the bandages firmly, knotting them on the uninjured side.

Use folded towel or clothing as padding

Narrow-fold bandage in figure-eight

2   3   4   1

Broad-fold bandage

Keep bandages clear of fracture site

SPECIAL CASE

SUSPECTED FRACTURE NEAR ANKLE
Place separate bandages above the ankle and around the feet to splint the injured ankle to the uninjured ankle.

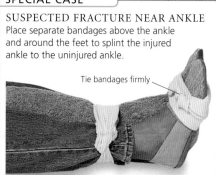

Tie bandages firmly

ANKLE INJURY

If the ankle is broken, treat it as a fracture of the lower leg (p.173). A more common injury is a sprain (p.154), usually caused by a wrench to the ankle. This problem can be treated by the RICE procedure: *rest* the affected part, apply *ice, compress* with bandaging, and *elevate*.

RECOGNITION

- Pain, increased either by movement or by putting weight on the foot.
- Swelling.

 See also STRAINS AND SPRAINS pp.154–155

YOUR AIMS

- To relieve pain and swelling.
- To obtain medical aid if necessary.

CAUTION

If you suspect a broken bone, tell the person not to put weight on the leg. Secure and support the lower leg (p.173), and arrange transport to a hospital.

1 Rest, steady, and support the ankle in the most comfortable position.

2 If the injury has only recently occurred, apply an ice pack or a cold compress (p.49) to the site to reduce swelling.

3 Wrap the ankle in thick padding and bandage firmly. Raise and support the injured limb. Advise the injured to rest the ankle and to see a doctor if pain persists.

FOOT AND TOE INJURIES

Fractures affecting the many small bones of the foot are usually caused by crushing injuries. These fractures are best treated at a hospital. When giving first aid, concentrate on relieving symptoms such as swelling.

RECOGNITION

- Difficulty walking.
- Stiffness of movement.
- Bruising and swelling.

YOUR AIMS

- To minimize swelling.
- To arrange transport to a hospital.

1 Quickly raise and support the foot to reduce blood flow to the area, which will minimize swelling.

2 Apply an ice pack or cold compress (p.49). This will also help relieve swelling.

3 Arrange to take or send the person to a hospital. If she is not being transported by ambulance, try to ensure that the foot remains elevated during travel.

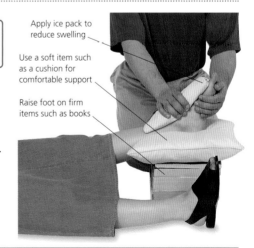

Apply ice pack to reduce swelling

Use a soft item such as a cushion for comfortable support

Raise foot on firm items such as books

8

THE NERVOUS SYSTEM is the most complex system in the body. Its control center, the brain, is the source of consciousness, thought, speech, and memory. It also receives and interprets sensory information, which is carried by the nerves, and controls other body systems. When we are fully conscious, we are awake, alert, and aware of our surroundings. However, if consciousness is impaired, even survival mechanisms, such as the cough reflex to keep the airway clear, may not function.

TREATMENT PRIORITIES
Because many of the problems described in this chapter can produce impaired consciousness, they need immediate attention. Your priority as a first aider is to monitor and maintain the vital functions of breathing and circulation.

CONTENTS

The nervous system 176

Impaired consciousness 178

Head injury 179

Concussion 180

Cerebral compression 181

Skull fracture 182

Stroke 183

Seizures in adults 184

Absence seizures 185

Seizures in children 186

Meningitis 187

Headache 188

Migraine 188

✚ FIRST-AID PRIORITIES

- Assess the victim's condition.
- Comfort and reassure the victim.
- Maintain an open airway, check breathing, and be prepared to resuscitate if necessary.
- Protect the victim from harm.
- Look for and treat any injuries associated with the condition.
- Obtain medical aid if necessary. Dial 9•1•1 or call EMS if you suspect a serious illness or injury.

THE NERVOUS SYSTEM

This is the body's information-gathering, storage, and control system. It consists of a central processing unit – the brain – and a complex network of nerve cells and fibers.

There are two main parts to the nervous system: the central nervous system, consisting of the brain and spinal cord, and the peripheral nervous system, which consists of all the nerves connecting the brain and the spinal cord to the rest of the body. In addition, the autonomic (involuntary) nervous system controls body functions such as digestion, heart rate, and breathing. The central nervous system receives and analyzes information from all parts of the body. The nerves carry messages, in the form of high-speed electrical impulses, between the brain and the rest of the nervous system.

Structure of the nervous system
The system consists of the brain, spinal cord, and a dense network of nerves that carry electrical impulses between the brain and the rest of the body.

Spinal cord carries nerve impulses between brain and rest of body

Spinal nerves (31 pairs) emerge from spinal cord and extend through vertebral column

Brain

Cranial nerves (12 pairs) extend directly from underside of the brain; most supply the head, face, neck, and shoulders

Vagus nerve, longest of the cranial nerves, supplies organs in chest and abdomen; it controls heart rate

Radial nerve controls muscles that straighten elbow and fingers

Sciatic nerve serves hip and hamstring muscles

Nerve fiber

Myelin sheath

Nerve fascicle

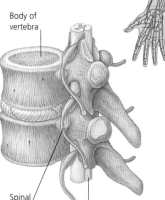

Body of vertebra

Spinal nerve

Spinal cord

Spinal cord protection
The spinal cord is protected by the bony vertebral (spinal) column. Nerves branching from the cord emerge between adjacent vertebrae.

Tibial nerve supplies calf muscles

Cross section of nerve
Each nerve is made up of bundles of nerve fibers called fascicles. A protective fatty substance called myelin surrounds and insulates larger nerve fibers.

Central nervous system

The brain and the spinal cord make up the central nervous system (CNS). This system contains billions of interconnected nerve cells (neurons) and is enclosed by three membranes (meninges). A clear fluid called cerebrospinal fluid flows around the brain and spinal cord. It functions as a shock absorber, provides oxygen and nutrients, and removes waste products.

The brain has three main structures: the cerebrum, which is concerned with thought, sensation, and conscious movement; the cerebellum, which coordinates movement, balance, and posture; and the brain stem, which controls basic functions such as breathing.

The main function of the spinal cord is to convey signals between the brain and the peripheral nervous system (below).

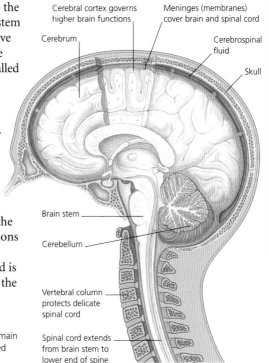

Cerebral cortex governs higher brain functions

Meninges (membranes) cover brain and spinal cord

Cerebrum

Cerebrospinal fluid

Skull

Brain stem

Cerebellum

Vertebral column protects delicate spinal cord

Spinal cord extends from brain stem to lower end of spine

Brain structure
The brain is enclosed within the skull. It has three main parts: the cerebrum, which has an outer layer called the cortex; the cerebellum; and the brain stem.

Peripheral nervous system

This part of the nervous system consists of two sets of paired nerves – the cranial and spinal nerves – connecting the CNS to the body. The cranial nerves emerge in 12 pairs from the underside of the brain. The 31 pairs of spinal nerves branch off at intervals from the spinal cord, passing into the rest of the body. Nerves comprise bundles of nerve fibers that can relay both incoming (sensory) and outgoing (motor) signals.

Autonomic nervous system

Some of the cranial nerves, and several small spinal nerves, work as the autonomic nervous system. This system is concerned with vital body functions such as heart rate and breathing. The system's two parts, the sympathetic and parasympathetic systems, counterbalance each other. The sympathetic system prepares the body for action by releasing hormones that raise the heart rate and reduce the blood flow to the skin and intestines. The parasympathetic system releases hormones with a calming effect.

IMPAIRED CONSCIOUSNESS

There is no absolute dividing line between consciousness and unconsciousness. People may be fully aware and awake (conscious), completely unresponsive to any stimulus (unconscious), or at any level between these two extremes. For example, someone may be "groggy" or respond only to loud sounds or to pain. Impaired consciousness is the term used when a person is anything less than fully conscious.

AVPU CODE

You can assess consciousness by checking the level of response to stimuli using the AVPU code.

A – Is the person *Alert*? Does he open his eyes and respond to questions?

V – Does the person respond to *Voice*? Does he answer simple questions and obey commands?

P – Does the person respond to *Pain*? Does he open his eyes or move if pinched?

U – Is the person *Unresponsive* to any stimulus?

You should record your findings on the observation charts (p.280).

CAUSES OF IMPAIRED CONSCIOUSNESS

The main causes of impaired consciousness are structural damage to the brain or a lack of nutrients – oxygen and glucose (sugar) – reaching the brain. Structural damage may occur with a head injury or a brain tumor. Low oxygen (hypoxia) or low blood sugar (hypoglyemia) may occur with any condition that reduces blood flow to the brain, such as stroke, shock, fainting, or a heart attack. It can also occur if blood flow is normal but there is insufficient oxygen or glucose in the blood – for example, due to poisoning, or a chemical imbalance caused by diabetes mellitus. Epilepsy can produce impaired consciousness due to abnormal electrical activity in the brain.

> ▶ See also DIABETES MELLITUS p.240
> ● HEAD INJURY opposite ● HYPOXIA p.106
> ● LIFE-SAVING PROCEDURES pp.71–102
> ● SPINAL INJURY pp.165–167

✚ YOUR AIMS

● To maintain an open airway.
● To assess and record level of response
● To arrange urgent transport to a hospital if necessary.

❶ WARNING

● If you suspect that someone may have a neck (spinal) injury, handle his head very carefully. To open the airway, use the jaw thrust method (p.167). kneel behind the head and place your hands on each side of the face, with your fingertips at the angles of the jaw; gently lift the jaw.
● Do not move the person unnecessarily.

1 Perform a quick check of consciousness by checking the level of response using the AVPU code (above). If the person is "groggy" but responds to sound or pain, support him in a comfortable resting position and watch for any change in his level of response.

2 If the person is unconscious, follow the procedure for treating an unconscious victim (*see* LIFE-SAVING PROCEDURES, pp.71–102).
DIAL 9•1•1 OR CALL EMS.

3 While waiting for medical help to arrive, monitor and record vital signs – level of response, pulse, and breathing (pp.42–43). Treat any associated injuries.

HEAD INJURY

All head injuries are potentially serious and require proper assessment because they can result in impaired consciousness (opposite). Injuries may be associated with damage to the brain tissue or to blood vessels inside the skull, or with a skull fracture.

A head injury may produce concussion, which is a brief period of unconsciousness followed by complete recovery. Some head injuries may produce compression of the brain (cerebral compression), which is life-threatening. It is therefore important to be able to recognize possible signs of cerebral compression (below) – in particular, a deteriorating level of response.

A head wound should alert you to the risk of deeper, underlying damage, such as a skull fracture, which may be serious. Bleeding inside the skull may also occur and lead to compression. Clear fluid or watery blood leaking from the ear or nose are signs of serious injury.

Any person with an injury to the head should be assumed to have a neck (spinal) injury as well and be treated accordingly (*see* SPINAL INJURY, p.165–167).

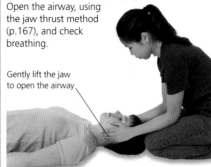

① WARNING

Handle the person's head very carefully because of the risk of neck (spinal) injury. Open the airway, using the jaw thrust method (p.167), and check breathing.

Gently lift the jaw to open the airway

If the position in which the person was found prevents maintenance of an open airway or you fail to open it using the jaw thrust, place her in the recovery position (pp.84–85). If you have helpers, use the "log-roll" technique (p.167).

⊙ See also CEREBRAL COMPRESSION p.181 ● CONCUSSION p.180 ● LIFE-SAVING PROCEDURES pp.71–102 ● SCALP AND HEAD WOUNDS p.137 ● SKULL FRACTURE p.182 ● SPINAL INJURY pp.165–167

RECOGNITION

Concussion	Cerebral compression	Skull fracture
● Brief period of impaired consciousness following a blow to the head.	● Deteriorating level of response – may progress to unconsciousness.	● Wound or bruise on the head.
There may also be:	*There may also be:*	● Soft area or depression on the scalp.
● Dizziness or nausea on recovery.	● History of recent head injury.	● Bruising/swelling behind one ear.
● Loss of memory of any events that occurred at the time of, or immediately preceding, the injury.	● Intense headache.	● Bruising around one or both eyes.
	● Noisy breathing, becoming slow.	● Loss of clear fluid or watery blood from the nose or an ear.
	● Slow, yet full and strong, pulse.	● Blood in the white of the eye.
● Mild, generalized headache.	● Unequal pupil size.	● Distortion or lack of symmetry of the head or face.
	● Weakness and/or paralysis down one side of the face and/or body.	● Deteriorating level of response – may progress to unconsciousness.
	● High temperature; flushed face.	
	● Drowsiness.	
	● Noticeable change in personality or behavior, such as irritability.	

CONCUSSION

The brain is free to move a little within the skull, so it can be "shaken" by a blow to the head. This shaking of the brain is called concussion. Among the more common causes of concussion are traffic accidents, sports injuries, falls, and blows received in fights.

Concussion produces widespread but temporary disturbance of normal brain activity. However, it is not usually associated with any lasting damage to the brain. A person will suffer impaired consciousness, but this only lasts for a short time (usually only a few minutes) and is followed by a full recovery. By definition, concussion can only be confidently diagnosed once the injured person has completely recovered.

Someone who has been concussed should be monitored and advised to seek a medical evaluation.

▶ **See also** CEREBRAL COMPRESSION opposite ● LIFE-SAVING PROCEDURES pp.71–102 ● SPINAL INJURY pp.165–167

opposite ● LIFE-SAVING PROCEDURES pp.71–102 ● SPINAL INJURY pp.165–167

RECOGNITION

● Brief period of impaired consciousness following a blow to the head.

There may also be:
● Dizziness or nausea on recovery.
● Loss of memory of events at the time of, or immediately preceding, the injury.
● Mild, generalized headache.

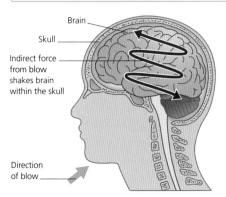

Mechanism of concussion
Concussion usually occurs as a result of a blow to the head. This "shakes" the brain within the skull, resulting in a temporary disturbance of brain function.

✚ YOUR AIMS

● To ensure the victim recovers fully and safely.
● To place the victim in the care of a responsible person.
● To obtain medical aid if necessary.

❶ WARNING

If the injured person does not recover fully, OR if there is a deteriorating level of response after an initial recovery

DIAL 9•1•1 OR CALL EMS.

❶ CAUTION

Anyone who has had a head injury should also be treated for a neck injury
(*see* SPINAL INJURY, pp.165–167).

1 Treat the victim as for impaired consciousness (p.178).

2 Monitor and record vital signs – level of response, pulse, and breathing (pp.42–43). Even if the victim appears to recover fully, watch him for subsequent deterioration in his level of response.

3 When the victim has recovered, place him in the care of a responsible person. If a victim has been injured on the sports field, never allow him to continue playing without first obtaining medical advice.

4 Advise the victim to go to a hospital if he later develops headache, nausea, vomiting, or excessive sleepiness following a blow to the head.

CEREBRAL COMPRESSION

Compression of the brain – a condition called cerebral compression – is very serious and almost invariably requires surgery. Cerebral compression occurs when there is a buildup of pressure on the brain. This pressure may be due to one of several different causes, such as an accumulation of blood within the skull or swelling of injured brain tissues.

Cerebral compression is usually caused by a head injury. However, it can also be due to other causes, such as a stroke (p.183), infection, or a brain tumor. The condition may develop immediately after a head injury, or it may appear a few hours or even days later. For this reason, you should always try to find out whether the person has a recent history of a head injury.

> ▶ **See also** LIFE-SAVING PROCEDURES pp.71–102 ● SPINAL INJURY pp.165–167

See also LIFE-SAVING PROCEDURES pp.71–102 ● SPINAL INJURY pp.165–167

Compression caused by bleeding
Bleeding may occur within the skull following a head injury or a disorder such as a stroke. The escaped blood may put pressure on tissues in the brain.

RECOGNITION

● Deteriorating level of response – person may become unconscious.

There may also be:
● History of a recent head injury.
● Intense headache.
● Noisy breathing, becoming slow.
● Slow, yet full and strong pulse.
● Unequal pupil size.
● Weakness and/or paralysis down one side of the face or body.
● High temperature; flushed face.
● Drowsiness.
● Noticeable change in personality or behavior, such as irritability or disorientation.

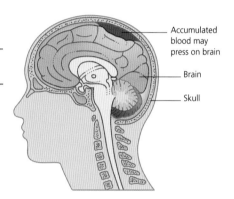

Accumulated blood may press on brain

Brain

Skull

+ YOUR AIM

● To arrange urgent transport of the injured person to a hospital.

ⓘ WARNING

If the person is unconscious, open the airway using the jaw thrust method (p.167) and check breathing; be prepared to give rescue breaths and chest compressions if necessary (*see* LIFE-SAVING PROCEDURES, pp.71–102).

DIAL 9·1·1 OR CALL EMS.

If the person is breathing, try to maintain the airway in the position in which he was found

1 DIAL 9·1·1 OR CALL EMS.
If the person is conscious, keep him supported in a comfortable resting position and reassure him.

2 Regularly monitor and record the vital signs – level of response, pulse, and breathing (pp.42–43) – until medical help arrives.

ⓘ CAUTION

Do not allow the person to eat, drink, or smoke because a general anesthetic may need to be given at the hospital.

SKULL FRACTURE

If someone has a head wound, be alert for a possible skull fracture. An affected person may have impaired consciousness.

A skull fracture is serious because there is a risk that the brain may be damaged either directly by fractured bone from the skull or by bleeding inside the skull. Clear fluid (cerebrospinal fluid) or watery blood leaking from the ear or nose are signs of serious injury.

You should suspect a skull fracture in anyone who has received a head injury resulting in impaired consciousness. Bear in mind that someone with a possible skull fracture may also have a neck (spinal) injury and should be treated accordingly (*see* SPINAL INJURY, pp.165–167).

RECOGNITION

- Wound or bruise on the head.
- Soft area or depression on the scalp.
- Bruising or swelling behind one ear.
- Bruising around one or both eyes.
- Clear fluid or watery blood coming from the nose or an ear.
- Blood in the white of the eye.
- Distortion or lack of symmetry of the head or face.
- Progressive deterioration in the level of response.

See also LIFE-SAVING PROCEDURES pp.71–102 ● SCALP AND HEAD WOUNDS p.137 ● SPINAL INJURY pp.165–167

YOUR AIMS

- To maintain an open airway.
- To arrange urgent transport of the injured person to a hospital.

WARNING

If the person is unconscious, open the airway using the jaw thrust method (p.167) and check breathing; be prepared to give rescue breaths and chest compressions if needed (see LIFE-SAVING PROCEDURES, pp.71–102).

DIAL 9•1•1 OR CALL EMS.

1 If the injured person is conscious, help her lie down. Do not turn the head in case there is a neck injury.

2 Control any bleeding from the scalp by applying pressure around the wound. Look for and treat any other injuries. DIAL 9•1•1 OR CALL EMS.

3 If there is discharge from an ear, cover the ear with a sterile dressing or clean pad, lightly secured with a bandage (*see* BLEEDING FROM THE EAR, p.138). Do not plug the ear.

4 Monitor and record vital signs – level of response, pulse, and breathing (pp.42–43) – until medical help arrives.

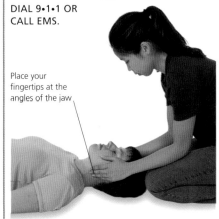

Place your fingertips at the angles of the jaw

If the position in which the person was found prevents maintenance of an open airway or you fail to open it using the jaw thrust, place her in the recovery position (pp.84–85). If you have helpers, use the "log-roll" technique (p.167).

STROKE

The term "stroke" describes a condition in which the blood supply to part of the brain is suddenly and seriously impaired by a blood clot or a ruptured blood vessel. It is vitally important that the victim is taken to a hospital quickly. If the stroke is due to a clot, drugs may then be given to limit the extent of the damage to the brain tissue and promote recovery.

Strokes occur more commonly in later life and in people who suffer from high blood pressure or some other circulatory disorder. The effect of a stroke depends on how much, and which part, of the brain is affected. In some cases, the condition can be fatal; however, many people make a complete recovery from a stroke.

RECOGNITION

There may be:
- Problems with speech and swallowing.
- If asked to show teeth, only one side of mouth will move or movement will be uneven.
- Loss of strength or movement in the limbs.
- Sudden, severe headache.
- Confused, emotional mental state that could be mistaken for drunkenness.
- Sudden or gradual loss of consciousness.

▶ See also LIFE-SAVING PROCEDURES pp.71–102

YOUR AIMS

- To maintain an open airway.
- To arrange urgent transport of the victim to a hospital.

WARNING

If the victim is unconscious, open the airway and check breathing; be prepared to give rescue breaths and chest compressions if necessary (see LIFE-SAVING PROCEDURES, pp.71–102).

If she is breathing, place her in the recovery position (pp.184–185).

DIAL 9·1·1 OR CALL EMS.

Monitor and record vital signs – level of response, pulse, and breathing (pp.42–43) – until medical help arrives.

CAUTION

Do not give the victim anything to eat or drink because a stroke may make it difficult to swallow.

1 If the victim is conscious, help her lie down with her head and shoulders slightly raised and supported. Incline her head to the affected side, and place a towel on her shoulder to absorb any dribbling.
DIAL 9·1·1 OR CALL EMS.

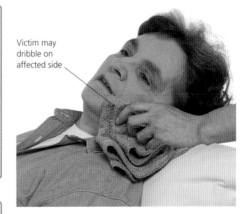

Victim may dribble on affected side

2 Loosen any clothing that might impair breathing. Continue to reassure her. Monitor and record vital signs – level of response, pulse, and breathing (pp.42–43) – until medical help arrives.

SEIZURES IN ADULTS

A seizure – also called a convulsion – consists of involuntary contractions of many of the muscles in the body. The condition is due to a disturbance in the electrical activity of the brain. Seizures usually result in loss or impairment of consciousness. The most common cause is epilepsy. Other causes include head injury, some brain-damaging diseases, shortage of oxygen or glucose in the brain, and the intake of certain poisons, including alcohol.

Epileptic seizures are due to recurrent, major disturbances of brain activity. These seizures can be sudden and dramatic. Just before a seizure, a person may have a brief warning period (aura) with, for example, a strange feeling or a special smell or taste.

No matter what the cause of the seizure, care must always include maintaining an open, clear airway and monitoring the vital signs – level of response, pulse, and breathing. You will also need to protect the person from further harm during a seizure and arrange appropriate aftercare once she has recovered.

RECOGNITION

Generally:
- Sudden unconsciousness.
- Rigidity and arching of the back.
- Convulsive movements.

In epilepsy the following sequence is common:
- The person suddenly falls unconscious, often letting out a cry.
- She becomes rigid, arching her back.
- Breathing may cease. The lips may show a gray–blue tinge (cyanosis) and the face and neck may become red and puffy.
- Convulsive movements begin. The jaw may be clenched and breathing may be noisy. Saliva may appear at the mouth and may be blood-stained if the lips or tongue have been bitten. There may be loss of bladder or bowel control.
- Muscles relax and breathing becomes normal; the person recovers consciousness, usually within a few minutes. She may feel dazed, or act strangely. She may be unaware of her actions.
- After a seizure, the person may feel tired and fall into a deep sleep.

▶ **See also** IMPAIRED CONSCIOUSNESS p.178
● LIFE-SAVING PROCEDURES pp.71–102

✚ YOUR AIMS

- To protect the person from injury.
- To give care when consciousness is regained.
- To arrange transport of the person to a hospital if necessary.

1 If you see the person falling, try to ease her fall (*see* CONTROLLING A FALL, p.66). Make space around her; ask bystanders to move away. Remove potentially dangerous items, such as hot drinks and sharp objects. Note the time when the seizure started.

2 If possible, protect the head by placing soft padding underneath it. Loosen clothing around her neck.

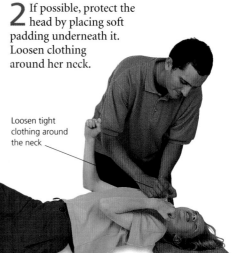

Loosen tight clothing around the neck

3 When the seizure has ceased, open the airway and check breathing; be ready to give rescue breaths and chest compressions if necessary (*see* LIFE-SAVING PROCEDURES, pp.71–102).

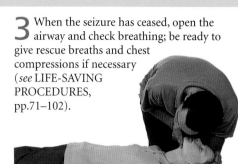

4 If she is breathing, place her in the recovery position. Monitor and record vital signs – level of response, pulse, and breathing (pp.42–43). Note the duration of the seizure.

ABSENCE SEIZURES

Some people experience a mild form of epilepsy, with small seizures during which they appear distant and unaware of their surroundings. These episodes, called "absence seizures," tend to affect children more than adults. There is unlikely to be any convulsive movement or loss of consciousness, but a full seizure may follow.

RECOGNITION

● Sudden "switching off"; the person may stare blankly ahead.

● Slight or localized twitching or jerking of the lips, eyelids, head, or limbs.

● Odd "automatic" movements, such as lip-smacking, chewing, or making noises.

✚ YOUR AIM

● To protect the person until she is fully recovered.

1 Help the person sit down in a quiet place. Make space around her; remove any potentially dangerous items, such as hot drinks and sharp objects.

2 Talk to the person in a calm and reassuring way. Do not pester her with questions. Stay with her until you are sure that she is fully recovered.

3 If the victim does not recognize or have any awareness of her condition, advise her to consult her own doctor as soon as possible.

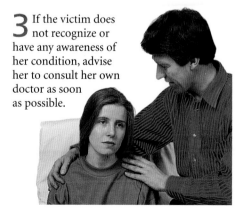

SEIZURES IN CHILDREN

In young children, seizures – sometimes called convulsions – are most often the result of a raised body temperature associated with a throat or ear infection or other infectious disease. This type of seizure is known as a febrile convulsion and is a reaction of the brain to high body temperature. Epilepsy is another possible cause of seizures in infants and children.

Although seizures can be alarming, they are rarely dangerous if properly dealt with. For safety's sake, however, the child should be seen at a hospital to rule out any serious underlying condition.

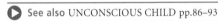

RECOGNITION
● Violent muscle twitching, with clenched fists and an arched back.

There may also be:
● Obvious signs of fever: hot, flushed skin, and perhaps sweating.
● Twitching of the face with squinting, fixed, or upturned eyes.
● Breath-holding, with red, "puffy" face and neck or drooling at the mouth.
● Loss or impairment of consciousness.

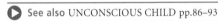

▶ **See also** UNCONSCIOUS CHILD pp.86–93

✚ YOUR AIMS
● To protect the child from injury.
● To cool the child.
● To reassure the parents or caregiver.
● To arrange transport to a hospital.

1 Position pillows or soft padding around the child so that even violent movement will not result in injury.

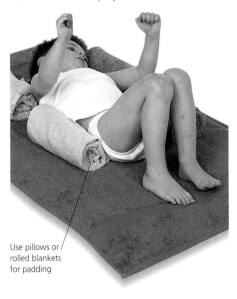

Use pillows or rolled blankets for padding

2 Remove any covering or clothes. Ensure a good supply of cool, fresh air (but be careful not to overcool the child).

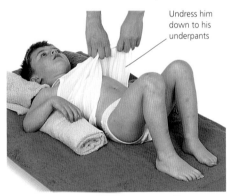

Undress him down to his underpants

3 Sponge the child's skin with tepid water to help cooling; start at his forehead and work down his body.

4 Once the seizures have stopped, keep the airway open by placing the child in the recovery position (pp.92–93) if necessary. DIAL 9·1·1 OR CALL EMS.

5 Reassure the child and parents or caregiver. Monitor and record vital signs – level of response, pulse, and breathing (pp.42–43) – until medical help arrives.

MENINGITIS

This is a disorder in which the linings that surround the brain and the spinal cord (the meninges) become inflamed. It can be caused by several different types of bacteria or viruses, and can occur at any age.

Meningitis is potentially a very serious illness, and the person may deteriorate very fast. Prompt treatment in a hospital with antibiotic drugs is vital. Without immediate treatment, meningitis may cause permanent disability, such as deafness or brain damage, and it can even be fatal.

For this reason, it is important that you are able to recognize the symptoms of meningitis – these may include high fever, stiff neck, severe headache, and possibly a rash. With early diagnosis and treatment, most people make a full recovery.

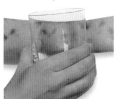

Testing for meningitis
Press a glass over a skin rash. If the rash does not fade under the glass, suspect meningitis.

RECOGNITION

The symptoms and signs include the following, but usually not all are present at the same time:
- High temperature or fever.
- Vomiting, which is often violent, or loss of appetite.
- Severe headache.
- Neck stiffness (the person cannot touch his chest with his chin).
- Joint or muscle pains.
- Drowsiness.
- Confusion or disorientation.
- Dislike of bright light.
- Seizures.
- Skin rash of small red/purple "pin prick" spots that may spread to look like fresh bruising. (The rash is more difficult to see on dark skin.) This rash does not fade when the side of a glass is pressed against it.

In babies and young children there may also be:
- Drowsiness or restlessness and high-pitched crying.
- Reluctance to feed.
- In babies, slight tenderness and swelling of the soft spot at the top of the skull.

YOUR AIM
- To obtain urgent medical aid.

⚠ WARNING

If a doctor cannot be contacted or is likely to be delayed

DIAL 9•1•1 OR CALL EMS.

If the person is ill and becoming worse, even if he has already seen a doctor, seek urgent medical attention again.

1 If you are concerned that an individual may have meningitis, seek medical advice immediately. Do not wait for all the symptoms and signs listed above to appear because victims with meningitis may not always develop all of these.

2 When calling the doctor or emergency services, describe the symptoms and say that you are concerned it may be meningitis. Be prepared to insist on medical attention.

3 While waiting for the doctor or ambulance, reassure the victim and keep him cool.

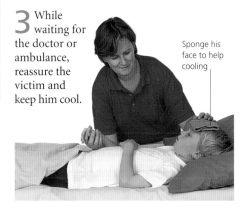

Sponge his face to help cooling

HEADACHE

A headache may accompany any illness, particularly a feverish ailment such as flu. It may develop for no reason but can often be traced to fatigue, tension, stress, or undue heat or cold. Mild "poisoning" caused by a stuffy or fume-filled atmosphere, or by excess alcohol or any other drug, can also induce a headache. However, a headache may also be the most prominent symptom of meningitis or stroke.

 See also MENINGITIS p.187 ● STROKE p.183

✚ YOUR AIMS
- To relieve the pain.
- To obtain medical aid if necessary.

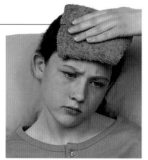

Cold compress may give relief

1 Help the person sit or lie down in a quiet place. Apply a cold compress to the head (p.49).

❗ CAUTION
Always seek urgent medical advice if the pain:
- Develops very suddenly.
- Is severe and incapacitating.
- Is accompanied by fever or vomiting.
- Is recurrent or persistent.
- Is accompanied by loss of strength or sensation or by impaired consciousness.
- Is accompanied by a stiff neck.
- Follows a head injury.

2 An adult may take two acetaminophen pills, a child the recommended dose of acetaminophen syrup. Do not give a child aspirin.

MIGRAINE

Many people are prone to migraine attacks – severe, "sickening" headaches. Attacks can be triggered by a variety of causes, such as allergy, stress, or tiredness. Other triggers include lack of sleep, missed meals, alcohol, and some foods, such as cheese or chocolate. Migraine sufferers usually know how to recognize and deal with attacks. They may carry their own medication.

RECOGNITION
- Before the attack there may be a warning period, with disturbance of vision in the form of flickering lights and/or a "blind patch."
- Intense throbbing headache, which is sometimes on just one side of the head.
- Abdominal pain, nausea, and vomiting.
- Inability to tolerate bright light or loud noise.

✚ YOUR AIMS
- To relieve the pain.
- To obtain medical aid if necessary.

1 Help the person take any medication that she may have for migraine attacks.

2 Advise the person to lie down or sleep for a few hours in a quiet, dark room. Provide towels and a container in case she vomits.

3 If this is the first attack or the headache is different from a usual headach, advise the person to see her doctor or seek medical care.

9

THIS CHAPTER DEALS with the effects of injuries and illnesses caused by environmental factors such as extremes of heat and cold.

The skin protects the body and helps maintain body temperature within a normal range. It can be damaged by fire, hot liquids, or caustic substances. Such injuries are often sustained in incidents such as explosions or chemical spills.

The effects of temperature extremes can also impair skin and other body functions. Injuries may be localized – as in frostbite or sunburn – or generalized, as in heat exhaustion or hypothermia. Very young children and elderly people are most susceptible to problems caused by extremes of temperature.

CONTENTS

The skin.....................................190

Assessing a burn.......................192

Severe burns and scalds............194

Minor burns and scalds............196

Burns to the airway.................197

Electrical burn...........................198

Chemical burn...........................199

Chemical burn to the eye.........200

Flash burn to the eye...............201

Tear gas or
      pepper spray injury..............201

Sunburn....................................202

Prickly heat..............................202

Heat exhaustion.......................203

Heatstroke...............................204

Frostbite..................................205

Hypothermia...........................206

ENVIRONMENTAL INJURIES

✚ FIRST-AID PRIORITIES

● Assess the victim's condition.

● Comfort and reassure the victim.

● Obtain medical aid if necessary. Call 9•1•1 or EMS if you suspect a serious illness or injury.

BURNS
● Protect yourself and the victim from danger.

● Assess the burn, prevent further damage, and relieve symptoms.

EXTREME TEMPERATURES
● Protect the victim from heat or cold.

● Restore normal body temperature.

THE SKIN

One of the largest organs, the skin plays key roles in protecting the body from injury and infection and in maintaining a constant body temperature.

The skin consists of two layers of tissue – an outer layer (epidermis) and an inner layer (dermis) – which lie on a layer of fatty tissue (subcutaneous fat). The top part of the epidermis is made up of dead, flattened skin cells, which are constantly shed and replaced by new cells made in the lower part of this layer. The epidermis is protected by an oily substance called sebum, secreted from glands called sebaceous glands, which keeps the skin supple and waterproof.

The lower layer of the skin, the dermis, contains the blood vessels, nerves, muscles, sebaceous glands, sweat glands, and hair roots (follicles). The ends of sensory nerves within the dermis register sensations from the body's surface, such as heat, cold, pain, and even the slightest touch. Blood vessels supply the skin with nutrients and help to regulate body temperature by preserving or releasing heat (opposite).

Structure of the skin
The skin is made up of two layers: the thin, outer epidermis and the thicker dermis beneath it. Most of the structures of the skin, such as blood vessels, nerves, and hair roots, are contained within the dermis.

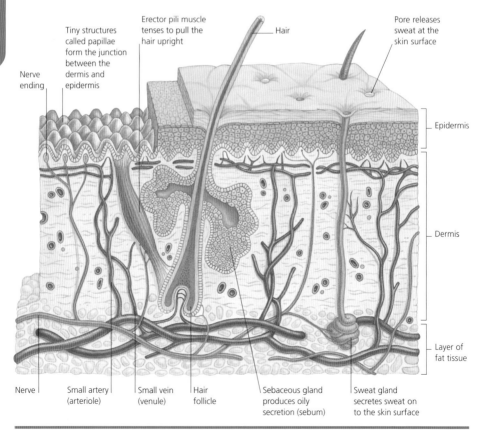

Nerve ending

Tiny structures called papillae form the junction between the dermis and epidermis

Erector pili muscle tenses to pull the hair upright

Hair

Pore releases sweat at the skin surface

Epidermis

Dermis

Layer of fat tissue

Nerve

Small artery (arteriole)

Small vein (venule)

Hair follicle

Sebaceous gland produces oily secretion (sebum)

Sweat gland secretes sweat on to the skin surface

Maintaining body temperature

One of the major functions of the skin is to help maintain the body temperature within its optimum range of 97–99°F (36–37°C). Body temperature is constantly monitored by a "thermostat" that lies deep within the brain. If the temperature of blood passing through this thermostat falls or rises to a level outside the optimum range, various mechanisms are activated to either warm or cool the body as necessary.

HOW THE BODY KEEPS WARM

When the body becomes too cold, changes take place to prevent heat from escaping. Blood vessels at the body surface narrow (constrict) to keep warm blood in the main part (core) of the body. The activity of the sweat glands is reduced, and hairs stand on end to "trap" warm air close to the skin.

In addition to the mechanisms that prevent heat loss, other body systems act to produce more warmth. The rate of metabolism is increased. Heat is also generated by muscle activity, which may be either voluntary (for example, during physical exercise) or, in cold conditions, involuntary (shivering).

HOW THE BODY LOSES HEAT

In hot conditions, the body activates a number of mechanisms to encourage heat loss and thus prevent the body temperature from becoming too high. Blood vessels that lie in or just under the skin widen (dilate). As a result, blood flow to the body surface increases and more heat is lost. In addition, the sweat glands become more active and secrete more sweat. This sweat then cools the skin as it evaporates.

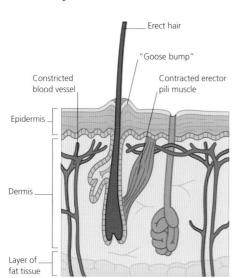

How skin responds to low body temperature
Blood vessels narrow (constrict) to reduce blood flow to the skin. The erector pili muscles contract, making the hairs stand upright and trap warm air close to the skin.

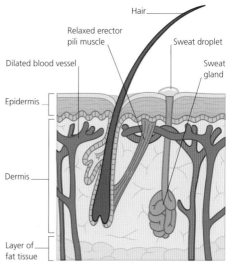

How skin responds to high body temperature
Blood vessels widen (dilate), making the skin look flushed, and heat is lost. Sweat glands become active and produce sweat, which evaporates to cool the skin.

ASSESSING A BURN

When skin is damaged by burning, it can no longer function effectively as a natural barrier against infection. In addition, body fluid may be lost because tiny blood vessels in the skin leak tissue fluid (serum). This fluid either collects under the skin to form blisters or leaks through the skin surface.

By assessing a burn before you start treatment, you can judge whether there are likely to be any related injuries, significant fluid loss, or infection.

WHAT TO ASSESS

When assessing a burn, it is important to consider the circumstances in which the burn has occurred; whether or not the airway is likely to have been affected; and the extent, location, and depth of the burn.

There are many possible causes of burns (below). By establishing the cause of the burn, the first aider may be able to identify any other potential problems that could result from the incident. For example, a fire in an enclosed space is likely to have produced poisonous carbon monoxide gas; other toxic fumes may have been released

if burning material was involved. If the victim's airway has been affected in any way, he may have difficulty breathing and will need urgent medical attention and admission to a hospital.

The extent of the burn will indicate whether or not shock is likely to develop. Shock is a life-threatening condition and occurs whenever there is a major loss of body fluids. In a burn over a large area of the body, fluid loss will be significant and the risk of shock high.

If the burn is on a limb, fluid may collect in the tissues, causing swelling and pain. This buildup of fluid is particularly serious if the limb is being constricted, for example, by clothing or footwear.

Burns allow germs to enter the skin and thus carry a serious risk of infection. To determine the degree of risk, you need to assess the depth of the burn (opposite): the deeper the burn, the higher the risk.

▶ See also BURNS TO THE AIRWAY p.197
● INHALATION OF FUMES pp.110–111
● SHOCK pp.120–121

TYPES OF BURN AND POSSIBLE CAUSES

Type of burn	Causes
Dry burn	Flames ● Contact with hot objects, such as domestic appliances or cigarettes ● Friction – for example, in rope burns
Scald	Steam ● Hot liquids, such as tea and coffee, or hot fat
Electrical burn	Low-voltage current, as used by domestic appliances ● High-voltage currents, as carried in mains overhead cables ● Lightning strikes
Cold injury	Frostbite ● Contact with freezing metals ● Contact with freezing vapors, such as liquid oxygen or liquid nitrogen
Chemical burn	Industrial chemicals, including inhaled fumes and corrosive gases ● Domestic chemicals and agents, such as paint stripper, caustic soda, weedkillers, bleach, oven cleaner, or any other strong acid or alkali
Radiation burn	Sunburn ● Overexposure to ultraviolet rays from a sunlamp ● Exposure to a radioactive source, such as an X ray

Depth of burns

There are three types of burn injury: first-degree (superficial), second-degree (partial-thickness), and third-degree (full-thickness). Burns are classified by the depth of skin damage. A person may suffer one or more depths of burn in a single incident.

A first-degree burn involves only the outermost layer of skin, the epidermis. This type of injury usually heals well if first aid is given promptly and if blisters do not form. Sunburn is one of the most common types of superficial burn.

Second-degree burns destroy the epidermis and are very painful. The skin becomes red and blistered. These burns usually heal well, but they can be serious if large areas of the body are affected.

In third-degree burns, pain sensation is usually lost, which may mislead you and the victim about the severity of the injury. The skin may look waxy, pale, or charred. These burns need urgent medical attention.

Burn | Tissue fluid | Blister | Damaged tissues

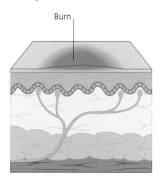 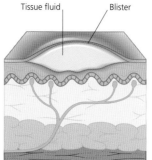 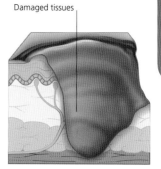

First-degree burn
This type of burn involves only the outermost layer of skin. First-degree burns are characterized by redness, swelling, and tenderness.

Second-degree burn
This affects the epidermis, and the skin becomes red and raw. Blisters form over the skin due to fluid released from the damaged tissues.

Third-degree burn
With this type of burn, all the layers of the skin are affected; there may be some damage to nerves, fat tissue, muscles, and blood vessels.

Burns that need hospital treatment

If the victim is a child, call a doctor or take the child to a hospital, however small the burn appears. For other people, medical attention should be sought for any serious burn. Such burns include:
- All third-degree burns.
- All burns involving the face, hands, feet, or genital area.
- All burns that extend right around an arm or a leg.

- All second-degree burns larger than 1 percent of the body surface (an area the size of the palm of the victim's hand).
- All first-degree burns larger than 5 percent of the body surface (equivalent to five palm areas).
- Burns with a mixed pattern of varying depths.

If you are unsure about the severity of any burn, seek medical attention.

SEVERE BURNS AND SCALDS

Take great care when treating burns that are deep or extensive. The longer the burning continues, the more severe the injury will be. If the victim has been burned in a fire, you should assume that smoke or hot air has also affected the respiratory system (*see* BURNS TO THE AIRWAY, p.197).

The priorities are to begin rapid cooling of the burn and to check breathing. A victim with a severe burn or scald injury will almost certainly be suffering from shock and will need hospital care.

The possibility of nonaccidental injury must always be considered, no matter what the age of the victim. Ensure you record all details accurately. Retain any removed clothing in case of future investigation.

▶ **See also** BURNS TO THE AIRWAY p.197
● FIRES pp.24–25 ● LIFE-SAVING PROCEDURES pp.71–102 ● SHOCK pp.120–121

RECOGNITION

There may be:
● Pain.
● Difficulty breathing.
● Signs of shock (pp.120–121).

✛ YOUR AIMS

● To stop the burning and relieve pain.
● To maintain an open airway.
● To treat associated injuries.
● To minimize the risk of infection.
● To arrange urgent transport to a hospital and to gather information for emergency services.

❗ WARNING

Watch for signs of difficulty breathing; be prepared to give rescue breaths and chest compressions if necessary (*see* LIFE-SAVING PROCEDURES, pp.71–102).

1 Help the person lie down. If possible, try to prevent the burned area from coming into contact with the ground.

2 Douse the burn with plenty of cold liquid for at least 10 minutes, but do not delay transport to a hospital.
DIAL 9·1·1 OR CALL EMS.

3 Continue cooling the affected area until the pain is relieved.

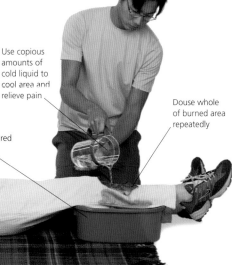

Use copious amounts of cold liquid to cool area and relieve pain

Douse whole of burned area repeatedly

Place bowl under injured leg to catch water

4 Put on disposable gloves if available. Gently remove any rings, watches, belts, shoes, or smoldering clothing before the tissues begin to swell. Carefully remove burned clothing, unless it sticks to the burn.

Remove clothing around site of burn | Use blunt-tipped scissors to cut clothing

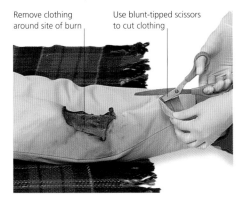

5 Cover the injured area with a sterile dressing to protect it from infection. If a sterile dressing is not available, use a folded triangular bandage, part of a sheet, or plastic wrap (discard the first two turns from the roll and apply it lengthwise over the burn). A clean plastic bag can be used to cover a hand or foot; secure it with a bandage or adhesive tape applied over the plastic, not the skin.

❶ CAUTION

● Do not overcool the victim because you may lower the body temperature to a dangerous level. This is a particular hazard for babies and elderly people.

● Do not remove anything sticking to the burn; you may cause further damage and introduce infection into the burned area.

● Do not touch or otherwise interfere with the burned area.

● Do not burst any blisters.

● Do not apply lotions, ointment, fat, or adhesive tape to the burned area.

SPECIAL CASE

BURNS TO THE FACE
If the victim has a facial burn, do not cover the injury; you could cause distress and obstruct the airway. Cool the area with water to relieve the pain until help arrives. Suspect airway burns.

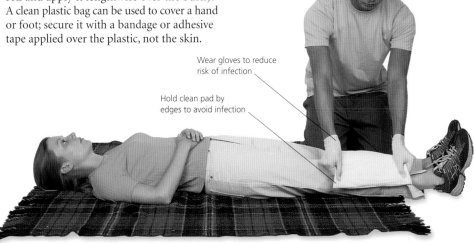

Wear gloves to reduce risk of infection

Hold clean pad by edges to avoid infection

6 Gather and record details of the injuries. Regularly monitor and record vital signs – level of response, pulse, and breathing (pp.42–43).

7 While waiting for help to arrive, reassure the victim and treat her for shock (pp.120–121) if necessary.

MINOR BURNS AND SCALDS

Small, superficial burns and scalds are often due to domestic incidents, such as touching a hot iron or spilling boiling water on the skin. Most minor burns can be treated successfully by first aid and will heal naturally. However, you should advise the victim to see a doctor if you are at all concerned about the severity of the injury (*see* ASSESSING A BURN, pp.192–193).

Some time after a burn, blisters may form. These thin "bubbles" are caused by tissue fluid (serum) leaking into the burned area just beneath the skin's surface. You should never break a blister because you may introduce infection into the wound.

See also ASSESSING A BURN pp.192–193

RECOGNITION

- Reddened skin.
- Pain in the area of the burn.

Later there may be:

- Blistering of the affected skin.

YOUR AIMS

- To stop the burning.
- To relieve pain and swelling.
- To minimize the risk of infection.

! CAUTION

- Do not break blisters or otherwise interfere with the injured area.
- Do not apply adhesive dressings or adhesive tape to the skin; the burn may be more extensive than it first appears.
- Do not apply butter, oils, or fats; they may damage tissues and increase the risk of infection.

1 Flood the injured part with cold water for at least 10 minutes to stop the burning and relieve the pain. This is more effective than using sprays. If water is not available, any cold, harmless liquid, such as milk or canned drinks, can be used.

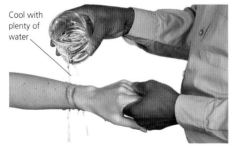

Cool with plenty of water

2 Put on disposable gloves if available. Gently remove any jewelry, watches, belts, or constricting clothing from the injured area before it begins to swell.

3 Cover the area with a sterile dressing or a clean, nonfluffy pad, and bandage loosely in place. A plastic bag or plastic wrap makes a good temporary covering. Apply plastic wrap lengthwise to prevent constriction of the area if the tissues swell.

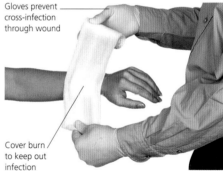

Gloves prevent cross-infection through wound

Cover burn to keep out infection

SPECIAL CASE

BLISTERS

A blister usually needs no treatment. However, if the blister breaks or is likely to burst, apply a nonadhesive dressing that extends well beyond the edges of the blister. Leave in place until the blister subsides.

BURNS TO THE AIRWAY

Burns to the face, and within the mouth or throat, are very serious because the air passages rapidly become swollen. Usually, signs of burning will be evident. However, you should always suspect damage to the airway if burns have been sustained in a confined space because the victim is likely to have inhaled hot air or gases.

There is no specific first-aid treatment for an extreme case; the swelling will rapidly block the airway, and there is a serious risk of suffocation. Immediate and specialized medical aid is required.

▶ **See also** LIFE-SAVING PROCEDURES pp.71–102 ● SHOCK pp.120–121

YOUR AIMS
● To maintain an open airway.
● To arrange urgent transport to a hospital.

⚠ WARNING
If the victim becomes unconscious, open the airway and check breathing; be prepared to give rescue breaths and chest compressions if necessary (*see* LIFE-SAVING PROCEDURES, pp.71–102). If he is breathing, place him in the recovery position (pp.84–85).

1 DIAL 9·1·1 OR CALL EMS.
Tell the dispatcher that you suspect burns to the airway.

2 Take any steps possible to improve the victim's air supply, such as loosening clothing around his neck.

3 Offer ice or small sips of cool water to reduce swelling and/or pain.

4 Reassure the victim. Monitor and record his vital signs – level of response, pulse, and breathing (pp.42–43) – until help arrives.

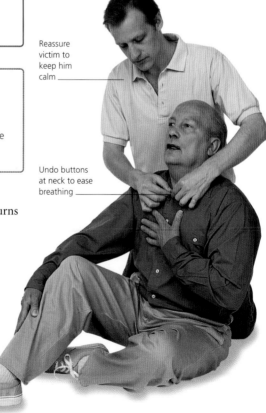

Reassure victim to keep him calm

Undo buttons at neck to ease breathing

ELECTRICAL BURN

Burns may occur when electricity passes through the body. Much of the visible damage occurs at the points of entry and exit of the current. However, there may also be a track of internal damage. The position and direction of entry and exit wounds will alert you to the likely site and extent of hidden injury, and to the degree of shock that the person may suffer.

Burns may be caused by a lightning strike or by low- or high-voltage electric current. An electric shock can also cause cardiac arrest. If the victim is unconscious, your immediate priority, once you are sure the area is safe, is to open the airway and check for breathing and circulation.

See also ELECTRICAL INJURIES pp.26–27
● LIFE-SAVING PROCEDURES pp.71–102
● SEVERE BURNS AND SCALDS pp.194–195
● SHOCK pp.120–121

RECOGNITION

There may be:
● Unconsciousness.
● Burns, with swelling, scorching, and charring, at the points of entry and exit.
● Signs of shock.
● A brown, coppery residue on the skin if the injured person has been a victim of "arcing" high-voltage electricity. (Do not mistake this residue for injury.)

YOUR AIMS

● To treat the burns and shock.
● To arrange urgent transport to a hospital.

WARNING

If the victim is unconscious, open the airway and check breathing; be prepared to give rescue breaths and chest compressions if necessary (*see* LIFE-SAVING PROCEDURES, pp.71–102).

1 Before touching the person, you must make sure that contact with the electrical source is broken (pp.26–27).

2 Flood the sites of injury, at the entry and exit points of the current, with plenty of cold water to cool the burns.

3 Put on disposable gloves if available. Place a sterile dressing, a clean, folded triangular bandage, or some other clean, nonfluffy material over the burns to protect them against airborne infection. DIAL 9·1·1 OR CALL EMS.

4 Reassure the person and treat him for shock (pp.120–121).

CAUTION

Do not approach a victim of high-voltage electricity until you are officially informed that the current has been switched off and isolated.

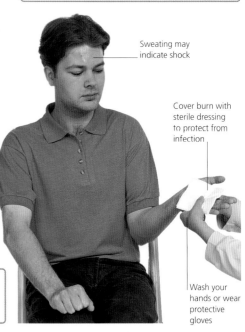

Sweating may indicate shock

Cover burn with sterile dressing to protect from infection

Wash your hands or wear protective gloves

CHEMICAL BURN

Certain chemicals may irritate, burn, or penetrate the skin, causing widespread and sometimes fatal damage. Unlike burns caused by heat, signs of chemical burns develop slowly, but the first aid is similar.

Most strong, corrosive chemicals are found in industry, but chemical burns can also occur in the home, especially from dishwasher products (the most common cause of alkali burns in children), oven cleaners, and paint stripper.

Chemical burns are always serious, and the victim may need urgent hospital treatment. If possible, note the name or

RECOGNITION

There may be:
- Evidence of chemicals in the vicinity.
- Intense, stinging pain.
- Later, discoloration, blistering, peeling, and swelling of the affected area.

brand of the burning substance. Before treating the victim, ensure your own safety and that of others because some chemicals give off poisonous fumes.

▶ See also CHEMICALS ON THE SKIN p.221 ● INHALATION OF FUMES pp.110–111

✚ YOUR AIMS
- To make the area safe and inform the relevant authority.
- To disperse the harmful chemical.
- To arrange transport to a hospital.

❶ CAUTION
- Never attempt to neutralize acid or alkali burns; only dilute them with water.
- Do not delay starting treatment by searching for an antidote.

1 Make sure that the area around the victim is safe. Ventilate the area to disperse fumes, and, if possible, seal the chemical container. Remove the victim if necessary.

2 Flood the burn with water for at least 20 minutes to disperse the chemical and stop the burning. If treating someone on the ground, ensure that the water does not collect underneath her.

3 Gently remove any contaminated clothing while flooding the injury.

4 Arrange transport to a hospital. Make sure that the airway is open. Monitor vital signs – level of response, pulse, and breathing (pp.42–43). Pass on details of the chemical to medical staff. If in the workplace, notify the safety department and/or EMS.

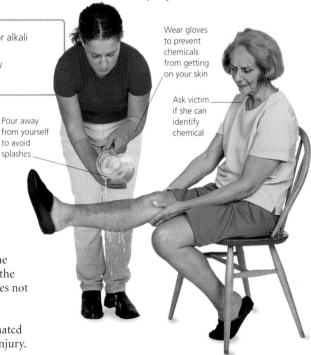

Pour away from yourself to avoid splashes

Wear gloves to prevent chemicals from getting on your skin

Ask victim if she can identify chemical

CHEMICAL BURN TO THE EYE

Splashes of chemicals in the eye can cause serious injury if not treated quickly. They can damage the surface of the eye, resulting in scarring and even blindness.

The priority for the first aider is to wash out (irrigate) the eye so that the chemical is diluted and dispersed. When irrigating the eye, be careful that the contaminated rinsing water does not splash you or the victim. Before beginning to treat the victim, put on protective gloves if available.

RECOGNITION

There may be:
- Intense pain in the eye.
- Inability to open the injured eye.
- Redness and swelling around the eye.
- Copious tearing of the eye.
- Evidence of chemical substances or containers in the immediate area.

YOUR AIMS
- To disperse the harmful chemical.
- To arrange transport to a hospital.

ⓘ CAUTION
Do not allow the victim to touch the injured eye or forcibly remove a contact lens.

1 Put on protective gloves if available. Hold the affected eye under gently running cold water for at least 10 minutes. Take care to irrigate the eyelid thoroughly both inside and out. You may find it easier to pour the water over the eye using an eye irrigator or a glass.

2 If the eye is shut in a spasm of pain, gently but firmly pull the eyelids open. Be careful that contaminated water does not splash the uninjured eye.

3 Ask the victim to hold a sterile eye dressing or a clean, nonfluffy pad over the injured eye. If it will be some time before she receives medical attention, bandage the pad loosely in position.

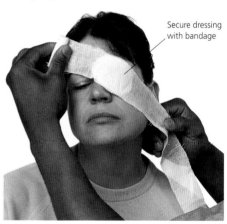

Secure dressing with bandage

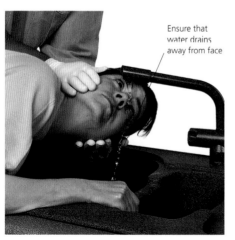

Ensure that water drains away from face

4 Identify the chemical if possible. Then arrange to take or send the victim to a hospital.

FLASH BURN TO THE EYE

This condition occurs when the surface (cornea) of the eye is damaged by exposure to ultraviolet light, such as prolonged glare from sunlight reflected off snow. It can also be caused by glare from a welder's torch. Symptoms usually develop gradually, and recovery can take up to several days.

RECOGNITION
- Intense pain in the affected eye(s).

There may also be:
- A "gritty" feeling in the eye(s).
- Sensitivity to light.
- Redness and tearing of the eye(s).

+ YOUR AIMS
- To prevent further damage.
- To arrange transport to a hospital.

⊘ CAUTION
Do not remove any contact lenses.

1 Reassure the victim. Ask him to hold an eye pad to each injured eye. If it is likely to take some time to obtain medical attention, lightly bandage the pad(s) in place.

2 Arrange to take or send the victim to a hospital.

TEAR GAS OR PEPPER SPRAY INJURY

These solvent sprays are used by police forces for riot control and self-protection, and may be used by unauthorized people as a weapon in assaults. It irritates the eyes and upper airways and may cause vomiting.

The effects usually wear off within about 15 minutes, although the eyes may remain sore for longer than this.

If tear gas or pepper spray is used on an asthmatic person, it may induce an attack.

RECOGNITION
There may be:
- Tearing of the eyes.
- Uncontrollable coughing and sneezing.
- Burning sensation in the skin and throat.
- Chest tightness and difficulty with breathing.

▶ **See also** ASTHMA p.115

+ YOUR AIM
- To get the victim into fresh air.

⊘ CAUTION
- Washing out (irrigating) the eyes is not usually necessary and may prolong the irritation.
- Do not rub any area affected by the spray.

1 Move the victim to a well-ventilated area and reassure him that the symptoms will soon disappear – he may be very agitated. Try to stop him from rubbing his eyes.

2 If the victim's eyes are painful, fan them to help speed up the vaporization of any remaining chemical.

3 If a large amount of the chemical is inhaled at close quarters, arrange to take or send the victim to a hospital.

SUNBURN

This type of burn can be caused by over-exposure to the sun or a sunlamp. At high altitudes, it can occur even on an overcast summer day. Some medicines trigger severe sensitivity to sunlight. Rarely, sunburn can be caused by exposure to radioactivity.

Most sunburn is superficial; in severe cases, the skin is lobster-red and blistered and the victim may suffer heatstroke.

RECOGNITION
- Reddened skin.
- Pain in the area of the burn.

Later there may be:
- Blistering of the affected skin.

 See also HEATSTROKE p.204

YOUR AIMS
- To move the victim out of the sun.
- To relieve discomfort and pain.

⚠ WARNING
If there is extensive blistering, or other skin damage, seek medical advice.

1 Cover the person's skin with light clothing or a towel. Help her move into the shade or, preferably, indoors.

2 Cool her skin by sponging with cold water, or by soaking the affected area in a cold bath, for 10 minutes.

3 Encourage her to have frequent sips of cold water.

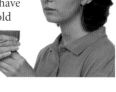

Tell victim to sip water

4 If the burns are mild, calamine or a sunburn preparation may soothe them. For severe sunburn, obtain medical aid.

PRICKLY HEAT

This is a highly irritating, prickly red rash that most commonly occurs in hot weather. It develops when sweat glands are blocked by bacteria and dead skin cells. The rash particularly affects areas where sweat is trapped and cannot evaporate, such as the feet. People who often have prickly heat also tend to be susceptible to heatstroke.

RECOGNITION
There may be:
- Prickling or burning sensation.
- Rash of tiny red spots or blisters.

 See also HEATSTROKE p.204

YOUR AIM
- To relieve discomfort and pain.

1 Encourage the person to stay in cool conditions as much as possible.

2 Cool the skin by gently sponging with cold water.

HEAT EXHAUSTION

This disorder is caused by loss of salt and water from the body through excessive sweating. It usually develops gradually. Heat exhaustion usually affects people who are not acclimatized to hot, humid conditions. People who are unwell, especially those with illnesses that cause vomiting and diarrhea, are more susceptible than others to developing heat exhaustion.

A dangerous and common cause of heat exhaustion is the excessively high body temperature, and other physical changes, that result from certain drugs taken for pleasure, such as Ecstasy. The user sweats profusely, due to prolonged overactivity, then dehydration develops, leading to heat exhaustion. These effects, coupled with the drug's effect on the temperature-regulating center in the brain, can lead to heatstroke and even cause death.

⏵ See also HEATSTROKE p.204 ● LIFE-SAVING PROCEDURES pp.71–102

RECOGNITION

As the condition develops, there may be:
- Headache, dizziness, and confusion.
- Loss of appetite and nausea.
- Sweating, with pale, clammy skin.
- Cramps in the arms, legs, or the abdominal wall.
- Rapid, weakening pulse and breathing.

YOUR AIMS

- To replace lost body fluids and salt.
- To cool the victim down if necessary.
- To obtain medical aid if necessary.

1 Help the victim to a cool place. Get him to lie down with raised legs.

2 Give him plenty of water or, if possible, a weak salt solution (one teaspoon of salt per quart of water).

3 Even if the victim recovers quickly, ensure that he sees a doctor. If his responses deteriorate, place him in the recovery position (pp.84–85). DIAL 9·1·1 OR CALL EMS.

4 Monitor and record vital signs – level of response, pulse, and breathing (pp.42–43). Be prepared to give rescue breaths and chest compressions if necessary (see LIFE-SAVING PROCEDURES, pp.71–102).

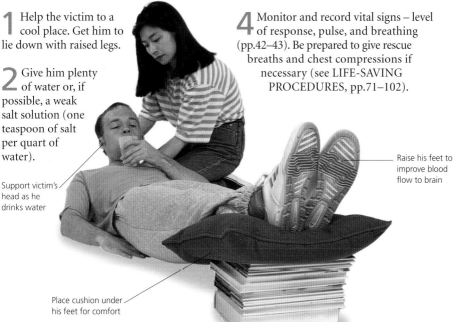

Raise his feet to improve blood flow to brain

Support victim's head as he drinks water

Place cushion under his feet for comfort

HEATSTROKE

This condition is caused by a failure of the "thermostat" in the brain, which regulates body temperature. The body becomes dangerously overheated, usually due to a high fever or prolonged exposure to heat. Heatstroke can also result from use of drugs such as Ecstasy. In some cases, heatstroke follows heat exhaustion when sweating ceases, and the body then cannot be cooled by the evaporation of sweat.

Heatstroke can develop with little warning, causing unconsciousness within minutes of the victim feeling unwell.

RECOGNITION

There may be:
- Headache, dizziness, and discomfort.
- Restlessness and confusion.
- Hot, flushed, and dry skin.
- Rapid deterioration in the level of response.
- Full, bounding pulse.
- Body temperature above 104°F (40°C).

● **See also** DRUG POISONING p.222
- LIFE-SAVING PROCEDURES pp.71–102
- CHECKING TEMPERATURE p.43

YOUR AIMS
- To lower the victim's body temperature as quickly as possible.
- To arrange urgent transport to a hospital.

1 Quickly move the person to a cool place. Remove as much of his outer clothing as possible.
DIAL 9·1·1 OR CALL EMS.

2 Wrap the person in a cold, wet sheet and keep the sheet wet until his temperature falls to 100.4°F (38°C) under the tongue, or 99.5°F (37.5°C) under the armpit. If no sheet is available, fan him, or sponge him with cold water.

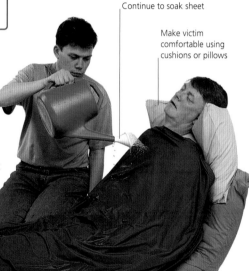

Continue to soak sheet

Make victim comfortable using cushions or pillows

Wrap victim in wet sheet

3 Once the his temperature appears to have returned to normal, replace the wet sheet with a dry one.

4 Monitor and record vital signs – level of response, pulse, and breathing (pp.42–43) – until help arrives. If his temperature rises again, repeat the cooling process.

❶ WARNING

If the victim becomes unconscious, open the airway and check breathing; be prepared to give rescue breaths and chest compressions if necessary (see LIFE-SAVING PROCEDURES, pp.71–102). If the victim is breathing, place him in the recovery position (pp.84–85).

FROSTBITE

With this condition, the tissues of the extremities – usually the fingers and toes – freeze due to low temperatures. In severe cases, this freezing can lead to permanent loss of sensation and, eventually, gangrene (tissue death) as the blood vessels become permanently damaged.

Frostbite usually occurs in freezing or cold and windy conditions. People who cannot move around are particularly susceptible. In many cases, frostbite is accompanied by hypothermia (pp.206–208), and this should be treated accordingly.

RECOGNITION

There may be:
- At first, "pins-and-needles."
- Pallor, followed by numbness.
- Hardening and stiffening of the skin.
- A color change to the skin of the affected area: first white, then mottled and blue. On recovery, the skin may be red, hot, painful, and blistered. Where gangrene occurs, the tissue may become black due to loss of blood supply.

See also HYPOTHERMIA pp.206–208

+ YOUR AIMS
- To warm the affected area slowly to prevent further tissue damage.
- To arrange transport to a hospital.

1 If possible, move the person into warmth before you thaw the affected part (*see* VICTIM HANDLING, pp.63–64).

2 Gently remove gloves, rings, and any other constrictions, such as boots. Warm the affected part with your hands, in your lap, or in the person's armpits. Avoid rubbing the affected area because this can damage skin and other tissues.

3 Place the affected part in warm water at around 104°F (40°C). Dry carefully, and apply a light dressing of fluffed-up, dry gauze bandage.

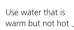
Use water that is warm but not hot

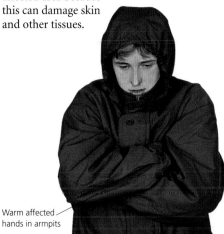
Warm affected hands in armpits

4 Raise and support the affected limb to reduce swelling. An adult victim may take two acetaminophen pills for intense pain. Take or send him to a hospital.

⊘ CAUTION
- Do not put the affected part near direct heat.
- Do not attempt to thaw the affected part if there is danger of it refreezing.
- Do not allow the victim to smoke.

HYPOTHERMIA

This develops when the body temperature falls below 95°F (35°C). The effects vary depending on the speed of onset and the level to which the body temperature falls. Moderate hypothermia can usually be completely reversed. Severe hypothermia – when the core body temperature falls below 86°F (30°C) – is often, although not always, fatal. However, no matter how low body temperature is, it is always worth persisting with life-saving procedures until a doctor evaluates the victim.

WHAT CAUSES HYPOTHERMIA
Hypothermia may develop over several days in poorly heated houses. Infants, homeless people, elderly people, and those who are thin and frail are particularly vulnerable. Lack of activity, chronic illness, and fatigue all increase the risk; alcohol and drugs can exacerbate the condition.

Hypothermia can also be caused by prolonged exposure to cold out of doors

(p.208). Moving air has a much greater cooling effect than still air so a high "wind-chill factor" can substantially increase the risk of a person developing hypothermia.

Death from immersion in cold water may be caused by hypothermia, not drowning. When surrounded by cold water, the body cools 30 times faster than in dry air, and body temperature falls rapidly.

▶ **See also** ● DROWNING p.109 ● LIFE-SAVING PROCEDURES pp.71–102

TREATMENT WHEN INDOORS

1 For someone who has been brought in from outside, quickly replace any wet clothing with warm, dry garments.

2 The person can be rewarmed by bathing if she is young, fit, and able to climb into the bath unaided. The water should be warm but not too hot – about 104°F (40°C).

3 Put the person in a bed and ensure that she is well covered. Give her warm drinks, soup, or high-energy foods to help rewarm her.

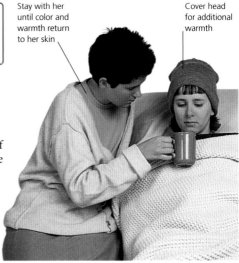

Stay with her until color and warmth return to her skin

Cover head for additional warmth

SPECIAL CASE

HYPOTHERMIA IN THE ELDERLY

An elderly person may develop hypothermia slowly over a number of days. Elderly people often have inadequate food or heating and are more likely to suffer from chronic illness that impairs their mobility.

When treating an elderly person with hypothermia, be careful to warm her slowly. Cover her with layers of blankets in a room at about 77°F (25°C). If she is warmed too rapidly, blood may be diverted suddenly from the heart and brain to the body surfaces.

Always seek medical care because hypothermia may disguise the symptoms of, or accompany, a stroke, a heart attack, or an underactive thyroid gland (hypothyroidism).

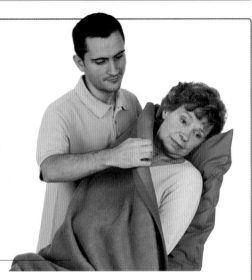

Warm an elderly person gradually

❶ CAUTION

● Do not allow an elderly person to have a bath to warm her up – the sudden warming may cause blood to divert suddenly from the heart and brain to the body surfaces.

● Do not place any heat sources, such as hot water bottles or fires, next to her because these may also mobilize blood too rapidly. In addition, they may burn the person.

● Do not give her alcohol because this will worsen the hypothermia.

● Handle the person gently because, in severe cases, rushed treatment or movement may cause the heart to stop.

4 Regularly monitor and record vital signs – level of response, pulse, breathing, and temperature (pp.42–43).

5 It is important to seek medical care if you have any doubts about the person's condition. Always obtain medical aid if an elderly person or a baby is affected.

SPECIAL CASE

HYPOTHERMIA IN INFANTS

A baby's mechanisms for regulating body temperature are underdeveloped, so she may develop hypothermia in a cold room. The baby's skin may look healthy but feel cold, and she may be limp and unusually quiet, and refuse to feed. Rewarm a cold baby gradually, by wrapping her in blankets and warming the room. You should always seek medical care if you suspect a baby has hypothermia.

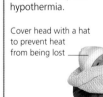

Cover head with a hat to prevent heat from being lost

Wrap the baby in a blanket

Continued on next page

HYPOTHERMIA (continued)

TREATMENT WHEN OUTDOORS

1 Take the person to a sheltered place as quickly as possible.

2 Remove wet clothing. Shield the person from the wind. Insulate him with extra clothing or blankets and cover his head. Do not give him your clothes.

3 Protect him from the ground and the elements. Put him in a dry sleeping bag, cover him with blankets or newspapers and enclose him in a plastic or foil survival bag, if available.

Lay victim on a thick layer of dry insulating material, such as pine branches, heather, or bracken

Protect him from wind and rain with survival bag

Shelter and warm him with your body

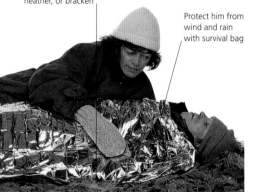

4 Send for help. In an ideal situation, two people should go together for help. However, it is important that you do not leave the person alone; someone must remain with him at all times.

5 To help rewarm someone who is conscious, give him warm drinks and high-energy foods if you have such drinks or foods available.

6 When help arrives, the person should be taken to a hospital by stretcher.

SPECIAL CASE

WHEN NO HELP IS AVAILABLE
If you are alone with the victim, try to attract attention by using a whistle, waving a flashlight, or lighting a fire.

10

OBJECTS THAT FIND their way into the body, either through a wound in the skin or via an orifice (such as the ear, nose, or eye), are known as "foreign objects." Such items range from specks of dirt or grit in the eye to small objects that young children may push into their noses and ears. Foreign objects do not usually cause serious problems for the victim, but they can be painful and distressing. Calm, reassuring treatment from the first aider is essential.

TREATMENT PROCEDURES

This chapter begins with an overview of the structure of the sensory organs: the skin, eyes, ears, mouth, and nose. This is followed by advice on how to remove objects from the skin and orifices, including what to do when something has been swallowed or inhaled. First aid for a person with an object embedded in a wound is given in Chapter 6, Wounds and Bleeding (pp.127–144).

CONTENTS

The sensory organs.................. 210

Splinter......................................212

Embedded fishhook............... 213

Foreign object in the eye..........214

Foreign object in the ear...........215

Foreign object in the nose........215

Inhaled foreign object.............. 216

Swallowed foreign object..........216

✚ FIRST-AID PRIORITIES

- Assess the victim's condition.
- Comfort and reassure the victim.
- Establish whether or not a foreign object can be removed safely.
- Prevent further damage.
- Obtain medical aid if necessary. Call 9•1•1 or EMS if you suspect a serious illness or injury.

THE SENSORY ORGANS

The skin

The body is covered and protected by the skin. This is one of the body's largest organs and is made up of two layers: the outer epidermis and an inner layer, the dermis. The skin forms a barrier against harmful substances and germs. It is also an important sense organ, containing nerves that ensure the body is sensitive to heat, cold, pain, and touch.

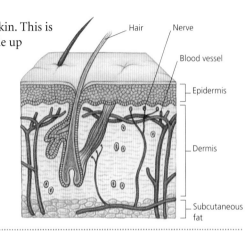

Hair   Nerve

Blood vessel

Epidermis

Dermis

Subcutaneous fat

Structure of the skin
The skin consists of the thin epidermis and the thicker dermis, which sit on a layer of fat (subcutaneous fat). Blood vessels, nerves, muscles, oil (sebaceous) glands, sweat glands, and hair roots (follicles) lie in the dermis.

The eyes

These complex organs allow us to see the world around us. Each eye consists of a colored part (iris) with a small opening (pupil) that allows rays of light to enter the eye. The size of the pupil changes according to the amount of light entering the eye.

Light rays are focused by the transparent lens on to a "screen" (retina) at the back of the eye. Cells in the retina convert this information into electrical impulses that travel, via the optic nerve, to the part of the brain where the impulses are analyzed.

The eyes are protected by the bony sockets in the skull. The eyelids, and delicate membranes called conjunctiva, protect the front of the eyes.

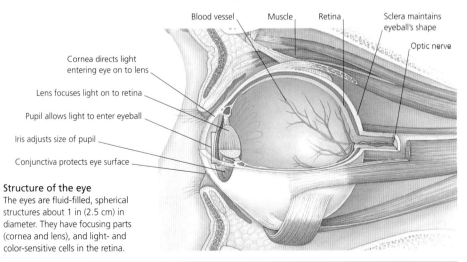

Blood vessel   Muscle   Retina   Sclera maintains eyeball's shape

Optic nerve

Cornea directs light entering eye on to lens

Lens focuses light on to retina

Pupil allows light to enter eyeball

Iris adjusts size of pupil

Conjunctiva protects eye surface

Structure of the eye
The eyes are fluid-filled, spherical structures about 1 in (2.5 cm) in diameter. They have focusing parts (cornea and lens), and light- and color-sensitive cells in the retina.

The ears

As well as being the organs of hearing, the ears also play an important role in balance. The visible part of each ear is the auricle, which funnels sounds into the ear canal to vibrate the eardrum. Fine hairs in the ear canal filter out dust, and glands secrete earwax to trap any other small particles. The vibrations of the eardrum pass across the middle ear to the hearing apparatus (cochlea) in the inner ear. This structure converts the vibrations into nerve impulses and transmits them to the brain via the auditory nerve. The vestibular apparatus within the inner ear is involved in balance.

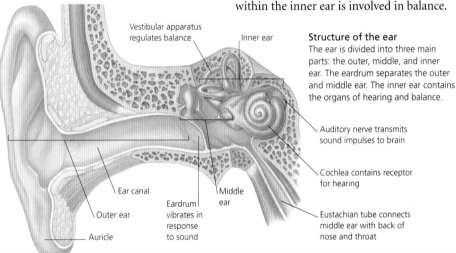

Structure of the ear
The ear is divided into three main parts: the outer, middle, and inner ear. The eardrum separates the outer and middle ear. The inner ear contains the organs of hearing and balance.

Vestibular apparatus regulates balance

Inner ear

Auditory nerve transmits sound impulses to brain

Cochlea contains receptor for hearing

Eustachian tube connects middle ear with back of nose and throat

Ear canal

Eardrum vibrates in response to sound

Middle ear

Outer ear

Auricle

The mouth and nose

These cavities form the entrances to the digestive and respiratory tracts respectively. The nasal cavities connect with the throat. They are lined with blood vessels and with membranes that secrete mucus to trap debris as it enters the nose. Food enters the digestive tract via the mouth, which leads into the esophagus. The epiglottis, a flap at the back of the throat, prevents food from entering the windpipe (trachea).

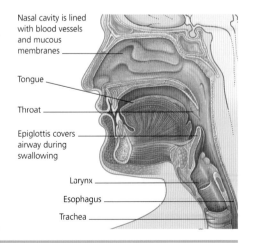

Nasal cavity is lined with blood vessels and mucous membranes

Tongue

Throat

Epiglottis covers airway during swallowing

Larynx

Esophagus

Trachea

Structure of the nose and mouth
The nostrils lead into the two nasal cavities, which are lined with mucous membranes and blood vessels. The nasal cavities connect directly with the top of the throat.

SPLINTER

Small splinters of wood, metal, or glass may enter the top layer of skin. They carry a risk of infection because they are rarely clean. The areas most frequently affected are the hands, knees, and feet. Usually, a splinter can be successfully withdrawn from the skin using sterile tweezers. However, if the splinter is deeply embedded in the skin, lies over a joint, or is difficult to remove, you should leave it in place and advise the person to consult a doctor.

▶ **See also** FOREIGN OBJECT IN A CUT p.135
● INFECTED WOUND p.136

✚ YOUR AIMS

● To remove the splinter.
● To minimize the risk of infection.

---

1 Sterilize a pair of tweezers by holding them in a flame and then letting them cool. Put on disposable gloves if available. Gently clean around the splinter with soap and warm water.

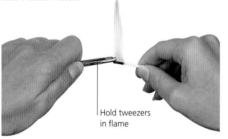

Hold tweezers in flame

2 Grasp the splinter with the tweezers as close to the skin as possible, and draw it out at the angle at which it went in.

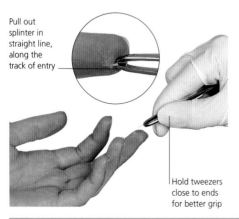

Pull out splinter in straight line, along the track of entry

Hold tweezers close to ends for better grip

SPECIAL CASE

EMBEDDED SPLINTER
If a splinter is embedded or difficult to dislodge, do not probe the area with a sharp object such as a needle or you may introduce infection. Pad around the splinter until you can bandage over it without pressing down, and seek medical advice.

---

3 Carefully squeeze the wound to encourage a little bleeding. This will help flush out any remaining dirt.

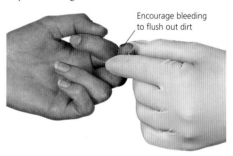

Encourage bleeding to flush out dirt

4 Clean the area, pat it dry, and apply an adhesive dressing to minimize the risk of infection.

---

❶ CAUTION

Always ask about tetanus immunization.

Seek medical advice if:
● The person has never been immunized.
● The person is uncertain about the timing and number of injections that have been given.
● It is more than 10 years since the person's last injection.

EMBEDDED FISHHOOK

A fishhook that is embedded in the skin is difficult to remove because of the barb at the end of the hook. If possible, you should ensure that the hook is removed by a health professional. Only attempt to remove a hook yourself if medical aid is not readily available. Embedded fishhooks may carry a risk of infection, including tetanus.

WHEN MEDICAL AID IS NOT READILY AVAILABLE

➕ YOUR AIM

● To remove the fishhook without causing any further injury and pain.

❶ WARNING

Do not try to pull out a fishhook unless you can cut off the barb. If you cannot, seek medical help.

1 Put on disposable gloves if available. If the barb is visible, use wirecutters to cut it away; carefully withdraw the hook by its eye.

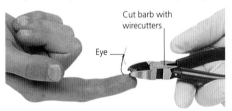

Cut barb with wirecutters

Eye

2 Clean the wound, then pad around it with gauze and bandage it.

SPECIAL CASE

BARB NOT VISIBLE
Push the hook further in until the barb emerges. Cut off the barb, and remove the hook (*see left*). If you cannot do this, seek medical help.

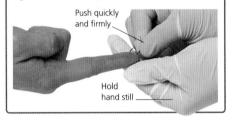

Push quickly and firmly

Hold hand still

❶ CAUTION

Always ask about tetanus immunization.

Seek medical advice if:
● The person has never been immunized.
● The person is uncertain about the timing and number of injections that have been given.
● It is more than 10 years since the person's last injection.

WHEN MEDICAL AID IS READILY AVAILABLE

➕ YOUR AIMS

● To obtain medical aid.
● To minimize the risk of infection.

1 Put on disposable gloves if available. Ask the person to sit down and support the injured area. Cut off the fishing line as close as possible to the hook.

2 Build up pads of gauze around the hook until you can bandage over it without pushing it in further.

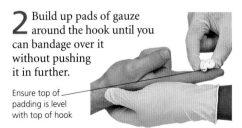

Ensure top of padding is level with top of hook

3 Bandage over the padding and the hook; take care not to press down on the hook. Ensure that the person receives medical attention as soon as possible.

FOREIGN OBJECT IN THE EYE

A speck of dust, a loose eyelash, or even a contact lens can float on the white of the eye. Usually, such objects can easily be rinsed off. However, you must not touch anything that sticks to the eye, penetrates the eyeball, or rests on the colored part of the eye (iris and pupil) because this may damage the eye. Instead, make sure that the person gets medical attention quickly.

See also EYE WOUND p.138

RECOGNITION

There may be:
- Blurred vision.
- Pain or discomfort.
- Redness and tearing of the eye.
- Eyelids closed in spasms.

YOUR AIM

- To prevent injury to the eye.

CAUTION

Do not touch anything that is sticking to, or embedded in, the eyeball or over the colored part of the eye. Cover the eye (*see* EYE WOUND, p.138) and take or send the victim to a hospital.

1 Ask the person to sit down facing the light; tell her not to rub her eye.

2 Stand behind the person. Gently separate her eyelids with your finger and thumb. Examine every part of her eye.

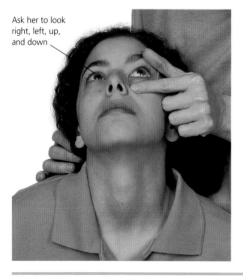

Ask her to look right, left, up, and down

3 If you can see a foreign object on the white of the eye, wash it out by pouring clean water from a glass or by using a sterile eyewash.

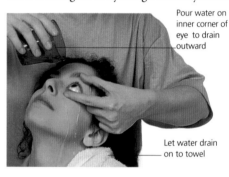

Pour water on inner corner of eye to drain outward

Let water drain on to towel

4 If this is unsuccessful, lift the object off with a moist swab or the damp corner of a tissue or clean handkerchief. If you still cannot remove the object, seek medical help.

SPECIAL CASE

OBJECT UNDER UPPER EYELID

Ask the person to grasp her lashes and pull the upper lid over the lower lid. Blinking under water may also make the object float off.

Lower lashes may brush particle clear

FOREIGN OBJECT IN THE EAR

If a foreign object becomes lodged in the ear, it may cause temporary deafness by blocking the ear canal. In some cases, a foreign object may damage the eardrum.

Young children frequently push objects into their ears; adults may leave cotton padding in an ear after cleaning it. Insects can fly or crawl into the ear and may cause alarm.

YOUR AIMS

- To prevent injury to the ear.
- To remove a trapped insect if it is moving.
- To arrange transport to a hospital if a foreign object is lodged in the ear.

1 Arrange to take or send the person to a hospital as soon as possible. Do not try to remove a lodged foreign object yourself.

2 Reassure the person during the journey or until medical help arrives.

CAUTION

Do not attempt to remove any object that is lodged in the ear. You may cause serious injury and push the foreign object in even further.

SPECIAL CASE

INSECT INSIDE THE EAR
Reassure the person, and ask her to sit down. Gently flood the ear with tepid water so that the insect floats out. If this flooding does not remove the insect, take or send the person to a hospital.

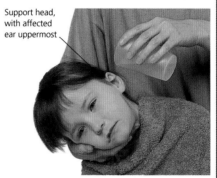

Support head, with affected ear uppermost

FOREIGN OBJECT IN THE NOSE

Young children may push small objects up their noses. Foreign objects can block the nose and cause infection. Sharp objects may damage the tissues, and button batteries can cause burns and bleeding. Do not try to remove a foreign object; you may cause injury or push it further into the airway.

RECOGNITION

There may be:
- Difficult or noisy breathing through the nose.
- Swelling of the nose.
- Smelly or blood-stained discharge, indicating that an object may have been lodged for a while.

YOUR AIM

- To arrange transport to a hospital.

CAUTION

Do not attempt to remove the foreign object, even if you can see it.

1 Try to keep the person quiet and calm. Tell him to breathe through his mouth at a normal rate. Advise him not to poke inside his nose to try to remove the object himself.

2 Arrange transport to a hospital, where the object can safely be removed by hospital staff.

INHALED FOREIGN OBJECT

Small, smooth objects can slip past the protective mechanisms in the throat and enter the air passages leading to the lungs (*see* THE RESPIRATORY SYSTEM, p.104).

Dry peanuts, which can swell up when in contact with body fluids, pose a particular danger in young children. Peanuts can be inhaled into the lungs, resulting in serious damage. In addition, some individuals are allergic to nuts, and may suffer anaphylactic shock (p.123) after swallowing them.

RECOGNITION

There may be:
- Some sign or noise of choking, which quickly passes.
- Persistent dry coughing.
- Difficulty breathing.

▶ **Treat as for** CHOKING ADULT p.100
● CHOKING CHILD p.101 ● CHOKING INFANT p.102

SWALLOWED FOREIGN OBJECT

Small objects such as coins, safety pins, or buttons are most commonly swallowed by young children. Often they travel straight through the digestive tract, but there is a risk that they may enter the respiratory tract and cause choking. Button batteries, which are used in some toys, watches, and hearing aids, are dangerous if swallowed because they contain corrosive chemicals. They can cause severe damage, and even death, if not removed. A large or sharp object may damage the digestive tract.

＋YOUR AIM
- To obtain medical aid if necessary.

1 Reassure the person and try to find out exactly what she has swallowed.

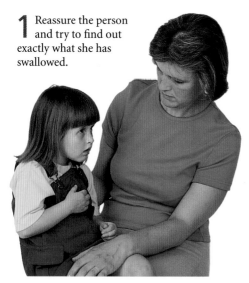

❶WARNING

If the person has swallowed something large or sharp, or has difficulty breathing or swallowing

DIAL 9•1•1 OR CALL EMS.

Reassure the person while waiting for medical help to arrive.

❶CAUTION

Do not allow the person to eat, drink, or smoke because a general anesthetic may need to be given at the hospital.

2 If the swallowed object is small and smooth, take or send the person to a hospital or to a doctor. Always seek urgent medical advice if you know or suspect that she has swallowed a battery.

11

POISONING IS USUALLY unintentional. It may result from exposure to or ingestion of toxic substances, including drugs and alcohol, chemicals, and contaminated food. Some cases of poisoning are intentional, as in cases of attempted suicide. The effects of a poison vary depending on the type and amount of the substance absorbed. However, in most cases of poisoning, medical aid will be needed.

BITES AND STINGS
Although insect stings and stings from marine creatures such as jellyfish can spoil a picnic or seaside outing, they are often minor injuries that can be treated successfully with first aid. However, multiple insect stings can produce a serious reaction that requires urgent medical help. Animal and human bites also always require medical attention because the mouth harbors many types of microorganisms (germs).

CONTENTS

How poisons affect the body.... 218

Swallowed poisons.................. 220

Chemicals on the skin.............. 221

Inhaled gases.......................... 221

Poisons in the eye................... 221

Drug poisoning....................... 222

Alcohol poisoning................... 223

Food poisoning....................... 224

Poisonous plants and fungi...... 225

Insect sting............................. 226

Other bites and stings............. 227

Tick bite................................. 227

Snake bite.............................. 228

Stings from sea creatures......... 229

Marine puncture wound.......... 229

Animal bite............................. 230

✚ FIRST-AID PRIORITIES

- Assess the victim's condition.
- Identify the poisonous substance.
- Ensure the safety of yourself and the victim.
- Comfort and reassure the victim.
- Obtain medical aid if necessary. Call 9•1•1 or EMS if you suspect a serious illness or injury.

POISONING, BITES, AND STINGS

HOW POISONS AFFECT THE BODY

A poison – also called a toxin – is a substance that, if taken into the body in sufficient quantity, may cause temporary or permanent damage.

Poisons can be swallowed, absorbed through the skin, inhaled, splashed into the eyes, or injected. Once in the body, they may enter the bloodstream and be carried swiftly to all organs and tissues. Signs and symptoms of poisoning vary with the poison – they may develop quickly or over a number of days. Vomiting is common, especially when the poison has been ingested. Inhaled poisons often cause breathing difficulties.

Effects of poisons on the body
Poisons can enter the body through the skin, digestive system, lungs, or bloodstream. Once in the bloodstream, poisons can be carried to all parts of the body and have multiple effects.

Poisons reaching the brain may cause confusion, delirium, seizures, and unconsciousness

Swallowed corrosive chemicals can burn the mouth, lips, and food passages

Poisonous gases, solvents, vapors, or fumes can be inhaled and affect the airways and lungs, causing severe breathing problems

Some poisons disturb the action of the heart by interrupting its normal electrical activity

Overload of poisons can seriously damage the liver, which acts as a "poison filter"

Poisons reaching the kidneys from the bloodstream can cause serious damage to these organs

Poisons in the digestive system can cause vomiting, abdominal pain, and diarrhea

Corrosive chemicals can burn the skin. Pesticides and plant toxins may be absorbed through the skin, causing local or general reactions

Injected poisons and drugs rapidly enter the bloodstream; some poisons prevent the blood cells from carrying oxygen to body tissues

Types of poison

Some poisons are man-made – for example, chemicals and drugs – and these are found in the home as well as in industry. Almost every household contains substances that are potentially poisonous, such as bleach and paint stripper, as well as prescribed or over-the-counter medicines, which may be dangerous if taken in excessive amounts.

Other poisons occur in nature: for example, plants produce poisons that may irritate the skin or cause more serious symptoms if ingested, and various insects and creatures produce venom in their bites and stings. Contamination of food by bacteria may result in food poisoning – one of the most common forms of poisoning.

RECOGNIZING AND TREATING THE EFFECTS OF POISONING

Route of entry to the body	Poison	Possible effects	Action
Swallowed (ingested)	• Drugs and alcohol • Cleaning products • Home repair and gardening products • Plant poisons • Bacterial (food) poisons • Viral (food) poisons	Nausea and vomiting; abdominal pain; seizures; irregular, or fast or slow heartbeat; impaired consciousness	• Monitor victim • Seek medical help • Resuscitate if necessary (pp.71–102)
Absorbed through the skin	• Cleaning products • Gardening and home repair products • Industrial poisons • Plant poisons	Pain; swelling; rash; redness; itching	• Remove contaminated clothing • Wash area for at least 10 minutes • Seek medical help • Resuscitate if necessary (pp.71–102)
Inhaled	• Cleaning and home repair product fumes • Industrial poisons • Fumes from fires	Difficulty breathing; hypoxia; cyanosis (gray-blue skin coloration)	• Help victim into fresh air • Seek medical help • Resuscitate if necessary (pp.71–102)
Splashed in the eye	• Cleaning products • Home repair and gardening products • Industrial poisons • Plant poisons	Pain and watering of the eye; blurred vision	• Irrigate the eye • Seek medical help • Resuscitate if necessary (pp.71–102)
Injected through the skin	• Venom from stings and bites • Drugs	Pain, redness and swelling at injection site Blurred vision; nausea and vomiting; difficulty breathing; seizures; impaired consciousness; anaphylactic shock	*For sting/venom:* • Remove sting, if possible • Seek medical help • Resuscitate if necessary (pp.71–102) *For injected drugs:* • Seek medical help • Resuscitate if necessary (pp.71–102)

SWALLOWED POISONS

Chemicals that are swallowed may harm the digestive tract, or cause more widespread damage if they enter the bloodstream and are transported to other parts of the body.

Hazardous chemicals include common household substances. For example, bleach, dishwasher detergent, and paint stripper are poisonous or corrosive if swallowed. Drugs, whether they are prescribed or bought over the counter, are also potentially harmful if they are taken in overdose. The effects of poisoning depend on the substance that has been swallowed.

RECOGNITION

Depends on the poison, but there may be:
- Vomiting, sometimes bloodstained.
- Impaired consciousness.
- Pain or burning sensation.
- Empty containers in the vicinity.
- History of ingestion/exposure.

▶ See also CHEMICAL BURN p.199 ● DRUG POISONING p.222 ● INHALATION OF FUMES p.110 ● LIFE-SAVING PROCEDURES pp.71–102

✚ YOUR AIMS
- To maintain airway, breathing, and circulation.
- To remove any contaminated clothing.
- To call the local poison control center.
- To identify the poison.
- To arrange urgent transport to a hospital.

1 If the person is conscious, ask her what she has swallowed, and try to reassure her.

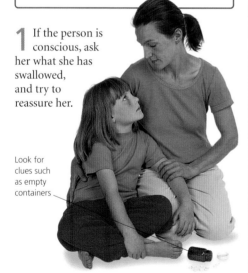

Look for clues such as empty containers

2 CALL YOUR LOCAL POISON CONTROL CENTER (800-222-1222). Give as much information as possible about the swallowed poison. If the person is unconscious, call 9·1·1 or EMS.

SPECIAL CASE

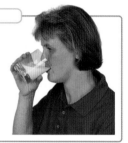

BURNED LIPS
If the person's lips are burned by corrosive substances, give her frequent sips of cold milk or water while waiting for medical help to arrive.

❶ WARNING
- Never attempt to induce vomiting.
- If the person becomes unconscious, open the airway and check breathing; be prepared to give rescue breaths and chest compressions if necessary (*see* LIFE-SAVING PROCEDURES, pp.71–102). If she is breathing, place her in the recovery position (pp.92–93).

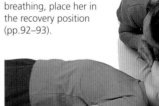

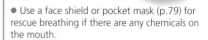

- Use a face shield or pocket mask (p.79) for rescue breathing if there are any chemicals on the mouth.

CHEMICALS ON THE SKIN

Hazardous chemicals that are spilled on the skin can cause irritation or burns. In addition, certain substances are absorbed through the skin and may cause widespread damage inside the body.

The most dangerous chemicals are found in industry, but domestic items such as dishwasher products, oven cleaners, and paint strippers are also harmful.

Burns caused by chemicals may require urgent hospital treatment.

RECOGNITION

There may be:
- Intense, stinging pain.
- Evidence of chemical substances or containers in the immediate area.
- Discoloration, blistering, peeling, and swelling of the affected area occurring at once or some time later.

▶ Treat as for CHEMICAL BURN p.199

INHALED GASES

Inhaling chemical fumes or sprays is potentially harmful and may lead to breathing problems, confusion, and collapse. Some factories use gases that are harmful if they are inhaled accidentally. Chlorine gas is stored at swimming pools and is hazardous if released. Poisonous gases may also be released in the chemical reaction that occurs when different cleaning products are used together, for example bleach and disinfectant.

RECOGNITION

Depends on the gas but there may be:
- Headache.
- Noisy, distressed breathing.
- Confusion.
- Impaired consciousness.

▶ Treat as for TEAR GAS OR PEPPER SPRAY INJURY p.201 or INHALATION OF FUMES p.110

POISONS IN THE EYE

Many chemicals – both liquids and gases – used in the home and the workplace can irritate the eyes. The membranes covering the eye absorb chemicals rapidly, and this can lead to damage to the eyes within minutes of a chemical being in contact.

Particular chemicals can damage the surface of the eye, and these may cause permanent scarring of the eye and even blindness. For these reasons, immediate first aid is needed to wash out any chemicals splashed in the eye. This should be followed by medical treatment.

RECOGNITION

There may be:
- Intense pain in the eye.
- Inability to open the injured eye.
- Redness and swelling around the eye.
- Copious watering of the eye.

▶ Treat as for CHEMICAL BURN TO THE EYE p.200 or TEAR GAS OR PEPPER SPRAY INJURY p.201

DRUG POISONING

Poisoning can result from an overdose of either prescribed drugs or drugs that are bought over the counter. It can also be caused by drug abuse or drug interaction. The effects vary depending on the type of drug and how it is taken (below). When you call emergency services, give as much information as possible. While waiting for help to arrive, look for containers that might help you to identify the drug.

▶ **See also** LIFE-SAVING PROCEDURES pp.71–102

RECOGNITION

Category	Drug	Effects of poisoning
Painkillers	Aspirin (swallowed)	Upper abdominal pain, nausea, and vomiting ● Ringing in the ears ● "Sighing" when breathing ● Confusion and delirium ● Dizziness
	Acetaminophen (swallowed)	Little effect at first, but abdominal pain, nausea, and vomiting may develop ● Irreversible liver damage may occur within 3 days (malnourishment and alcohol increase the risk)
Nervous system depressants and tranquillizers	Barbiturates and benzodiazepines (swallowed)	Lethargy and sleepiness, leading to unconsciousness ● Shallow breathing ● Weak, irregular, or abnormally slow or fast pulse
Stimulants and hallucinogens	Amphetamines (including Ecstasy) and LSD (swallowed); cocaine (inhaled)	Excitable, hyperactive behavior, wildness, and frenzy ● Sweating ● Tremor of the hands ● Hallucinations, in which the victim may claim to "hear voices" or "see things"
Narcotics	Morphine, heroin (commonly injected)	Small pupils ● Sluggishness and confusion, possibly leading to unconsciousness ● Slow, shallow breathing, which may stop altogether ● Needle marks, which may be infected
Solvents	Glue, lighter fuel (inhaled)	Nausea and vomiting ● Headaches ● Hallucinations ● Possibly, unconsciousness ● Rarely, cardiac arrest

✚ YOUR AIMS

● To maintain breathing and circulation.
● To arrange transport to a hospital.

❶ WARNING

● If the victim is unconscious, open the airway and check breathing; be prepared to give rescue breaths and chest compressions if necessary (see LIFE-SAVING PROCEDURES, pp.72–p.102). If breathing, place in recovery position (pp.84–85).

DIAL 9•1•1 OR CALL EMS.

● Do not induce vomiting.

1 If the victim is conscious, help him into a comfortable position and ask what he has taken. Reassure him while you talk to him.

2 DIAL 9•1•1 OR CALL EMS. Monitor and record vital signs – level of response, pulse, and breathing (pp.42–43) – until medical help arrives.

3 Keep samples of any vomited material. Look for evidence that might help to identify the drug, such as empty containers. Give these samples and containers to the paramedic or ambulance crew.

ALCOHOL POISONING

Alcohol (chemical name, ethanol) is a drug that depresses the activity of the central nervous system – in particular, the brain. Prolonged or excessive intake can severely impair all physical and mental functions, and the person may sink into deep unconsciousness.

There are several risks to the victim from alcohol poisoning:
- An unconscious person risks inhaling and choking on vomit.
- Alcohol widens (dilates) the blood vessels. This means that the body loses heat, and hypothermia may develop.
- Someone who smells of alcohol may be misdiagnosed and not receive appropriate treatment for an underlying cause of unconsciousness, such as a head injury, stroke, or heart attack.

RECOGNITION

There may be:
- A strong smell of alcohol
- Empty bottles or cans.
- Impaired consciousness: the victim may respond if roused, but will quickly relapse.
- Flushed and moist face.
- Deep, noisy breathing.
- Full, bounding pulse.
- Unconsciousness.

In the later stages of unconsciousness:
- Dry, bloated appearance to the face.
- Shallow breathing.
- Weak, rapid pulse.
- Dilated pupils that react poorly to light.

See also HYPOTHERMIA p.206 • LIFE-SAVING PROCEDURES pp.72–102

YOUR AIMS
- To maintain an open airway.
- To assess for other conditions.
- To seek medical help if necessary.

WARNING
- If the victim is unconscious, open the airway and check breathing; be prepared to give rescue breaths and chest compressions if necessary (*see* LIFE-SAVING PROCEDURES, pp.72–p.102). If the victim is breathing, place him in the recovery position (pp.84–85).

DIAL 9•1•1 OR CALL EMS.
- Do not induce vomiting.

1 Cover the person with a coat or blanket to protect him from the cold.

2 Assess the person for any injuries, especially head injuries, or other medical conditions.

3 Monitor and record vital signs – level of response, pulse, and breathing (pp.42–43) – until the person recovers or is placed in the care of a responsible caretaker.

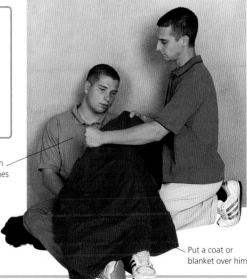

Watch victim in case he becomes unconscious

Put a coat or blanket over him

FOOD POISONING

This is usually caused by consuming food or drink that is contaminated with bacteria or viruses. Some food poisoning is caused by poisons (toxins) from bacteria already in the food. The salmonella or *E. coli* group of bacteria, which are found mainly in meat, are common causes of food poisoning. Symptoms may develop rapidly (within hours), or they may not occur until a day or so after eating contaminated food.

Toxic food poisoning is frequently caused by poisons produced by the staphylococcus group of bacteria. Symptoms usually develop rapidly, possibly within 2–6 hours of eating the affected food.

One of the dangers of food poisoning is loss of body fluids. The dehydration that results from this fluid loss can be serious if the fluids are not replaced quickly enough. Dehydration is especially serious in the very young and the very old, and, in some cases, treatment may be required in a hospital.

▶ **See also** SHOCK pp.120–121 ● VOMITING AND DIARRHEA p.247

RECOGNITION

There may be:
- Nausea and vomiting.
- Cramping abdominal pains.
- Diarrhea (possibly bloodstained).
- Headache or fever.
- Features of shock (p.120).
- Impaired consciousness.

✚ YOUR AIMS

- To encourage the person to rest.
- To give the person plenty of bland fluids to drink.
- To obtain medical aid if necessary.

❶ WARNING

If the condition worsens,

DIAL 9•1•1 OR CALL EMS.

1 Advise the person to lie down and rest. Help her if necessary.

2 Give the person plenty of bland fluids to drink and a bowl to use if she vomits. Call a doctor for advice.

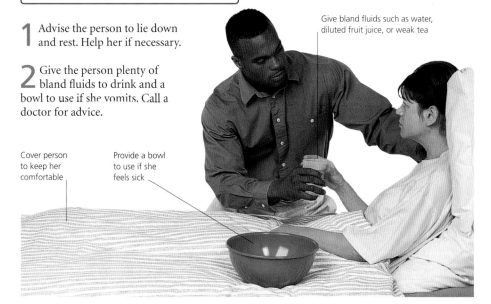

Give bland fluids such as water, diluted fruit juice, or weak tea

Cover person to keep her comfortable

Provide a bowl to use if she feels sick

POISONOUS PLANTS AND FUNGI

Many young children eat plant leaves or brightly colored berries, but serious poisoning rarely occurs as a result. However, ingesting even small amounts of foxglove or wild arum can cause nausea, vomiting, and stomach cramps; and large amounts are potentially fatal. Seizures may occur after ingesting laburnum seeds.

Serious poisoning as a result of eating mushrooms is also rare. Mushrooms found in the garden may cause nausea, vomiting, and, occasionally, hallucinations. Death cap mushrooms cause vomiting and severe, watery diarrhea between 6 and 12 hours after ingestion and can be fatal.

Mushrooms and plants that cause severe poisoning
Death cap mushrooms and wild arum berries grow in woodland and hedges during late summer and autumn. Foxgloves flower in spring, and laburnum produces seed pods in summer.

RECOGNITION
There may be:
● Nausea and vomiting.
● Cramping abdominal pains.
● Diarrhea.
● Seizures.
● Impaired consciousness.

▶ **See also** LIFE-SAVING PROCEDURES pp.71–102 ● SEIZURES pp.184–186 ● VOMITING AND DIARRHEA p.247

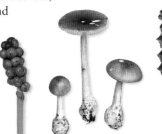
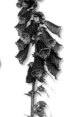
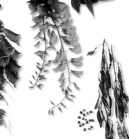

WILD ARUM   DEATH CAP MUSHROOMS   FOXGLOVE   LABURNUM

✚ YOUR AIMS
● To identity the poisonous plant, if possible.
● To manage any seizures.
● To obtain medical aid if necessary.

❶ WARNING
● If the person is unconscious, open the airway and check breathing. Be prepared to give rescue breaths and chest compressions, if necessary (*see* LIFE-SAVING PROCEDURES, pp.71–102). If the person is breathing, put him in the recovery position (pp.84–85).
DIAL 9•1•1 OR CALL EMS.
Monitor person until medical help arrives.
● Do not induce vomiting.

1 If the person is conscious, ask him what he has eaten and reassure him.

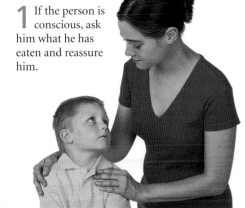

2 Try to identify the poisonous plant, and find out which part of it has been eaten. Get medical advice at once so that the appropriate treatment can be given.

3 Keep any small pieces of the plant that you have found, together with samples of vomited material, to show to the doctor or to send with the person to a hospital.

INSECT STING

Usually, a sting from a bee, wasp, or hornet is painful rather than dangerous. An initial sharp pain is followed by mild swelling, redness, and soreness.

However, multiple insect stings can produce a serious reaction. A sting in the mouth or throat is potentially dangerous because swelling can obstruct the airway. With any bite or sting, it is important to watch for signs of an allergic reaction, which may lead to anaphylactic shock (p.123).

RECOGNITION

- Pain at the site of the sting.
- Redness and swelling around the site of the sting.

▶ See also ANAPHYLACTIC SHOCK p.123
- LIFE-SAVING PROCEDURES pp.71–102

✚ YOUR AIMS

- To relieve swelling and pain.
- To arrange transport to a hospital if necessary.

⚠ WARNING

If the victim shows signs of anaphylactic shock, such as impaired breathing or swelling of the face and neck,

DIAL 9•1•1 OR CALL EMS.

SPECIAL CASE

STINGS TO THE MOUTH AND THROAT
If a victim has been stung in the mouth, there is a risk that swelling of tissues in the mouth and/or throat may occur, causing the airway to become blocked. To help prevent this from happening, give the victim an ice cube to suck or a glass of cold water to sip. If swelling starts to develop,

DIAL 9•1•1 OR CALL EMS.

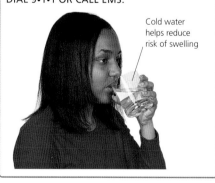

Cold water helps reduce risk of swelling

1 Reassure the person. If the sting is visible, brush or scrape it off sideways with your fingernail or the blunt edge of a knife. Do not use tweezers because more poison may be injected into the person.

Brush stinger off with a fingernail or blunt edge

2 Raise the affected part if possible, and apply an ice pack or cold compress (p.49). Advise the person to see her doctor if the pain and swelling persist.

Advise her to hold compress or ice pack against affected area for at least 10 minutes

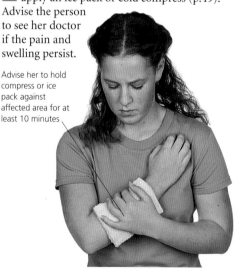

OTHER BITES AND STINGS

Bites from certain species of scorpions and spiders can cause serious illness and may even be fatal if not treated promptly.

Bites or stings in the mouth or throat are dangerous because swelling can obstruct the airway. Be alert to an allergic reaction, which may lead to anaphylactic shock (p.123).

RECOGNITION

Depends on the species but generally:
- Pain, redness, and swelling at site of sting.
- Nausea and vomiting.
- Headache.

▶ **See also** ANAPHYLACTIC SHOCK p.123
● LIFE-SAVING PROCEDURES pp.71–102

YOUR AIMS
- To relieve the pain and swelling.
- To arrange transport to a hospital, if necessary.

⚠ WARNING

If the person has been stung by a scorpion or a black widow or brown recluse spider, or if the person is showing signs of anaphylactic shock,

DIAL 9•1•1 OR CALL EMS.

1 Help the person sit or lie down, and reassure her.

2 Raise the affected part if possible. Apply an ice pack or cold compress (p.49).

3 Monitor vital signs – level of response, pulse, and breathing (pp.42–43). Watch for signs of an allergy, such as wheezing.

SPECIAL CASE

STINGS TO THE MOUTH AND THROAT
Give the person an ice cube to suck or cold water to drink. If swelling starts to develop,

DIAL 9•1•1 OR CALL EMS.

TICK BITE

Ticks are tiny, spiderlike creatures found in grass or woodlands. They attach themselves to passing animals (including humans) and bite into the skin to suck blood. When sucking blood, a tick swells to about the size of a pea, and it can then be seen easily. Ticks can carry disease and cause infection, so they should be removed as soon as possible.

YOUR AIM
- To remove the tick.

1 Using fine-pointed tweezers, grasp the tick's head close to the skin.

2 Use a back-and-forth action to lever the head out. Try to avoid breaking the tick and leaving the buried head behind.

Lever tick out carefully

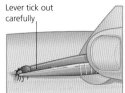

3 Advise the person to see a doctor. Take the tick; it may be required for analysis.

SNAKE BITE

The only poisonous snakes native to the US are pit vipers (rattlesnakes, copperheads, and cottonmouth moccasins) and coral snakes. However, exotic snakes – some of them poisonous – are kept as pets. A snake bite can be frightening, but it is not usually serious. Reassurance is vital; keeping the victim still may delay the spread of venom (poison) through the body. Note the snake's appearance to help doctors give the correct antivenin. If it is safe to do so, put the snake in a secure container; but bear in mind that venom is active even if the snake is dead. If the snake is not captured, notify the police.

See also LIFE-SAVING PROCEDURES pp.71–102

RECOGNITION

Depends on the species, but there may be:
- A pair of puncture marks.
- Severe pain, redness, and swelling at the site of the bite.
- Nausea and vomiting.
- Disturbed vision.
- Increased salivation and sweating.
- Labored breathing; in extreme cases, breathing may stop altogether.

YOUR AIMS
- To prevent the spread of venom in the body.
- To arrange urgent transport to a hospital.

WARNING
- Do not apply a tourniquet, slash the wound with a knife, or suck out the venom.
- If the victim become unconscious, open the airway and check breathing; be prepared to give rescue breaths and chest compressions if necessary (*see* LIFE-SAVING PROCEDURES, pp.71–102).

1 Help the person lie down. Reassure her, and tell her to keep calm and still. DIAL 9·1·1 OR CALL EMS.

2 Gently wash the wound and pat dry with clean swabs.

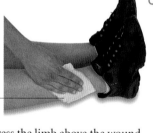

Clean wound with gauze swab

3 Lightly compress the limb above the wound with a roller bandage. Use triangular bandages to immobilize the affected area (p.57).

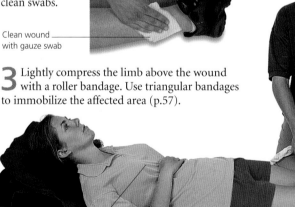

Tie narrow-fold bandage in figure eight around feet

Leave bite exposed

Keep heart above the level of wounded part

Broad-fold bandage

Soft padding

Roller bandage

STINGS FROM SEA CREATURES

Jellyfish, Portuguese man-of-war, corals, and sea anemones cause painful stings. Their venom is contained in stinging cells that stick to the skin. Most marine species found in temperate regions of the world are not dangerous, but some tropical species can cause severe poisoning. Occasionally, death results from paralysis of the chest muscles, and, very rarely, from anaphylaxis.

 See also ANAPHYLACTIC SHOCK p.269

YOUR AIMS
- To relieve pain and discomfort.
- To arrange transport to a hospital if necessary.

1 Reassure the person and encourage him to sit or lie down.

2 Hold an ice pack or cold compress (p.49) against the skin for 10 minutes to relieve pain and swelling; raise the affected part.

⚠ WARNING
If the injury is severe or there is a serious reaction, **DIAL 9•1•1 OR CALL EMS.**

SPECIAL CASE
TROPICAL JELLYFISH
Pour copious amounts of vinegar or ocean water over the injury to incapacitate the stinging cells. Lightly compress the limb above the sting with a roller bandage, and immobilize the injured limb (opposite).

DIAL 9•1•1 OR CALL EMS.

Keep the victim completely still until help arrives.

Pour vinegar directly onto wound

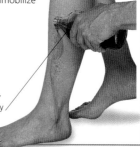

MARINE PUNCTURE WOUND

Many marine creatures have spines, which provide a mechanism against attack from predators, but which can cause painful wounds in humans if they are stepped on.

Sea urchins have sharp spines that can become embedded in the sole of the foot. Wounds may become infected if the spines are not removed.

YOUR AIMS
- To relieve pain and discomfort.
- To minimize the risk of infection.
- To arrange transport to a hospital.

⚠ CAUTION
Do not bandage the wound.

1 Help the person immerse the injured part in water as hot as he can tolerate for about 30 minutes.

2 Take or send the person to a hospital so that the spines can be safely removed.

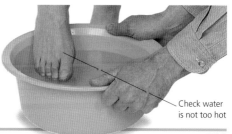

Check water is not too hot

ANIMAL BITE

Bites from sharp, pointed teeth cause deep puncture wounds that can carry bacteria and other microorganisms (germs) far into the tissues. Human bites also crush the tissue. Hitting someone's teeth with a bare fist can produce a bite. Any bite that breaks the skin needs prompt first aid and medical attention because of the risk of infection.

The most serious infection risk is rabies, a potentially fatal viral infection of the nervous system. The virus is carried in the saliva of infected animals. If bitten by a domestic animal behaving unusually or any wild animal, the victim must receive anti-rabies injections. Tetanus is also a potential risk. There is probably only a small risk of hepatitis B or C viruses being transmitted through a human bite – and an even smaller risk of transmission of the HIV (AIDS) virus. However, seek medical advice if you are concerned.

▶ See also CUTS AND ABRASIONS p.134 ● INFECTED WOUND p.136 ● SEVERE BLEEDING pp.130–131 ● SHOCK pp.120–121

✚ YOUR AIMS

- To control bleeding.
- To minimize the risk of infection, both to the victim and yourself.
- To obtain medical aid if necessary.

❶ CAUTION

Always ask about tetanus immunization.
Seek medical advice if:
- The person has never been immunized.
- The person is uncertain about the timing or number of injections that have been given.
- It is more than 10 years since the person's last injection.

1 Put on disposable gloves, if available. Wash the bite wound thoroughly with soap and warm water in order to minimize the risk of infection.

2 Pat dry with clean gauze swabs and cover with an adhesive dressing or a small sterile dressing.

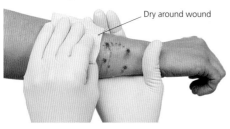

Dry around wound

3 Arrange to take or send the person to a hospital if the wound is large or deep.

❶ WARNING

If you suspect rabies, arrange immediate transport to a hospital.

SPECIAL CASE

DEEP WOUND

If the wound is deep, control bleeding by applying direct pressure and raising the injured part. Cover the wound with a nonfluffy pad, or a sterile dressing, and bandage firmly in place to control bleeding. Arrange to take or send the victim to a hospital.

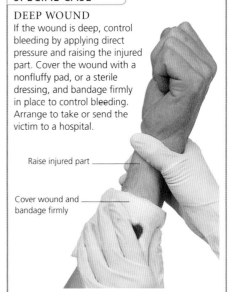

Raise injured part

Cover wound and bandage firmly

12

CHILDBIRTH is a natural and often lengthy process: when a woman goes into labor, there is usually plenty of time to get her to a hospital before her baby arrives. In the rare event of a baby arriving quickly, a first aider should not try to deliver the baby – the birth will happen naturally without intervention. Your role is to comfort and listen to the wishes of the mother and care for her and her newborn baby.

Miscarriage, however, is a potentially serious problem because there is a risk of severe bleeding. A woman who is miscarrying needs urgent medical help.

MEDICAL PROBLEMS include everyday conditions, such as fever and cramp, and more serious ones, such as diabetes-related hypoglycemia, which develop quickly. They need prompt treatment and respond well to first aid. However, a minor complaint can be the start of serious illness, so you should always consult a doctor if you are in doubt about someone's condition.

✚ FIRST-AID PRIORITIES

- Assess the victim's condition.
- Comfort and reassure the victim.
- Obtain medical aid if necessary. Call 9•1•1 or EMS if you suspect a serious illness.

CONTENTS

CHILDBIRTH

Childbirth..................................232

Childbirth: first stage...............233

Childbirth: second stage..........234

Childbirth: third stage.............236

MEDICAL PROBLEMS

Miscarriage 237

Allergy....................................238

Hiccups...................................238

Fever......................................239

Vertigo....................................239

Diabetes mellitus....................240

Hyperglycemia........................240

Hypoglycemia.........................241

Panic attack............................242

Disturbed behavior.................242

Earache..................................243

Toothache...............................244

Sore throat.............................244

Abdominal pain.......................245

Hernia....................................246

Vomiting and diarrhea.............247

Stitch.....................................247

Cramp....................................248

Overseas travel health............249

CHILDBIRTH AND MEDICAL PROBLEMS

CHILDBIRTH AND MEDICAL PROBLEMS

CHILDBIRTH

The process of giving birth normally begins at about the 40th week of pregnancy. The entire process is called labor, and there are three distinct stages: in the first, the uterus contracts and the baby gets in position for birth; in the second, the baby is born; in the third, the afterbirth (placenta and umbilical cord) is expelled.

FIRST STAGE OF LABOR
In the first stage of labor, the woman's body prepares for the birth. A mucus plug, which protects the uterus from infection, is expelled. This is called the "show." It occurs some time before contractions of the uterus begin. The start of the contractions, together with the pressure of the baby's head, causes the cervix (neck of the uterus) to widen (dilate). The contractions become stronger and more frequent until the cervix is fully dilated – about 4 in (10 cm) in diameter. This process may take several hours. At some point in this stage of labor, the amniotic sac breaks and the "water" (amniotic fluid) leaks out from the vagina.

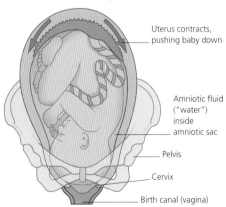

Uterus contracts, pushing baby down

Amniotic fluid ("water") inside amniotic sac

Pelvis

Cervix

Birth canal (vagina)

Preparations for birth
Muscular contractions begin to spread through the uterus as waves every 2–5 minutes. The intervals between the contractions become shorter as the first stage progresses. At the same time, the cervix gradually widens.

SECOND STAGE OF LABOR
Once the cervix is fully dilated, the baby's head presses down on the mother's pelvic floor, triggering an urge for the mother to push. The birth canal (vagina) stretches as the baby travels through it. The head emerges and the baby is delivered. This stage usually lasts for up to 1 hour.

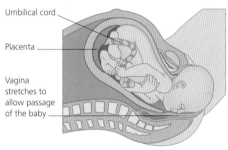

Umbilical cord

Placenta

Vagina stretches to allow passage of the baby

The birth
With the cervix fully dilated, the flexible tissues of the vagina (birth canal) stretch to allow the head to emerge. In most cases, the baby turns to face the mother's back as it travels down the vagina.

THIRD STAGE OF LABOR
The placenta (the organ that nourishes an unborn baby) and the umbilical cord are expelled from the uterus a short time after the baby's birth. The uterus contracts, closing down the area where the placenta was attached; this reduces bleeding.

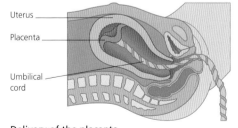

Uterus

Placenta

Umbilical cord

Delivery of the placenta
The placenta comes away from the wall of the uterus 10–30 minutes after the birth of the baby. It moves down the vagina and is pushed out of the mother's body by contractions of the uterus.

CHILDBIRTH: FIRST STAGE

In the first stage of labor, the woman will begin to have contractions – waves of intense pain that peak and then gradually fade away. The amniotic fluid ("water") that cushioned the baby will be discharged at some point during this stage.

Although most pregnant women are aware of what happens during labor, a woman who goes into labor unexpectedly may be very anxious. You will need to reassure her; she will then be more able to remember any coping techniques that she has learned. If you think that the baby may be born before any other help can be summoned, try to gather together a few essential items of equipment for the birth:

RECOGNITION

There may be:

● Contractions, occurring at shortening intervals.

● Bloodstained discharge (the "show") when the mucus plug is expelled.

● Discharge of clear fluid (amniotic fluid). This is known as the water breaking; fluid may flow out from the vagina in a trickle or a rush, depending on the position of the baby.

disposable gloves, mask to cover your mouth and nose (a handkerchief or similar can be used), a plastic sheet, a bowl of hot water for washing, sanitary napkins, clean, warm towels, and a blanket.

✚ YOUR AIMS

● To obtain medical aid or arrange for the woman to be taken to a hospital.

● To reassure the woman and make her comfortable.

1 Call for a doctor or a midwife. If the contractions are rapidly becoming more frequent, or if the hospital is some distance away and cannot be reached quickly DIAL 9·1·1 OR CALL EMS.
Give the dispatcher any information that you have that may affect the labor, and any details of the place where the mother had planned to give birth.

2 Help the mother sit or lie on the floor in a position that is comfortable for her. Lay cushions or pillows on the floor to support her body if necessary.

3 Stay calm and encourage the mother to breathe deeply, or to use any other methods that she prefers, to cope with the pain. Massaging her lower back can help.

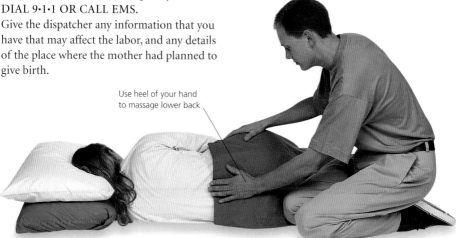

Use heel of your hand to massage lower back

CHILDBIRTH: SECOND STAGE

During the second stage of labor, the baby is delivered (born). At the start of this stage, the cervix (neck of the womb) will be fully dilated (open) and the mother will begin to feel an overwhelming urge to push.

You need to have prepared a comfortable, clean environment for the delivery (*see* CHILDBIRTH: FIRST STAGE, p.233). You also need to take measures to ensure hygiene and prevent infection.

The number of people present at the delivery should be kept to a minimum, but do not exclude anyone whom the mother wishes to be present. You may want to enlist the help of a female friend or relative.

The delivery usually happens naturally. However, as a first aider it will be your responsibility to ensure the baby's comfort and protection once it has been born.

PREVENTING INFECTION

It is extremely important to ensure good hygiene before and during the delivery in order to reduce the risk of the mother, the baby, or yourself contracting an infection. The following precautions should be taken if possible:

RECOGNITION

- Mother experiences an urge to push.
- Strong, frequent contractions due to activity of the uterus.
- Stinging or burning sensation in the vagina as the walls are stretched.
- Emergence of the baby's head at the vaginal opening.
- Rapid delivery of the baby's body.

- Keep anyone with a sore throat, cold, or any other infection well away.
- Wear a mask to cover your mouth and nose. If you do not have a mask, you can improvise by tying a piece of clean fabric, such as a clean handkerchief or a folded triangular bandage, over your face.
- If you are wearing a jacket, remove it. Roll up long sleeves. Wear a plastic apron to cover your clothes if possible.
- Wash your hands and forearms, and scrub your nails thoroughly, for about 5 minutes.
- Put on disposable gloves, if these are available.
- After the baby has been delivered, wash your hands again.

+ YOUR AIMS

- To ensure that the mother is comfortable.
- To prevent infection in the mother, baby, and yourself.
- To care for the baby during and after delivery.

ⓘ CAUTION

- Do not allow the mother to eat because there is a risk that she may vomit. If she is thirsty, allow her to take sips of water.
- Do not pull on the baby's head or shoulders during delivery.
- Do not pull on or cut the umbilical cord.
- Do not smack the baby.

1 Cover the area beneath the mother's body with plastic sheets, newspaper, or towels for warmth and to absorb body fluids.

2 Help her into a comfortable position; a half-sitting position, with the knees raised, may be best. Make sure that her back and shoulders are well supported.

3 If you called 9·1·1 or EMS, check that all important details have been passed on to emergency services, such as the expected delivery date, any medical needs, and the name of the hospital where the mother had planned to give birth.

4 Check that the mother has removed any items of clothing that might interfere with the birth. Cover her lower body with a sheet or blanket if she prefers.

5 Check the position of the baby's head during each contraction.

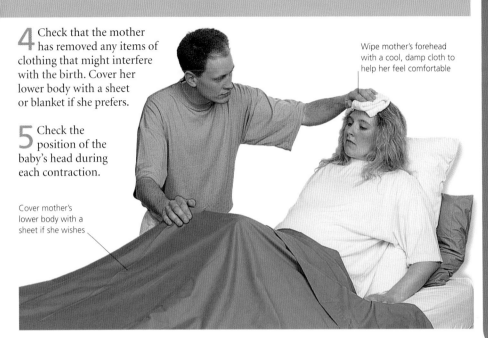

Wipe mother's forehead with a cool, damp cloth to help her feel comfortable

Cover mother's lower body with a sheet if she wishes

6 Once the widest part of the baby's head has emerged at the mother's vaginal opening, advise the mother to stop pushing and start panting.

7 If there is a membrane covering the baby's face, gently move it aside so that he can breathe normally.

8 The baby's shoulders will soon appear. Allow the baby to be expelled naturally. This happens quickly, and you should be ready to hold the baby.

9 Lift the baby away from the vaginal opening. Handle the baby carefully, since newborn babies are very slippery. Pass him to the mother, and lay him on her stomach.

> **❶ WARNING**
>
> If the umbilical cord is wrapped around the baby's neck, you should first check that it is loose, then very carefully pull it over the head to protect the baby from strangulation.

10 The baby may start to cry at this point. If this does not happen, you must check the airway, breathing, and circulation; be prepared to give the baby rescue breaths and chest compressions if necessary (*see* UNCONSCIOUS INFANT, pp.95–98).

11 Dry the baby with a clean cloth. Wrap him carefully in another cloth or a blanket, and give him back to the mother. When laying the baby down, keep him on his side so that any fluid or mucus can drain easily from his nose and mouth.

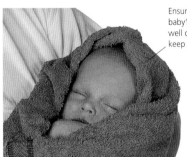

Ensure that baby's head is well covered to keep him warm

CHILDBIRTH: THIRD STAGE

In the third stage of labor, the afterbirth (the placenta and the umbilical cord) is delivered. This stage usually takes place 10–30 minutes after the baby has been born. As the placenta comes away from the wall of the uterus, further contractions occur to constrict the blood vessels in the uterus lining and minimize bleeding. Although the baby has been delivered, the mother still needs your help.

You should collect the afterbirth in a plastic bag so that the medical staff can examine it. The umbilical cord, which may continue to pulsate, should be left uncut until medical help arrives. At the end of the third stage, you should encourage the mother to put the baby to her breast and begin feeding him. This action will also help reduce blood loss by stimulating uterine contractions.

 See also SHOCK pp.120–121

RECOGNITION

- Mild contractions before the afterbirth is expelled.
- Some bleeding from the uterus once the afterbirth has been delivered.

+ YOUR AIMS

- To support the mother while she is delivering the afterbirth.
- To preserve the afterbirth.

❶ WARNING

- Do not pull on the umbilical cord as the afterbirth is being expelled.
- Do not cut the umbilical cord, even when the afterbirth has been delivered.
- Severe bleeding (postpartum or after-delivery hemorrhage) can occur if the uterus does not contract sufficiently when the placenta is detached. Tell emergency services, and treat the mother for shock (pp.120–121).

1 Reassure the mother while she is delivering the afterbirth.

2 Keep the placenta and umbilical cord intact, preferably in a plastic bag. EMS personnel will cut the umbilical cord. The doctor will examine the afterbirth to check that all of it has been expelled; if even a small piece of afterbirth remains inside the uterus, bleeding may continue and infection may develop.

3 It is normal for the mother to bleed slightly as the placenta is expelled. Gently massaging her abdomen, just below the navel, aids the expulsion of the afterbirth, helps the uterus contract, and stops the bleeding.

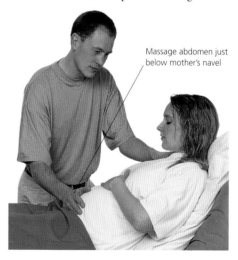

Massage abdomen just below mother's navel

4 Provide warm water, clean towels, and sanitary napkins for the mother. Help her use them if necessary.

5 If bleeding from the uterus is severe, DIAL 9·1·1 OR CALL EMS and treat the mother for shock (pp.120–121).

MISCARRIAGE

A miscarriage is the loss of an unborn baby (fetus or embryo) before the 24th week of pregnancy. The main symptoms are lower abdominal pain and vaginal bleeding. There is a risk of severe bleeding and shock. Some pregnant women experience a "threatened miscarriage," with vaginal bleeding but no loss of the baby; but any woman who seems to be miscarrying must be seen by a doctor.

An affected woman may be frightened and very distressed. Offer as much help as you can without being intrusive. A woman who suspects that she is miscarrying may feel reluctant to confide in a stranger, particularly a man, so a male first aider should seek help from a female assistant.

RECOGNITION

There may be:
● Cramplike pains in the lower abdomen or pelvic area.
● Vaginal bleeding, which may possibly be sudden and profuse.
● Signs of shock (pp.120–121).
● Passage of the fetus or embryo and other tissue from the uterus.

▶ **See also** SHOCK pp.120–121 ● VAGINAL BLEEDING p.143

✚ YOUR AIMS
● To reassure and comfort the woman.
● To obtain medical aid.

1 Reassure the woman. Help her into a comfortable lying or sitting position, with legs bent up. Support her body and legs with pillows.

2 Give the woman a sanitary napkin or a clean towel for the bleeding. Even if the bleeding or pain is only slight, call a doctor.

3 Monitor and record vital signs – level of response, pulse, and breathing (pp.42–43).

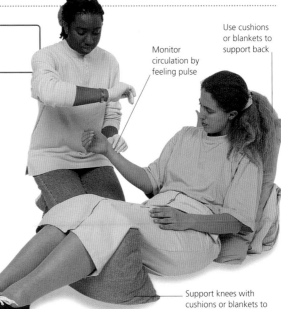

Monitor circulation by feeling pulse

Use cushions or blankets to support back

Support knees with cushions or blankets to ease strain on abdomen

4 If any material is expelled from the vagina, collect it in a plastic bag and give it to the medical services so that it can be examined by a doctor. Keep the material out of the woman's sight, if possible, unless she specifically asks to see it.

⊘ WARNING

If the bleeding or pain is severe,

DIAL 9•1•1 OR CALL EMS.

While waiting for medical help, treat the woman for shock if necessary (pp.120–121).

ALLERGY

An allergic reaction is an abnormal physical sensitivity to a "trigger" substance that is usually harmless, such as a food, a chemical, a drug, or pollen. It occurs when the immune system, which normally fights infection, "attacks" the trigger substance. Allergies may produce various respiratory, digestive, and skin conditions. Examples include asthma (p.115); hay fever; abdominal pain (p.245); vomiting and diarrhea (p.247); "nettle rash" (urticaria); and dermatitis. Some people are at risk of a life-threatening reaction called anaphylactic shock (p.123).

RECOGNITION

Features vary depending on the trigger and the person. There may be one or more of the following symptoms:
- Red, itchy rash or raised areas of skin (wheals).
- Wheezing and difficulty in breathing.
- Abdominal pain.
- Vomiting and diarrhea.

▶ See also ANAPHYLACTIC SHOCK p.123
● ASTHMA p.115 ● VOMITING AND DIARRHEA p.247

YOUR AIMS
- To assess the severity of the allergic reaction.
- To treat symptoms if they are only mild.
- To obtain medical aid if necessary.

⚠ WARNING
If the afflicted person is distressed, or has difficulty breathing,

DIAL 9•1•1 OR CALL EMS.

1 Assess the person's signs and symptoms, and ask him whether he knows that he suffers from an allergy.

2 Treat any symptoms, and help the person take any medication that he has.

3 Advise the person to arrange to consult his doctor. If you are at all concerned about the person's condition, you should call a doctor or EMS.

HICCUPS

This condition is caused by repeated spasms in which the diaphragm (the sheet of muscle that separates the chest cavity from the abdominal cavity) contracts suddenly and, at the same time, the windpipe partially closes. Hiccups are a common problem.

Attacks usually last for only a few minutes, but occasionally they may be prolonged, tiring, and painful. To relieve hiccups, you need to raise the level of carbon dioxide in the blood for a few moments; this should cause normal breathing to resume.

YOUR AIMS
- To help normal breathing to resume.
- To obtain medical aid if necessary.

1 Advise the person to sit quietly and hold his breath for as long as possible.

2 If the hiccups persist, advise the person to place a paper (not plastic) bag over his nose and mouth and to rebreathe the expired air for a few minutes.

3 If the hiccups continue for more than a few hours, you should call a doctor for advice.

FEVER

A sustained body temperature above the normal level of 98.6°F (37°C) is known as fever. It is usually caused by a bacterial or viral infection, and may be associated with measles, chickenpox, meningitis, earache, sore throat, or local infections such as an abscess. Infection may have been acquired during recent travel.

Moderate fever is not harmful, but a fever above 104°F (40°C) can be dangerous and may trigger seizures in very young children (p.186). If you are in any doubt about a person's condition, call a doctor.

RECOGNITION
- Raised temperature.
- Initial pallor.
- A "chilled" feeling – goose bumps, shivering, and chattering teeth.
- Later, hot, flushed skin, and sweating.
- Headache.
- Generalized "aches and pains".

See also HEATSTROKE p.204 ● MENINGITIS p.187 ● OVERSEAS TRAVEL HEALTH pp.249–250 ● SEIZURES IN CHILDREN p.186

YOUR AIMS
- To bring down the fever.
- To obtain medical aid if necessary.

❶ CAUTION
If you are concerned about the person's condition, call a doctor.

1 Keep the person cool and comfortable, preferably in bed with a light covering. Give him plenty of cool, bland drinks to replace body fluids lost through sweating.

2 Adults may take acetaminophen, ibuprofen, or aspirin tablets. Give a child the recommended dose of acetaminophen or ibuprofen (*not* aspirin).

VERTIGO

This disorder is a disturbance of the sense of balance. Vertigo produces an abnormal sensation of movement: the person feels "giddy," as if he is spinning.

The usual causes include infections of the middle or inner ear, and psychological disorders such as acute anxiety. Occasionally, the cause is a more serious condition, such as Ménière's disease (an inner ear disorder).

RECOGNITION
- Sensation of spinning.
- Possible nausea and vomiting.

YOUR AIMS
- To relieve any symptoms.
- To obtain medical aid if necessary.

1 Advise the person to adopt a comfortable sitting or lying position, and note any change in his condition. Ask if he has had vertigo attacks before.

2 If the person has special medication prescribed for vertigo or nausea, advise him to take it; you may need to help him take the medication.

3 Call a doctor if the person is very distressed or if he requests it. Stay with the person and note any further changes in his condition.

DIABETES MELLITUS

In this condition, the body fails to produce sufficient amounts of insulin, a chemical that regulates blood sugar (glucose) levels. As a result, sugar builds up in the blood and can cause hyperglycemia (below). People with diabetes mellitus have to control their blood sugar with diet and insulin injections or pill; too much insulin or too little sugar can cause hypoglycemia (opposite). The chart below enables you to compare these two conditions. If a known diabetic appears unwell, give sugar. This will rapidly correct hypoglycemia and will do little harm in hyperglycemia. Always contact a doctor.

COMPARING HYPERGLYCEMIA AND HYPOGLYCEMIA

Category		Hyperglycemia	Hypoglycemia
History	Recent eating habits	Eaten excessively	Undereaten or missed meals
	Amount of insulin used food eaten	Not enough for amount	Too much for amount of of food eaten
	Speed of onset of symptoms	Gradual	Rapid
Symptoms	Thirst	Present	Absent
	Hunger	Absent	Present
	Vomiting	Common	Uncommon
	Urination	Excessive	Normal
Signs	Odor on the breath	Fruity/sweet	Normal
	Breathing	Rapid	Normal
	Pulse	Rapid and weak	Rapid and strong
	Skin	Warm and dry	Pale and cold, with sweating
	Seizures	Uncommon	Common
	Level of consciousness	Drowsy	Rapid loss of consciousness

HYPERGLYCEMIA

High blood sugar (hyperglycemia) over a long period can result in unconsciousness. Usually, the victim will drift into this state over a few days. Hyperglycemia requires urgent treatment in a hospital.

RECOGNITION

- Warm, dry skin; rapid pulse and breathing.
- Fruity/sweet breath and excessive thirst.
- If untreated, drowsiness, then unconsciousness.

+ YOUR AIM

- To arrange urgent transport of the victim to a hospital.

1 DIAL 9•1•1 OR CALL EMS.
If the victim is unconscious, place him in the recovery position (pp.84–85).

2 Monitor and record vital signs – level of response, pulse, and breathing (pp.42–43).

HYPOGLYCEMIA

When the blood-sugar level falls below normal (hypoglycemia), brain function is affected. This problem is characterized by a rapidly deteriorating level of response. Hypoglycemia can occur in people with diabetes mellitus and, more rarely, appear with an epileptic seizure or after an episode of binge drinking. It can also complicate heat exhaustion or hypothermia.

People with diabetes mellitus may carry their own blood-testing kits with which to check their blood-sugar levels, and are usually well prepared for emergencies. For example, many diabetic people carry sugar lumps or a tube of glucose in gel form in case they feel they are having a "hypo."

If the hypoglycemic attack is at an advanced stage, consciousness may be impaired or lost. Get emergency help.

RECOGNITION

There may be:
- A history of diabetes; the person may recognize the onset of a "hypo" attack.
- Weakness, faintness, or hunger.
- Palpitations and muscle tremors.
- Strange actions or behavior; the person may seem confused or belligerent.
- Sweating and cold, clammy skin.
- Pulse may be rapid and strong.
- Deteriorating level of response.
- Diabetic's medic-alert bracelet, glucose gel, tablets, or an insulin syringe in his possessions.

► See also HEAT EXHAUSTION p.203
● HYPOTHERMIA pp.206–208 ● LIFE-SAVING PROCEDURES pp.71–102 ● SEIZURES IN ADULTS pp.184–185

✚ YOUR AIMS

- To raise the sugar content of the blood as quickly as possible.
- To obtain medical aid if necessary.

❶ WARNING

- If consciousness is impaired, do not give the person anything to eat or drink.
- If the person is unconscious, open the airway and check breathing; be ready to give rescue breaths and chest compressions if necessary (*see* LIFE-SAVING PROCEDURES, pp.71–102). If he is breathing, place him in the recovery position.

DIAL 9•1•1 OR CALL EMS.

Monitor and record the vital signs – level of response, pulse, and breathing (pp.42–43).

1 Help the person to sit or lie down. Give her a sugary drink, sugar lumps, chocolate, or other sweet food; alternatively, if she has her own glucose gel, help her take it.

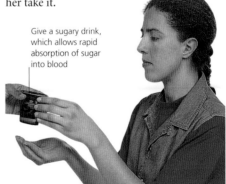

Give a sugary drink, which allows rapid absorption of sugar into blood

2 If she responds quickly, give more food or drink, and let her rest until she feels better. Advise her to see her doctor even if she feels fully recovered. If her condition does not improve, monitor level of response (p.42) and look for other possible causes. Call EMS.

PANIC ATTACK

A panic attack is a sudden bout of extreme anxiety. It produces severe physical symptoms, such as hyperventilation and palpitations (a feeling of an abnormal or fast heart rate), and a feeling of distress. Panic attacks may have no obvious cause or occur in situations that are not normally stressful. If someone is very anxious, check for a history of panic attacks, and ask about any intense fear (phobia), such as a terror of spiders or of being in a crowd.

RECOGNITION

There may be:
- Hyperventilation (over-breathing).
- Muscular tension, producing headache, backache, and a feeling of pressure in the chest.
- Extreme apprehension and fear of dying.
- Trembling, sweating, and dry mouth.
- High pulse rate and sometimes palpitations.

 See also HYPERVENTILATION p.114

YOUR AIMS
- To remove any obvious cause of panic.
- To help the person regain self-control.

CAUTION
- Do not slap the person's face.
- Do not try to restrain the person.

1 Try to find out and remove the cause of the fear. Take the person to a quiet area. Reassure him and explain that he is having a panic attack if he does not already know.

2 Encourage him to breathe more slowly. If he is hyperventilating, advise him to breathe into a paper bag (*see* HYPER-VENTILATION, p.114). Stay with him until he has recovered. Advise him to seek medical help. If you have any concerns, call EMS.

DISTURBED BEHAVIOR

There are many reasons why a person may behave in an abnormal or aggressive way. Some people become irrational in stressful situations. Disturbed behavior can also be due to alcohol or drug abuse; the use of certain prescribed drugs; or certain physical disorders, such as hypoglycemia, epilepsy, or head injuries. Other possible causes include mental disorders such as anxiety, psychosis, and dementia.

See also DRUG POISONING p.222
- HEAD INJURY p.179 - HYPOGLYCEMIA p.241

YOUR AIMS
- To help the person resume normal behavior.
- To obtain medical aid if necessary.

CAUTION
- If the person is aggressive, do not put yourself in danger. Make sure that you can retreat rapidly if necessary.
- Do not try to restrain the person.

1 Talk calmly to the person and, if you can, try to find out the cause of the problem. Do not argue with him, because this may worsen the situation.

2 Call a doctor (if possible, the person's own). If necessary, call the police.

EARACHE

This common condition results from inflammation of the tissues inside the ear or from blockage in the ear. It may be accompanied by partial or total hearing loss, which is usually temporary.

The most common cause of an earache, particularly in children, is an ear infection. Pain in the ear can also be caused by a boil, a foreign object stuck in the ear canal, or another condition such as an abscess in a nearby tooth. In addition, earaches often occur on airplane journeys due to changes in cabin air pressure during the plane's ascent and descent.

Occasionally, infection causes pus to collect in the middle ear. The eardrum may then rupture, allowing the pus to drain from the ear; this will temporarily ease the pain.

▶ **See also** FOREIGN OBJECT IN THE EAR p.215 ● TOOTHACHE p.244

✚ YOUR AIMS
- To relieve pain.
- To obtain medical aid if necessary.

❶ CAUTION
If there is a discharge, fever, or marked hearing loss, obtain medical help.

1 Adults may take acetaminophen, ibuprofen, or aspirin tablets. Give a child the recommended dose of acetaminophen or ibuprofen (*not* aspirin).

2 Make the victim comfortable. Give her a source of heat, such as a hot-water bottle wrapped in a towel, to hold against the affected ear. If lying flat makes the pain worse, prop her up with pillows.

SPECIAL CASE

AIR TRAVEL
If earache occurs during air travel, help the person to equalize the pressure in her ears by making the ears "pop." Advise her to swallow with her mouth open; alternatively, tell her to close her mouth, hold her nose tightly closed, and "blow" her nose. If this does not help, reassure the person that the pain will go away when the pressure inside the middle ear is reduced as the aircraft lands.

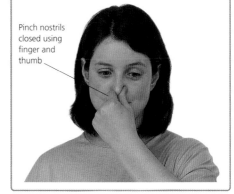

Pinch nostrils closed using finger and thumb

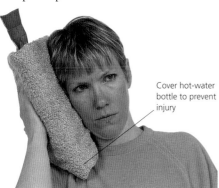

Cover hot-water bottle to prevent injury

3 Advise the person to see her doctor. If you are worried about her condition (particularly if the person is a child), obtain medical help.

TOOTHACHE

Pain may occur either in the teeth or in the gums. Persistent toothache is usually caused by a decayed tooth and can be made worse by hot or cold food or drinks.

Throbbing toothache indicates an infection at the root of a tooth. Infection can also cause swelling of the gums in the painful area and bad breath. Pain in the teeth can sometimes be due to disorders affecting the facial nerves, such as sinusitis, or an ear infection.

 See also EARACHE p.243

YOUR AIMS

- To relieve pain.
- To ensure that the person consults a dentist.

1 Adults may take acetaminophen, ibuprofen, or aspirin tablets. Give a child the recommended dose of acetaminophen or ibuprofen (*not* aspirin).

2 Make the person comfortable. If lying down makes the toothache worse, prop her up with pillows.

3 To help relieve pain, give the person a hot-water bottle wrapped in a towel to hold against her face, and/or give her a rolled-up plug of gauze soaked in oil of cloves to hold against the affected tooth.

Person should hold plug against affected tooth

4 Advise the person to make an appointment with her dentist.

SORE THROAT

The most common type of sore throat is a rough or "raw" feeling, which is caused by inflammation. This problem is often the first sign of a cough or cold, and usually passes within a day or two. A more serious condition, called tonsillitis, occurs when the tonsils, at the back of the throat, become infected with bacteria or a virus. The tonsils are swollen and red, and ulcers or white spots of pus may be seen. Swallowing may be difficult, and the glands at the angle of the jaw may be enlarged and sore.

See also FEVER p.239

YOUR AIMS

- To relieve pain.
- To obtain medical aid if necessary.

1 Give the person plenty of fluids to drink, to ease the pain and stop the throat from becoming dry.

2 Adults may take acetaminophen, ibuprofen, or aspirin tablets. Give a child the recommended dose of acetaminophen or ibuprofen (*not* aspirin).

3 If you suspect that the person has tonsillitis, advise her to see a doctor as soon as possible.

ABDOMINAL PAIN

Pain in the abdomen often has a relatively minor cause, such as food poisoning. However, it can occasionally be a sign of a serious disorder affecting the organs and other structures in the abdomen.

Distension (widening) or obstruction of the intestine causes colic – pain that comes and goes in "waves." It often makes the victim double up in agony and may be accompanied by vomiting. If the appendix bursts, or the intestine is damaged, the contents of the intestine can leak into the abdominal cavity, causing inflammation of the cavity lining. This life-threatening condition, called peritonitis, causes sudden, intense pain, which is made worse by movement or pressure on the abdomen, and will lead to shock (pp.120–121).

APPENDICITIS
An inflamed appendix (appendicitis) is especially common in children. Symptoms include pain (often starting in the center of the abdomen and moving to the lower right-hand side), nausea, vomiting, bad breath, and fever. If the appendix bursts, peritonitis will develop. The treatment is urgent surgical removal of the appendix.

 See also FOOD POISONING p.224

YOUR AIMS

- To relieve pain and discomfort.
- To obtain medical aid if necessary.

1 Make the victim comfortable, and prop her up if breathing is difficult. Give her a container to use if she is vomiting.

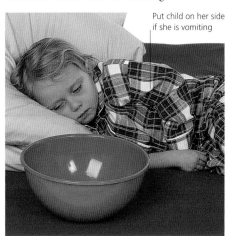

Put child on her side if she is vomiting

2 Give the victim a hot-water bottle wrapped in a towel for her to place against her abdomen.

SPECIAL CASE

WINDED VICTIM
A blow to the upper abdomen may stun a local nerve junction, causing a temporary breathing problem called "winding." To treat a winded victim, help him to sit down, and loosen clothing at the chest and waist. The victim should recover rapidly.

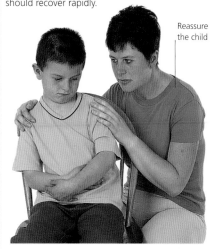

Reassure the child

3 If the pain is severe, or occurs with fever and vomiting, call a doctor. Do not give medicine or allow her to eat, drink, or smoke, because a general anesthetic may be needed.

HERNIA

A hernia, commonly called a rupture, is a soft swelling in the abdomen or the groin. It occurs when a small loop of intestine, or other tissue, pushes through a weak area of muscle in the abdominal wall. The disorder may result from increased muscle pressure due to persistent coughing, straining during bowel movements, or lifting heavy weights.

A hernia may or may not be painful. If the person has a painless lump, no first aid is necessary; simply reassure him and advise him to see a doctor as soon as possible. However, vomiting and severe pain indicate that part of the intestine has become trapped and deprived of blood (a condition called a strangulated hernia). This problem needs urgent surgery.

RECOGNITION

There may be:
- Bulge or swelling in abdominal wall or groin, which may disappear when the victim lies flat.
- Dragging or aching sensation in the abdomen or groin.
- Pain in the abdomen or groin.
- Vomiting.

✚ YOUR AIMS

- To reassure the person.
- To relieve any discomfort.
- To obtain medical aid.

❶ CAUTION

- Do not attempt to push the swelling back or allow the person to do so. This may increase the risk of damage to the intestine.
- Do not give the person any medicines or allow him to eat, drink, or smoke, because a general anesthetic may need to be given in hospital.

1 If the person is in pain, help him to sit down, and support him in the position he finds most comfortable by propping him up with cushions or pillows.

2 Call a doctor or, if the pain is severe, DIAL 9·1·1 OR CALL EMS.

3 While you are waiting for medical aid, continue to reassure the casualty. Monitor his vital signs – level of response, pulse, and breathing (pp.42–43) – until help arrives.

Provide support from behind with a pillow

Person with abdominal pain may prefer to bend his knees

Support the knees with a folded pillow or rolled-up jacket

VOMITING AND DIARRHEA

These problems are usually due to irritation of the digestive system. This can be caused by unusual or rich foods; alcohol; certain medications; contaminated foods or drinks; or an allergic reaction.

Vomiting and diarrhea may occur either separately or together. Both conditions can cause the body to lose vital fluids and salts, resulting in dehydration. When they occur together, the risk of dehydration is increased and can be serious, especially in infants, young children, and elderly people.

The main aim of treatment is to help restore the lost fluids and salts. Water is sufficient in most cases, but nonfizzy, "isotonic" glucose drinks are ideal if they are available. Alternatively, add salt (1 teaspoonful per quart) and sugar (4–5 teaspoonfuls per quart) to water or to diluted orange juice.

See also DRUG POISONING p.222 ● FOOD POISONING p.224 ● SWALLOWED POISONS p.220

YOUR AIMS
● To reassure the person.
● To restore lost fluids and salts.

CAUTION
If you are worried about the person's condition, particularly if the vomiting or diarrhea is persistent, call a doctor.

1 Reassure the person if he is vomiting. Afterwards, give him a warm, damp cloth to wipe his face.

2 Give the person plenty of clear fluids to sip in small amounts slowly and often.

3 If the person's appetite returns, give only easily digested, nonspicy foods for the first 24 hours.

STITCH

This common condition is a form of cramp that occurs in the trunk or the sides of the chest. A stitch is usually associated with exercise. The most likely cause of the cramp is an accumulation of chemical waste products, such as lactic acid, in the muscles during physical exertion. The pain of a stitch can be like that of angina pectoris (p.124), but it is usually sharper.

RECOGNITION
● Cramplike pains in the side of the chest and muscles of the trunk.
● History of recent physical exertion.

See also ABDOMINAL PAIN p.245 ● ANGINA PECTORIS p.124

YOUR AIM
● To help relieve the symptoms.

1 Help the person to sit down, and reassure him. The pain will usually ease quickly.

2 If the pain does not disappear within a few minutes, or if you are concerned about the person's condition, call a doctor.

CRAMP

This condition is a sudden, painful spasm (contraction) in one or more muscles. It commonly occurs during sleep. It can also develop after strenuous exercise, due to a buildup of chemical waste products in the muscles, or to excessive loss of salt and fluids from the body through sweating. A cramp can often be relieved by stretching and massaging the affected muscle.

▶ **See also** HEAT EXHAUSTION p.203
● STITCH p.247

CRAMP IN THE FOOT

+ YOUR AIM
● To help relieve the spasm and pain.

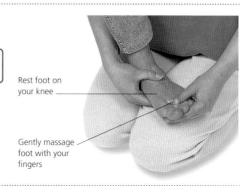

Rest foot on your knee

Gently massage foot with your fingers

1 Help the person stand with her weight on the front of her foot.

2 Once the first spasm has passed, massage the affected area of the foot.

CRAMP IN THE CALF

+ YOUR AIM
● To help relieve the spasm and pain.

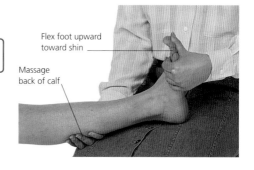

Flex foot upward toward shin

Massage back of calf

1 Straighten the person's knee and support the foot.

2 Flex the foot toward the shin to stretch the calf muscles, then massage the area.

CRAMP IN THE THIGH

+ YOUR AIM
● To help relieve the spasm and pain.

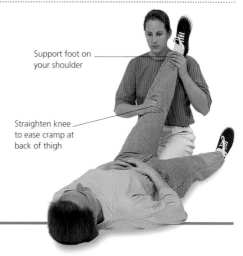

Support foot on your shoulder

Straighten knee to ease cramp at back of thigh

1 Help the person lie down. To ease a cramp in the back of the thigh, raise the leg and straighten the knee. For a cramp in the front of the thigh, bend the knee.

2 Support the leg and massage the affected thigh muscle gently but firmly with your fingers until the pain eases.

OVERSEAS TRAVEL HEALTH

With the increase in travel, many people are now at risk from diseases that are either not commonly encountered in their own country or pose a greater risk in other countries. Being in a hot climate can create problems such as heat exhaustion. It is important to understand any potential health risks, how they can be prevented or reduced, and how to respond to some of the medical emergencies that might arise.

PLANNING AHEAD

Many conditions can be avoided. You should consult your doctor well in advance of your planned departure – preferably at least 2 months – to allow sufficient time to arrange any immunizations that you may need. However, do see your doctor even if you have to travel abroad at short notice – some protection may be better than none. You should tell your doctor:

● Where you are going, including any countries that you may visit en route.
● If you are or may become pregnant, as some medicines will be unsuitable for you.
● If you are taking children with you. This is especially important if any of the children have not completed their full course of childhood immunizations.

▶ See also POISONING, BITES, AND STINGS pp.217–230 ● HEAT EXHAUSTION p.203 ● HEATSTROKE p.204 ● SUNBURN p.202 ● VOMITING AND DIARRHEA p.247

FOOD- AND WATERBORNE INFECTIONS

Infection due to consuming contaminated food or water is one of the most common problems affecting travelers. You can reduce the risk by taking the following precautions: wash your hands after using the toilet and before eating; avoid food that has been kept warm; do not eat raw vegetables, salads, shellfish, or ice cream; and peel all fruit yourself. If you are in any doubt about the safety of drinking water, boil it, sterilize it with disinfectant tablets, or use bottled water supplied in sealed containers.

RECOGNIZING AND TREATING FOOD- AND WATERBORNE INFECTIONS

Disorder	Recognition	Action
Traveler's diarrhea Spread through food and water that is contaminated with one of several disease-causing microorganisms.	● Nausea and vomiting ● Diarrhea ● Abdominal pain	● Restore lost body fluids ● Careful hygiene to prevent spread of infection ● Seek medical advice if symptoms persist
Hepatitis A Spread through contaminated food or water. The infection may spread from person to person, especially if sanitation is poor. Protection by immunization is available	● Abdominal pain ● Raised temperature ● Yellowing of the whites of the eyes (jaundice) and skin after several days	● Seek medical advice ● Relieve the fever, but do NOT give acetaminophen ● Careful hygiene to prevent spread of infection
Cholera Spread through contaminated water, this infection can cause fatal dehydration.	● Profuse diarrhea ● Weakness and dehydration ● Nausea and vomiting	● Seek urgent medical advice ● Restore lost body fluids ● Careful hygiene to prevent spread of infection

OVERSEAS TRAVEL HEALTH (continued)

OTHER INFECTIONS AND DISORDERS

In addition to water and food-borne infections, travelers may be at risk of diseases from insects and ticks, and from unprotected sex. Simple steps should help to prevent infection.

INSECT-BORNE DISEASES

Mosquitoes are carriers of infections such as malaria and yellow fever in certain areas. Protect yourself by covering arms and legs after sunset, using mosquito repellent, and sleeping under a mosquito net. Take antimalarial medication where advised.

BLOOD-BORNE INFECTION

Abstinence from sex with a new partner is the safest way to avoid the risk of sexually transmitted infections, but you can reduce the risk by using condoms.

Any procedure in which the skin is pierced may also carry the risk of infection. Do not have a tattoo, acupuncture, or body piercing when overseas. Try to avoid having injections or surgical or dental treatment, but if you cannot, ask about sterilization of equipment. If you need a blood transfusion, check that only screened blood is used.

RECOGNIZING AND TREATING INSECT- AND BLOOD-BORNE ILLNESSES

Disorder	Recognition	Action
Hepatitis B and C Both occur worldwide. Spread through unprotected sex; sharing contaminated needles or syringes; needle-stick injury; transfusions of contaminated blood; using inadequately sterilized medical, dental, tattooing, or piercing equipment.	• May be no immediate signs • Loss of appetite • Abdominal discomfort • Nausea and vomiting • Sometimes, jaundice (yellowing of the skin/whites of the eyes)	• Seek urgent medical aid • Restore lost body fluids • Careful hygiene to prevent spread of infection
Lyme disease Contracted from infected ticks. No evidence of transmission from person to person.	• Stiff neck • Fever • Severe headache	• Seek urgent medical aid • Relieve fever
Malaria The parasite is spread by the bites of infected mosquitoes. Antimalarial drugs must be taken as directed.	• Fever • Headache	• Seek urgent medical aid • Relieve fever
Rabies A serious viral infection that is transmitted via a bite from an infected dog, bat, or other animal. Immunization is available for workers in high-risk employment.	• Headache • Fever • Excitability • Fear – particularly of water • Seizures and delirium	• Immediate, thorough cleansing of wound • Seek urgent medical aid • Saliva is infective: wear gloves and masks and incinerate soiled items
Yellow fever Viral disease transmitted by the bites of infected mosquitoes. Immunization is available.	• Headache and fever • Jaundice (yellowing of the skin/whites of the eyes) • May progress to bleeding from nose, gums, and intestines	• Seek urgent medical aid • Relieve fever • Careful hygiene to prevent spread of infection

13

THIS SECTION is a quick-reference guide to first-aid measures for people with serious illnesses or injuries. It begins with a plan of action to help you determine how to deal with an emergency effectively. The section then describes resuscitation procedures for unconscious victims. It is followed by first-aid treatment for people with serious or potentially life-threatening conditions. Observation charts are included for you to complete when monitoring a person.

HOW TO USE THIS SECTION

Recognition lists help you to identify condition quickly

Cross-references direct you to extra useful information

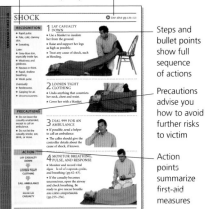

Steps and bullet points show full sequence of actions

Precautions advise you how to avoid further risks to victim

Action points summarize first-aid measures

CONTENTS

Action in an emergency 252

Unconscious adult 254

Unconscious child
(1–7 years) 258

Unconscious infant
(under 1 year) 262

Choking adult 264

Choking child
(1–7 years) 265

Choking infant
(under 1 year) 266

Asthma attack 267

Shock 268

Anaphylactic shock 269

Severe bleeding 270

Heart attack 271

Head injury 272

Spinal injury 273

Seizures in adults 274

Seizures in children 275

Broken bones 276

Burns 277

Eye injury 278

Swallowed poisons 279

Observation charts 280

ACTION IN AN EMERGENCY

1 ASSESS SITUATION
- Are there any risks to you or the victim?

`YES`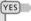

- Put your safety first. If possible, remove the danger from the victim or, if this is not possible, remove the victim from danger.
- If it is unsafe, call for emergency help and wait for it to arrive.

`NO`

2 CHECK VICTIM
- Is the victim visibly conscious?

`YES`

- Check for other conditions (opposite) and treat as necessary.
- Summon help if needed.

`NO`

3 CHECK RESPONSE
- Does the victim respond to your voice or to gentle stimulation?

`YES`

- Check for other conditions (opposite) and treat as necessary.
- Summon help if needed.

`NO`

4 OPEN AIRWAY; CHECK BREATHING
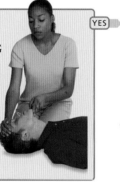
- Open and, if necessary, clear the victim's airway and check for breathing (see p.254 for an adult; p.258 for a child; p.262 for an infant).
- Is the victim breathing?

`YES`

- Place the victim in the recovery position (see p.257 for an adult; p.261 for a child; p.262 for an infant).

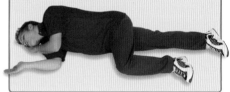

`NO`

ARE YOU ALONE?

`YES`

- Is the unconsciousness due to injury, drowning, or choking, or is the victim a child or an infant?

`NO`

`NO` / `YES`

- Ask a helper to call 9•1•1 or EMS and to pass on details of the victim's condition.

▶ Move on to STEP 5

- Call 9•1•1 or EMS immediately.

▶ Move on to STEP 5

▶ Move on to STEP 5 Carry out the resuscitation sequence for 1 minute before calling 9•1•1 or EMS.

5 RESCUE BREATHING

● Give two effective rescue breaths (*see* p.255 for an adult; p.259 for a child; p.263 for an infant).

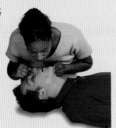

❶ WARNING

If at any stage the victim begins breathing, place him in the recovery position (*see* p.257 for an adult; p.261 for a child; p.262 for an infant).

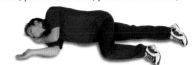

6 ASSESS FOR CIRCULATION

● Check for signs of circulation for no more than 10 seconds (*see* p.255 for an adult; p.259 for a child; p.263 for an infant).
● Are there any signs of circulation?

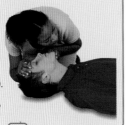

YES

● Continue with rescue breaths.
● Recheck for signs of circulation after every 10 breaths for an adult or 20 breaths for a child (about 1 minute).

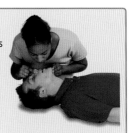

NO

7 BEGIN CPR

● ADULT: Alternate 15 chest compressions with two rescue breaths (p.256); repeat as needed.
● CHILD/INFANT: Give five compressions to one rescue breath (*see* p.260 for a child; p.263 for an infant).

● Continue CPR until emergency help takes over; the victim moves or takes a breath; or you are too exhausted to continue.

TREATMENTS FOR OTHER CONDITIONS

See the following pages for step-by-step treatments:

Anaphylactic shock..269	Choking adult........... 264	Head injury.................272	Severe bleeding.........270
Asthma attack...........267	Choking child............265	Heart attack................271	Shock 268
Broken bones............ 276	Choking infant..........266	Seizures in adults......274	Spinal injury...............273
Burns...........................277	Eye injury....................278	Seizures in children 275	Swallowed poisons...279

UNCONSCIOUS ADULT
ASSESS THE VICTIM

▶ See also pp.76–77

1 CHECK RESPONSE

• Ask a question, such as "What happened?", or give a command, such as "Open your eyes." Speak loudly and clearly.

• Gently shake the victim's shoulders.

• If there is a response, leave the victim in the position found and summon help, if needed. Treat any condition found.

• If there is no response, shout for help, then proceed to step 2.

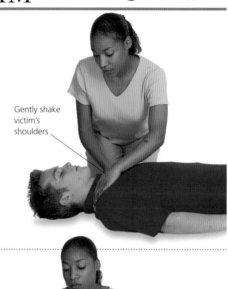

Gently shake victim's shoulders

2 OPEN AIRWAY

• Place one hand on the victim's forehead, and gently tilt his head back.

• Pick out any obvious obstructions from the victim's mouth. Do not do a finger sweep.

• Place the fingertips under the point of the victim's chin. Lift the chin.

• If you suspect a neck (spinal) injury, open the airway by gently lifting the jaw but not tilting the head (jaw thrust).

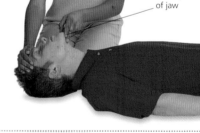

Place fingers under point of jaw

3 CHECK BREATHING

• Look for chest movement, listen for sounds of breathing, and feel for breath on your cheek. Do this for no more than 10 seconds.

• If the victim is not breathing, send a helper to
DIAL 9·1·1 OR CALL EMS.
Begin rescue breathing (opposite).

• If he is breathing, check for life-threatening conditions such as severe bleeding. Place him in the recovery position (p.257).

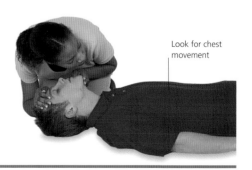

Look for chest movement

GIVE RESCUE BREATHS

See also pp.78–79

1 MAKE SURE THAT AIRWAY IS STILL OPEN

• Make sure that the victim's head remains tilted, by keeping one hand on his forehead and two fingers of the other hand under the tip of his chin.

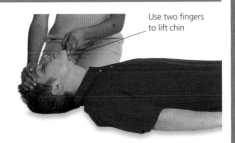

Use two fingers to lift chin

2 PINCH NOSE AND OPEN MOUTH

• Use your thumb and index finger to pinch the soft part of the victim's nose firmly.

• Make sure that his nostrils are closed to prevent air from escaping.

• Open his mouth.

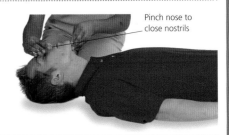

Pinch nose to close nostrils

3 GIVE RESCUE BREATHS

• Use a pocket mask or plastic face shield if possible. Take a deep breath to fill your lungs with air. Place your lips around the victim's lips, forming a good seal.

• Blow steadily into the mouth until the chest rises. This usually takes about 2 seconds. Maintaining head tilt and chin lift, take your mouth away and watch the chest fall. If the chest rises visibly and falls fully, you have given an effective breath. Give two effective breaths.

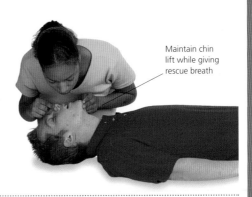

Maintain chin lift while giving rescue breath

4 ASSESS FOR SIGNS OF CIRCULATION

• Look, listen, and feel for signs of circulation, such as breathing, coughing, or movement, for no more than 10 seconds.

• If circulation is absent, perform CPR (p.256).

• If circulation is present, continue with rescue breaths. After every 10 breaths (about 1 minute), recheck for circulation.

• If the victim starts breathing but remains unconscious, place him in the recovery position (p.257).

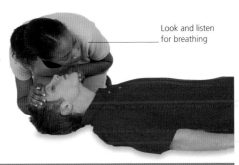

Look and listen for breathing

UNCONSCIOUS ADULT
COMMENCE CPR

▶ **See also** pp.80–81

1 POSITION HANDS FOR CHEST COMPRESSIONS

• Compressions are administered to the center of the chest. The following steps are the most accurate method for locating the best spot for compressions.

• With the index and middle fingers of your lower hand, locate one of the victim's lowermost ribs on the side nearest you. Slide your fingertips along the rib to where it meets the breastbone. Place your middle finger here and the index finger beside it on the breastbone.

• Place the heel of your other hand on the breastbone; slide it down to meet your index finger. This is the point at which you will apply pressure.

• Place the heel of your first hand on top of the other hand, and interlock your fingers.

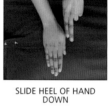

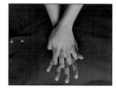

SLIDE HEEL OF HAND DOWN

INTERLOCK FINGERS

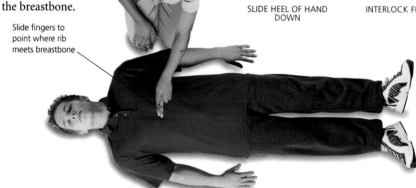

Slide fingers to point where rib meets breastbone

2 GIVE CHEST COMPRESSIONS AND RESCUE BREATHS

• Lean well over the victim, with your arms straight. Press down vertically on the breastbone, and depress the chest by about 1½–2in (4–5cm).

• Compress the chest 15 times, at a rate of 100 compressions per minute.

• Tilt the head, lift the chin, and give two rescue breaths (p.255).

• Alternate 15 chest compressions with two rescue breaths.

• Continue CPR until emergency help takes over; the victim makes a movement or takes a breath; or you are too exhausted to continue.

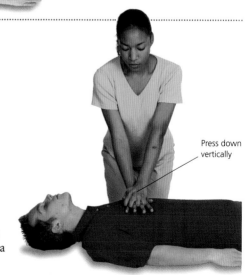

Press down vertically

RECOVERY POSITION

▶ **See also** pp.84–85

1 POSITION ARM AND STRAIGHTEN LEGS

- Kneel beside the victim.

- Remove glasses and any bulky objects (such as mobile phones or large bunches of keys) from the pockets. Straighten his legs.

- Place the arm nearest you at right angles to the victim's body, with the elbow bent and the palm facing upward.

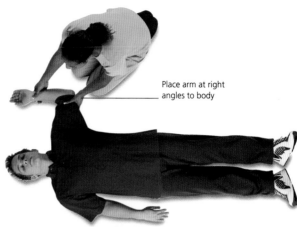

Place arm at right angles to body

2 POSITION FAR ARM, HAND, AND KNEE

- Bring the arm farthest from you across the victim's chest and hold the back of his hand against the cheek nearest you.

- Using your other hand, grasp the far leg just above the knee and pull it up until the foot is flat on the floor.

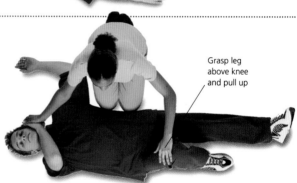

Grasp leg above knee and pull up

3 ROLL VICTIM TOWARD YOU

- Keeping the victim's hand pressed against his cheek, pull on the far leg and roll him toward you and onto his side.

- Adjust the upper leg so that both the hip and knee are bent at right angles.

- Tilt the head back to ensure that the airway remains open.

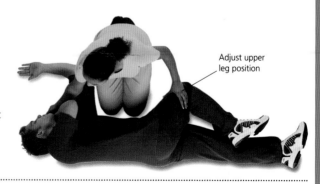

Adjust upper leg position

4 DIAL 9•1•1 OR CALL EMS, IF NOT ALREADY DONE

- Ideally, ask a helper to make the call while you wait with the victim.

- Monitor and record vital signs (pp.42–43) – level of response, pulse, and breathing.

ASSESS THE CHILD

▶ See also pp.87–88

1 CHECK RESPONSE

● Ask the child a question, such as "Can you hear me?" Speak loudly and clearly.

● Gently tap her on the shoulder.

● If there is a response, leave the child in the position found and summon help, if needed. Treat any condition found.

● If there is no response, shout for help, then proceed to step 2.

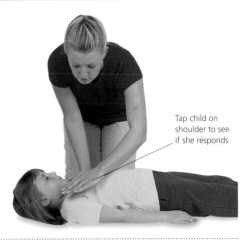

Tap child on shoulder to see if she responds

2 OPEN AIRWAY

● Place one hand on the child's forehead. Gently tilt the head back.

● Using your fingertips, pick out any obvious obstructions from the child's mouth. Do not do a finger sweep.

● Place the fingertips under the point of the child's chin. Lift the chin.

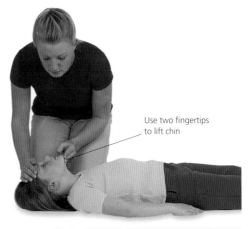

Use two fingertips to lift chin

3 CHECK BREATHING

● Look, listen, and feel for breathing: look for chest movement, listen for sounds of breathing, and feel for breath on your cheek. Do this for no more than 10 seconds.

● If the child is not breathing, send a helper to DIAL 9·1·1 OR CALL EMS. Begin rescue breathing (opposite).

● If she is breathing, check for life-threatening conditions such as severe bleeding. Place the child in the recovery position (p.261).

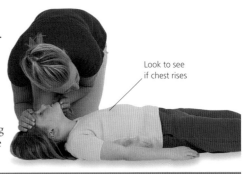

Look to see if chest rises

EMERGENCY FIRST AID

GIVE RESCUE BREATHS

 See also p.89

1 MAKE SURE THAT AIRWAY IS STILL OPEN

● Make sure that the child's head remains tilted, by keeping one hand on her forehead and two fingers of the other hand under her chin.

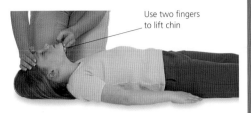

Use two fingers to lift chin

2 PINCH NOSE AND OPEN MOUTH

● Use your thumb and index finger to pinch the soft part of the child's nose firmly. Make sure that her nostrils are closed to prevent air from escaping.

● Open the child's mouth.

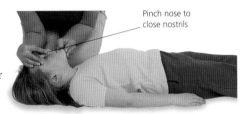

Pinch nose to close nostrils

3 GIVE RESCUE BREATHS

● Use a pocket mask or plastic face shield if available. Take a deep breath to fill your lungs with air. Place your lips around the child's lips, forming an airtight seal.

● Blow steadily into the mouth until the chest rises. Maintaining head tilt and chin lift, take your mouth away and watch the chest fall. If the chest rises visibly and falls fully, you have given an effective breath. Give two effective rescue breaths.

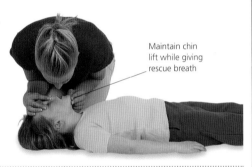

Maintain chin lift while giving rescue breath

4 ASSESS FOR SIGNS OF CIRCULATION

● Look, listen, and feel for signs of circulation, such as breathing, coughing, or movement, for no more than 10 seconds.

● If circulation is absent, perform CPR (p.260) for 1 minute, then DIAL 9·1·1 OR CALL EMS.

● If circulation is present, give 20 rescue breaths in 1 minute, then DIAL 9·1·1 OR CALL EMS.

● If the child starts breathing but remains unconscious, place her in the recovery position (p.261).

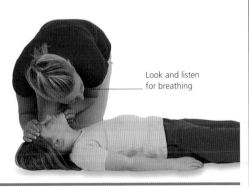

Look and listen for breathing

COMMENCE CPR

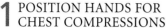 **See also** pp.90–91

1 POSITION HANDS FOR CHEST COMPRESSIONS

● Compressions are administered to the center of the chest. The following steps are the most accurate method for locating the best spot for compressions.

● With the index and middle fingers of your lower hand, locate one of the child's lowermost ribs on that side. Slide your fingertips along the rib to the point at which it meets the breastbone. Place your middle finger there and the index finger beside it.

● Place the heel of your other hand on the breastbone; slide it down to meet your index finger. You will apply pressure here.

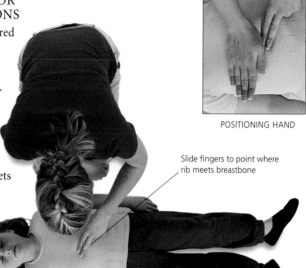

POSITIONING HAND

Slide fingers to point where rib meets breastbone

2 GIVE CHEST COMPRESSIONS AND RESCUE BREATHS

● Use the heel of only one hand to apply pressure. Lift your fingers to ensure that you do not apply pressure to the child's ribs.

● Lean well over the child, with your arm straight. Press down vertically on the breastbone, and depress the chest by 1–1½ in (2½–4 cm).

● Compress the chest five times, at a rate of 100 compressions per minute.

● Give one rescue breath (p.259).

● Continue to alternate five chest compressions with one rescue breath for 1 minute. Then DIAL 9·1·1 OR CALL EMS.

● Continue CPR until emergency help takes over; the child makes a movement or takes a spontaneous breath; or you become too exhausted to continue.

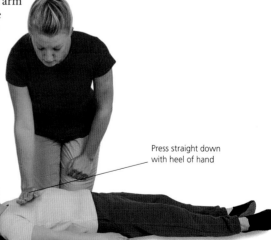

Press straight down with heel of hand

RECOVERY POSITION

● See also pp.92–93

1 POSITION ARM AND STRAIGHTEN LEGS

- Kneel beside the victim.

- Remove glasses and any bulky objects from the pockets.

- Straighten her legs.

- Place the arm nearest you at right angles to the child's body, with the elbow bent and the palm facing upward.

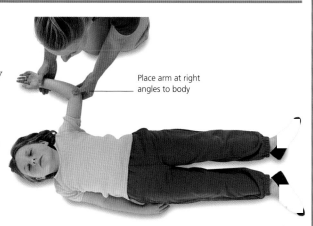

Place arm at right angles to body

2 POSITION FAR ARM, HAND, AND KNEE

- Bring the arm farthest from you across the child's chest.

- Hold the back of her hand against the cheek nearest you.

- Using your other hand, grasp the far leg just above the knee and pull it up until the foot is flat on the floor.

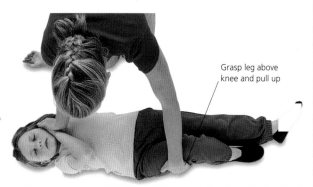

Grasp leg above knee and pull up

3 ROLL CHILD TOWARD YOU

- Keeping the child's hand pressed against her cheek, pull on the far leg and roll her toward you and onto her side.

- Adjust the child's upper leg so that both the hip and the knee are bent at right angles.

- Tilt her head back to ensure that the airway remains open.

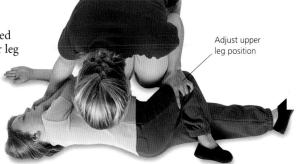

Adjust upper leg position

4 DIAL 9·1·1 OR CALL EMS, IF NOT ALREADY DONE

- Monitor and record vital signs – level of response, pulse, and breathing (pp.42–43).

UNCONSCIOUS INFANT (UNDER 1 YEAR)
ASSESS THE INFANT

▶ See also pp.95–96

1 CHECK RESPONSE

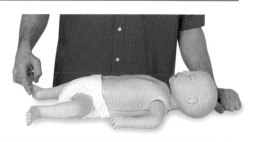

- Gently tap or flick the sole of the infant's foot. Never shake an infant.

- If there is a response, take the baby with you to summon help if needed.

- If no response, shout for help; go to step 2.

2 OPEN AIRWAY

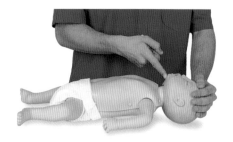

- Place one hand on the infant's forehead, and very gently tilt the head back.

- Using your fingertips, pick out any obvious obstructions. Do not do a finger sweep.

- Place one fingertip under the point of the infant's chin. Lift the chin.

3 CHECK BREATHING

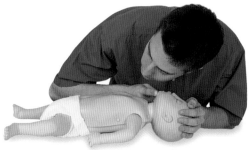

- Look for chest movement, listen for sounds of breathing, and feel for breath on your cheek. Do this for no more than 10 seconds.

- If the infant is not breathing, send a helper to DIAL 9·1·1 OR CALL EMS. Begin rescue breathing (opposite).

- If the infant is breathing, check for injuries and hold in the recovery position (below).

UNCONSCIOUS INFANT (UNDER 1 YEAR)
RECOVERY POSITION

▶ See also p.98

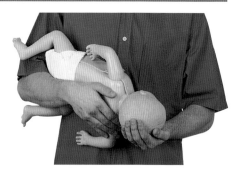

- Cradle the infant in your arms, with his head tilted downward to prevent him from choking on his tongue or inhaling vomit.

- Monitor and record vital signs – level of response, pulse, and breathing (pp.42–43) – until medical help arrives.

GIVE RESCUE BREATHS

▶ See also pp.96–97

1 GIVE RESCUE BREATHS

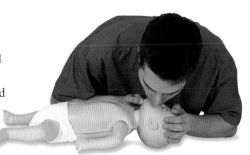

- Make sure that the airway remains open, by keeping the infant's head tilted back and the chin lifted.

- Take a deep breath. Place your lips around the infant's mouth and nose. Blow steadily until the chest rises. Take your mouth away and watch the chest fall. Give two effective breaths.

2 ASSESS FOR SIGNS OF CIRCULATION

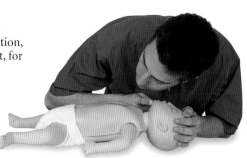

- Look, listen, and feel for signs of circulation, such as breathing, coughing, or movement, for no more than 10 seconds.

- If circulation is absent, perform CPR (below) for 1 minute, then DIAL 9·1·1 OR CALL EMS.

- If circulation is present, give 20 rescue breaths in 1 minute, then DIAL 9·1·1 OR CALL EMS.

COMMENCE CPR

▶ See also p.98

1 POSITION FINGERS FOR CHEST COMPRESSIONS

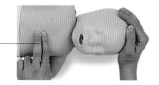

Place fingertips on lower breastbone

- With the baby on her back on a flat surface, place your index finger at the level of the nipples and your middle finger next to it.

2 GIVE CHEST COMPRESSIONS AND RESCUE BREATHS

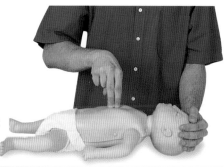

- Press down vertically on the chest, depressing it by ½–¾ in (1¼–2 cm). Do this five times, at a rate of 100 compressions a minute.

- Give one rescue breath. Alternate five chest compressions with one rescue breath. Continue CPR until emergency help takes over; the infant makes a movement or takes a breath; or you become too exhausted to continue.

CHOKING ADULT

▶ **See also** p.100

See also p.100

RECOGNITION

Partial obstruction
- Difficulty speaking and breathing.
- Coughing and distress.

Complete obstruction
- Inability to speak, breathe, or cough.
- Eventual loss of consciousness.

PRECAUTIONS

- If the victim loses consciousness, give rescue breaths and chest compressions (pp.255–256).
- Do not do a finger sweep of the mouth.

ACTION

DETERMINE IF PERSON IS CHOKING

POSITION HANDS TO GIVE ABDOMINAL THRUSTS

GIVE UP TO FIVE ABDOMINAL THRUSTS

REPEAT SEQUENCE UNTIL HELP ARRIVES

1 DETERMINE WHETHER THE PERSON IS CHOKING

- Ask the person "Are you choking?"
- If the person can speak or cough, do not interfere. If the person cannot speak or cough, proceed to Step 2.
- Encourage the victim to cough to try to remove the obstruction.
- If the victim is beginning to struggle, bend her forward.

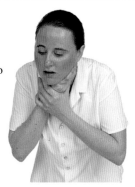

2 HOLD VICTIM FROM BEHIND

- Stand behind the victim.
- Put both arms around her, and put one fist between her navel and the bottom of her breastbone.

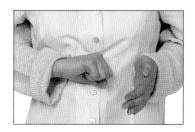

3 GIVE UP TO FIVE ABDOMINAL THRUSTS

- Grasp your fist with your other hand, and pull sharply inward and upward up to five times.
- If the obstruction is still not cleared, recheck the mouth for any object and remove it if possible.

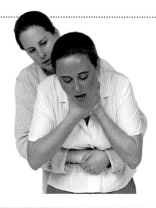

4 REPEAT ENTIRE SEQUENCE

- Repeat steps 1–3 until the obstruction clears. If after three cycles the obstruction still has not cleared, DIAL 9·1·1 OR CALL EMS.

- Continue the sequence until help arrives; the obstruction is cleared; or the victim becomes unconscious (*see* PRECAUTIONS, left).

CHOKING CHILD (1–7 years)

▶ **See also** p.101

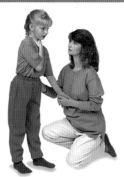

RECOGNITION

Partial obstruction
- Difficulty speaking and breathing.
- Coughing and distress.

Complete obstruction
- Inability to speak, breathe, or cough.
- Eventual loss of consciousness.

PRECAUTIONS

- If the child loses consciousness, give rescue breaths and chest compressions (pp.259–260).
- Do not do a finger sweep of the mouth.

ACTION

DETERMINE IF CHILD IS CHOKING

POSITION HANDS TO GIVE ABDOMINAL THRUSTS

GIVE UP TO FIVE ABDOMINAL THRUSTS

REPEAT SEQUENCE UNTIL HELP ARRIVES

1 DETERMINE WHETHER THE CHILD IS CHOKING

- Ask the child "Are you choking?"

- If the child can speak or cough, do not interfere. If the child cannot speak or cough, proceed to Step 2.

- Encourage the child to cough. If the child is beginning to struggle, bend him forward.

2 PREPARE TO GIVE ABDOMINAL THRUSTS

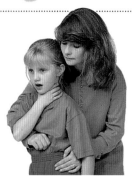

- Stand or kneel behind the child. Wrap your arms around her abdomen just above the line of the hips. Make a fist with one hand and place the thumb side of your fist against the middle of her abdomen, just above her navel.

3 GIVE UP TO FIVE ABDOMINAL THRUSTS

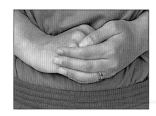

- Grasp your fist with your other hand. Pull sharply inward and upward up to five times. Check the child's mouth.

- If choking persists, proceed to step 4.

4 REPEAT ENTIRE SEQUENCE

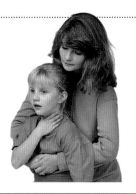

- Repeat steps 1–3 until the obstruction clears. If after three cycles the obstruction still has not cleared, DIAL 9·1·1 OR CALL EMS.

- Continue the sequence until help arrives; the obstruction is cleared; or the child becomes unconscious (*see* PRECAUTIONS, left).

CHOKING INFANT (under 1 year)

▶ See also p.102

RECOGNITION

- Difficulty breathing.
- Flushed face and neck.
- Strange noises or no sound.

Later:
- Gray–blue skin.

PRECAUTIONS

- If the infant loses consciousness, give rescue breaths and chest compressions (p.263).
- Do not do a finger sweep of the mouth.
- Do not use abdominal thrusts.

ACTION

GIVE UP TO FIVE
BACK SLAPS
CHECK MOUTH

GIVE UP TO FIVE
CHEST THRUSTS
CHECK MOUTH

REPEAT SEQUENCE
THREE TIMES THEN
CALL 9•1•1 OR EMS

REPEAT
SEQUENCE UNTIL
HELP ARRIVES

1 GIVE UP TO FIVE BACK SLAPS

- Check the infant's mouth, but do not do a finger sweep as you may make the obstruction worse.

- Lay the infant face down along your forearm, with his head low, and supporting his body and head.

- Give up to five back slaps between the shoulder blades. If choking persists, proceed to step 2.

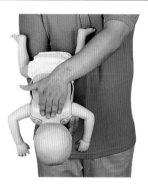

2 CHECK INFANT'S MOUTH

- Turn the infant face up along your other forearm.

- Use your fingertips to remove any obvious obstructions.

- If choking persists, proceed to step 3.

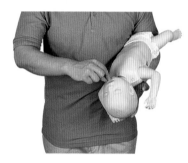

3 GIVE UP TO FIVE CHEST THRUSTS

- Place two fingertips on the breastbone between the nipples.

- Give up to five sharp thrusts inward at rate of one every 3 seconds.

- Check the mouth again.

- If choking persists, proceed to step 4.

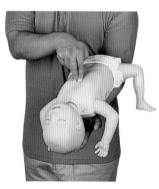

4 REPEAT ENTIRE SEQUENCE

- Repeat steps 1–3 three times.

- If the obstruction still does not clear, take the infant with you to DIAL 9•1•1 OR CALL EMS.

- Continue the sequence until help arrives; the obstruction is cleared from the airway; or the infant becomes unconscious (*see* PRECAUTIONS, left).

ASTHMA ATTACK

▶ See also p.115

RECOGNITION

- Difficulty breathing.

There may be:
- Wheezing.
- Difficulty speaking.
- Gray-blue skin.
- Exhaustion and possible loss of consciousness.

PRECAUTIONS

- Do not lay the victim down.
- Do not use a preventer inhaler.
- If the attack is severe, or if the inhaler has no effect after 5 minutes, or if the victim is getting worse

DIAL 9•1•1 OR CALL EMS.

- If the victim loses consciousness, open the airway and check breathing (p.252). Be prepared to give rescue breaths and chest compressions if needed.

ACTION

ALLOW VICTIM TO USE RELIEVER INHALER

MAKE VICTIM COMFORTABLE

ENCOURAGE VICTIM TO BREATHE SLOWLY

1 MAKE VICTIM COMFORTABLE

- Keep calm and reassure the victim.

- Help her into the position that she finds most comfortable; sitting slightly forward and supporting the upper body by leaning the arms on a firm surface is usually best.

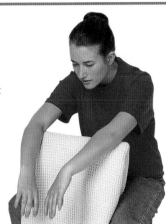

2 ALLOW VICTIM TO USE RELIEVER INHALER

- Help the victim find her reliever inhaler (it usually has a blue cap).

- Encourage the victim to use the inhaler; it should take effect within minutes.

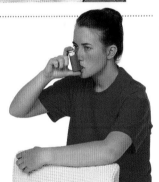

3 ENCOURAGE VICTIM TO BREATHE SLOWLY

- If the attack does not ease within 3 minutes, encourage the victim to take another dose from her inhaler and to breathe slowly and deeply.

- Tell the victim to inform her doctor of the attack if it is severe or if it is her first attack.

- If the attack is severe, if the inhaler has no effect after 5 minutes, or if the victim is getting worse, DIAL 9•1•1 OR CALL EMS.

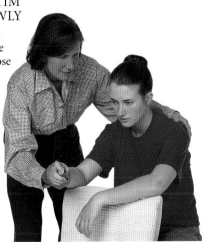

SHOCK

▶ See also pp.120–121

RECOGNITION

- Rapid pulse.
- Pale, cold, clammy skin.
- Sweating.

Later:
- Gray–blue skin, especially inside lips.
- Weakness and giddiness.
- Nausea or thirst.
- Rapid, shallow breathing.
- Weak pulse.

Eventually:
- Restlessness.
- Gasping for air.
- Unconsciousness.

PRECAUTIONS

- Do not leave the victim unattended, except to call 9•1•1 or EMS.
- Do not let the victim smoke, eat, drink, or move.

ACTION

HELP VICTIM LIE DOWN

LOOSEN TIGHT CLOTHING

CALL 9•1•1 OR EMS

MONITOR VICTIM

1 HELP VICTIM TO LIE DOWN

- Use a blanket to insulate the victim from the ground.
- Raise and support her legs as high as possible.
- Treat any cause of shock, such as bleeding.

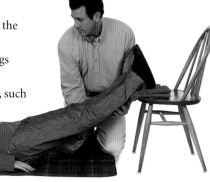

2 LOOSEN TIGHT CLOTHING

- Undo anything that constricts her neck, chest, or waist.
- Cover her with a blanket.

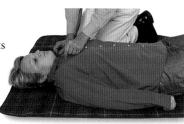

3 DIAL 9•1•1 OR CALL EMS

- If possible, send a helper to call 9•1•1 or EMS.
- The caller should give the dispatcher details about the cause of shock, if known.

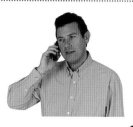

4 MONITOR BREATHING, PULSE, AND RESPONSE

- Monitor and record vital signs – level of response, pulse, and breathing (pp.42–43).
- If the victim becomes unconscious, open the airway and check breathing (p.252). Be ready to give rescue breaths and chest compressions.

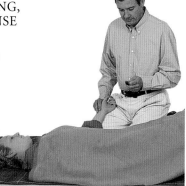

ANAPHYLACTIC SHOCK

▶ **See also** p.123

RECOGNITION

- Anxiety.
- Red, blotchy skin.
- Swelling of tongue and throat.
- Puffiness around eyes.
- Impaired breathing, possibly with wheezing and gasping for air.
- Signs of shock.

PRECAUTIONS

- Check to see if the victim is carrying an auto-injector or a syringe of epinephrine (adrenaline). If necessary, help the victim use it. It can save his life when given promptly.
- If the victim loses consciousness, open the airway and check breathing (p.252). If breathing, place him in the recovery position. Be prepared to give rescue breaths and chest compressions if needed.

ACTION

DIAL 9·1·1 OR
CALL EMS

⬇

HELP TO RELIEVE
SYMPTOMS

⬇

MONITOR
VICTIM

1 DIAL 9·1·1 OR CALL EMS

- Pass on as much information as possible about the cause of the allergy.

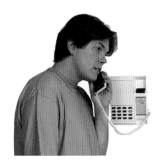

2 HELP RELIEVE SYMPTOMS

- Check whether the person is carrying a syringe or an auto-injector of epinephrine (adrenaline). Help him find and use it if necessary.
- Help the person sit in a position that eases any breathing difficulties.

3 MONITOR VICTIM

- Monitor and record vital signs – level of response, pulse, and breathing (pp.42–43) – until help arrives.

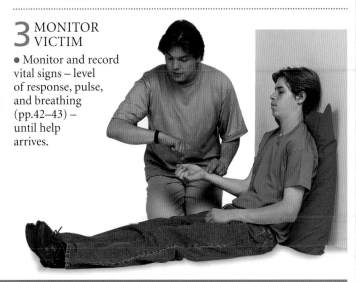

SEVERE BLEEDING

▶ See also pp.130–131

PRECAUTIONS

- Wear gloves, if available, to protect against infection.
- Do not apply a tourniquet.
- If there is an embedded object in the wound, apply pressure on either side of the wound, and pad around it before bandaging (p.131).
- If the victim loses consciousness, open the airway and check breathing (p.252). If breathing, place her in the recovery position. Be ready to give rescue breaths and chest compressions if needed.

ACTION

APPLY PRESSURE
TO WOUND

RAISE AND SUPPORT
INJURED PART

BANDAGE
WOUND

DIAL 9•1•1 OR
CALL EMS

TREAT FOR SHOCK
AND MONITOR
VICTIM

1 APPLY PRESSURE TO WOUND

- Put on disposable gloves if available. Remove or cut any clothing over the wound.
- Place a sterile dressing or nonfluffy pad over the wound. Apply firm pressure with the fingers or palm of your hand.

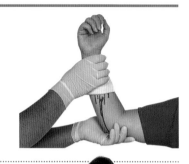

2 RAISE AND SUPPORT INJURED PART

- Raise the injured part above the level of the victim's heart.
- Handle the injured part gently if you suspect that the injury involves a fracture.
- Help the victim to lie down.

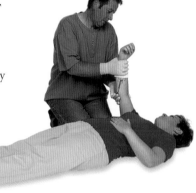

3 BANDAGE WOUND

- Apply a sterile dressing over the pad, and bandage firmly in place.
- Bandage another pad on top if blood seeps through. If blood seeps through the second pad, remove all dressings and apply a fresh one, ensuring that it exerts pressure on the bleeding area.
- Check the circulation beyond the bandages at intervals; loosen them if necessary.

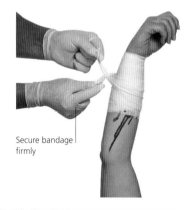

Secure bandage firmly

4 DIAL 9•1•1 OR CALL EMS

- Give details of the site of the injury and the extent of the bleeding when you telephone.

5 TREAT FOR SHOCK; MONITOR VICTIM

- Treat for shock (pp.120–121). Monitor and record vital signs – level of response, pulse, and breathing (pp.42–43).

HEART ATTACK

▶ See also p.125

RECOGNITION

There may be:

- Vicelike chest pain, spreading to one or both arms.
- Breathlessness.
- Discomfort, like indigestion, in upper abdomen.
- Sudden faintness.
- Sudden collapse.
- Sense of impending doom.
- Ashen skin and blueness at lips.
- Rapid, then weakening, pulse.
- Profuse sweating.

PRECAUTIONS

- Do not give fluids.
- If the victim loses consciousness, open the airway and check breathing (p.252). Be ready to give rescue breaths and chest compressions if needed.

ACTION

MAKE VICTIM COMFORTABLE

CALL 9•1•1 OR EMS

GIVE VICTIM ASPIRIN

MONITOR VICTIM

1 MAKE VICTIM COMFORTABLE

- Help the victim into a half-sitting position.
- Support his head, shoulders, and knees.
- Reassure the victim.

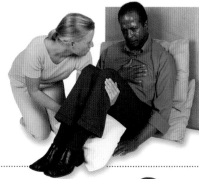

2 DIAL 9•1•1 OR CALL EMS

- Tell the dispatcher that you suspect a heart attack.
- Call the victim's doctor as well, if he asks you to do so.

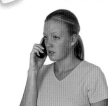

3 GIVE VICTIM MEDICATION

- If the victim is conscious, give one aspirin pill to be *chewed* slowly.
- If the victim is carrying pills or a puffer aerosol for angina, allow him to administer it himself. Help him if necessary.

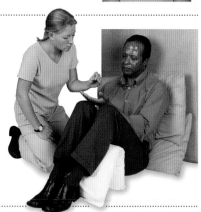

4 MONITOR VICTIM

- Encourage the victim to rest. Keep any bystanders at a distance.
- Monitor and record vital signs – level of response, pulse, and breathing (pp.42–43) – until help arrives.

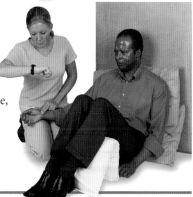

HEAD INJURY

▶ **See also** p.137 and p.179

RECOGNITION

There may be:
- Head wound.
- Impaired consciousness.

PRECAUTIONS

- Wear disposable gloves, if available, to protect against infection.
- If the victim loses consciousness, open the airway and check breathing (p.252). If she is breathing, place her in the recovery position. Be ready to give rescue breaths and chest compressions if needed.
- If the bleeding does not stop, re-apply pressure and add a second pad.
- Always suspect the possibility of a neck (spinal) injury (opposite).

ACTION

CONTROL BLEEDING

⬇

SECURE DRESSING
WITH BANDAGE

⬇

HELP VICTIM
TO LIE DOWN

⬇

DIAL 9•1•1 OR
CALL EMS

1 CONTROL BLEEDING

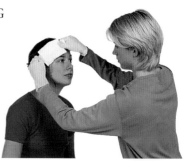

- Put on disposable gloves if available.
- Replace any displaced skin flaps over the wound.
- Place a sterile dressing or a clean, nonfluffy pad over the wound and apply firm, direct pressure with your hand.

2 SECURE DRESSING WITH BANDAGE

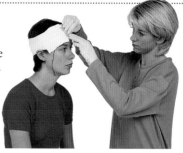

- Secure the dressing over the wound with a roller bandage.

3 HELP VICTIM LIE DOWN

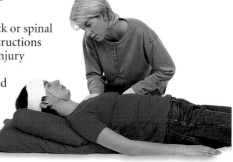

- If you suspect a neck or spinal injury, follow the instructions for treating a spinal injury (opposite).
- Ensure that her head and shoulders are slightly raised.
- Make sure that she is comfortable.

4 DIAL 9•1•1 OR CALL EMS

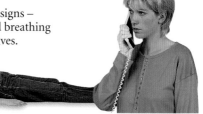

- Monitor and record vital signs – level of response, pulse, and breathing (pp.42–43) – until help arrives.

SPINAL INJURY

▶ See also pp.165–167

RECOGNITION

- Pain in neck or back.
- A step or twist in the curve of the spine.
- Tenderness over the spine.

There may be:
- Weakness or loss of movement in limbs.
- Loss of sensation, or abnormal sensation.
- Loss of bladder and/or bowel control.
- Difficulty breathing.

PRECAUTIONS

- Do not move the victim unless she is in danger.
- If the victim loses consciousness, open the airway by gently lifting the jaw but not tilting the head (*see* SPINAL INJURY, p.167), and check breathing. Be ready to give rescue breaths and chest compressions if needed. Put her into the recovery position only if the airway cannot be maintained using the jaw thrust method (p.167).

ACTION

STEADY AND SUPPORT HEAD

DIAL 9•1•1 OR CALL EMS

1 STEADY AND SUPPORT HEAD

- Reassure the victim and tell her not to move.

- Keep the head, neck, and spine aligned by placing your hands on the sides of the head to hold the head still.

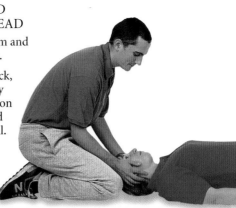

2 SUPPORT VICTIM'S NECK

- Ask a helper to place rolled towels or other padding around the victim's neck and shoulders.

- Keep holding her head throughout, until medical help arrives.

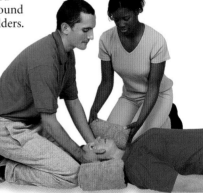

3 DIAL 9•1•1 OR CALL EMS

- If possible, ask a helper to call for help and say that a spinal injury is suspected.

- Monitor and record vital signs – level of response, pulse, and breathing (pp.42–43).

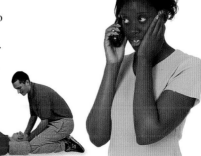

SEIZURES IN ADULTS

▶ **See also** pp.184–185

- Sudden loss of consciousness.
- Rigidity and arching of the back.
- Convulsive movements.
- Muscle relaxation.
- Regaining of consciousness.
- Gray–blue tinge to skin.

PRECAUTIONS

- Do not use force to restrain the victim.
- If the victim is unconscious for more than 10 minutes, is having repeated seizures, or it is her first seizure, DIAL 9•1•1 OR CALL EMS. Note the time when the seizure starts and the duration of the seizure.

ACTION

PROTECT VICTIM

PROTECT HEAD AND LOOSEN TIGHT CLOTHING

PLACE VICTIM IN RECOVERY POSITION

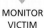

MONITOR VICTIM

1 PROTECT VICTIM

- Try to ease her fall.
- Talk to her calmly and reassuringly.
- Clear away any potentially dangerous objects to prevent injury to the victim.
- Ask bystanders to keep clear.

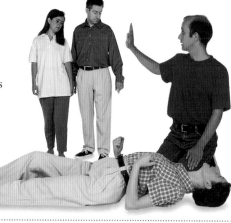

2 PROTECT HEAD AND LOOSEN TIGHT CLOTHING

- If possible, cushion the victim's head with soft material until the convulsions cease.
- Undo any tight clothing around the victim's neck.

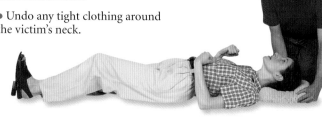

3 PLACE VICTIM IN RECOVERY POSITION

- Once the convulsions have stopped, open the airway and check breathing (p.254); then place the victim in the recovery position (p.257).
- Monitor and record vital signs – level of response, pulse, and breathing (pp.42–43).

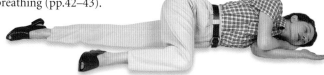

SEIZURES IN CHILDREN

▶ See also p.186

RECOGNITION

- Violent muscle twitching, clenched fists, and arched back.

There may be:

- Fever.
- Twitching of the face.
- Breath-holding.
- Drooling at the mouth.
- Loss of, or impaired, consciousness.

PRECAUTIONS

- Do not let the child become chilled.
- If the child loses consciousness, open the airway and check breathing (p.258, p.262). Be ready to give rescue breaths and chest compressions if needed (p.260, p.263).

ACTION

PROTECT CHILD FROM INJURY

COOL CHILD IF FEBRILE

SPONGE WITH TEPID WATER IF FEBRILE

PUT CHILD IN RECOVERY POSITION

CALL 9•1•1 OR EMS; MONITOR CHILD

1 PROTECT CHILD FROM INJURY

- Clear away any nearby objects.
- Surround the child with soft padding.

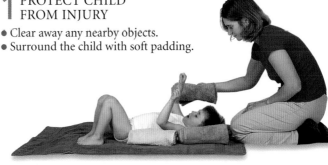

2 COOL CHILD IF FEBRILE

- Remove his clothing.
- Ensure a good supply of cool air.

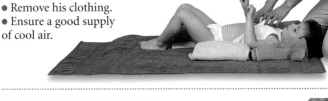

3 SPONGE WITH TEPID WATER IF FEBRILE

- Start at his head and work down.

4 PUT CHILD IN RECOVERY POSITION

- Once the convulsions have stopped, open the airway and check breathing (p.258, p.262), then put the child in the recovery position (p.261, p.263).

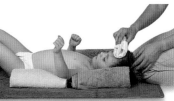

5 DIAL 9•1•1 OR CALL EMS AND MONITOR CHILD

- Monitor and record vital signs – level of response, pulse, and breathing (pp.42–43) – until help arrives.

BROKEN BONES

▶ See also pp.150–174

RECOGNITION

- Distortion, swelling, and bruising at the injury site.
- Pain and difficulty moving the injured part.

There may be:

- Bending, twisting, or shortening of a limb.
- A wound, possibly with bone ends protruding.

PRECAUTIONS

- Do not attempt to bandage the injury if medical assistance is on its way.
- Do not attempt to move an injured limb unnecessarily.
- Do not allow a victim with a suspected fracture to eat, drink, or smoke.

ACTION

STEADY AND SUPPORT INJURED PART

⬇

PROTECT INJURY WITH PADDING

⬇

TAKE OR SEND VICTIM TO A HOSPITAL

1 STEADY AND SUPPORT INJURED PART

- Help the victim to support the affected part, above and below the injury, in the most comfortable position.

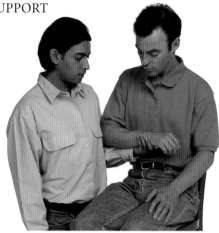

2 PROTECT INJURY WITH PADDING

- Place padding, such as towels or cushions, around the affected part, and support it in position.

- If there is an open wound, cover it with a large, sterile dressing or a clean, nonfluffy pad and bandage it in place (p.231).

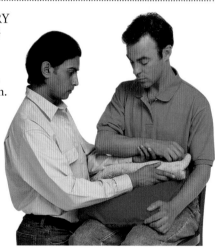

3 TAKE OR SEND VICTIM TO A HOSPITAL

- Dial 9·1·1 or call EMS if necessary.

- Treat the victim for shock (p.268) if necessary.

- Monitor and record vital signs – level of response, pulse, and breathing (pp.42–43).

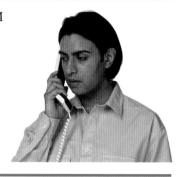

BURNS

RECOGNITION

- Reddened skin.
- Pain in the area of the burn.
- Swelling and blistering of the skin.

PRECAUTIONS

- Do not apply lotion, ointment, butter, or other fat to a burn.
- Do not touch the burn or burst any blisters.
- Do not remove anything sticking to the burn.
- If the burn is to the face, do not cover it. Keep cooling with water until help arrives.
- If the burn is caused by chemicals, cool for at least 20 minutes.

ACTION

COOL BURN

REMOVE ANY CONSTRICTIONS

COVER BURN

TAKE OR SEND VICTIM TO A HOSPITAL

1 COOL BURN

- Make the victim comfortable.
- Pour cold liquid on the burn for at least 10 minutes.
- Watch for signs of smoke inhalation, such as difficulty breathing.

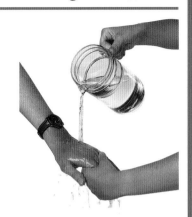

2 REMOVE ANY CONSTRICTIONS

- Put on disposable gloves if available.
- Carefully remove any clothing or jewelry from the area before it starts to swell. However, do not try to remove any clothing that is sticking to the burn.

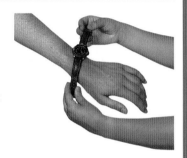

3 COVER BURN

- Cover the burn and the surrounding area with a sterile dressing, clean nonfluffy material, plastic wrap, or a plastic bag.
- Reassure the victim.

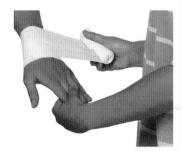

4 TAKE OR SEND VICTIM TO A HOSPITAL

- Dial 9·1·1 or call EMS if necessary.
- Treat the victim for shock (p.268) if necessary.
- Monitor and record vital signs – level of response, pulse, and breathing (pp.42–43).

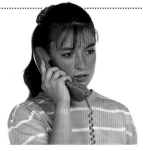

EYE INJURY

▶ **See also** p.138 and pp.200–201

RECOGNITION

- Intense pain in the affected eye.
- Spasm of the eyelids.

There may also be:
- A visible wound.
- A bloodshot eye, even if wound is not visible.
- Partial or total loss of vision.
- Leakage of blood or clear fluid from the injured eye.

PRECAUTIONS

- Do not touch the eye or any contact lens in it, and do not allow the victim to rub the eye.
- Do not try to remove any object embedded in the eye.
- If it will be some time before medical aid is available, bandage an eye pad in place over the injured eye.

ACTION

SUPPORT VICTIM'S HEAD

⬇

GIVE EYE DRESSING TO VICTIM

⬇

TAKE OR SEND VICTIM TO A HOSPITAL

1 SUPPORT VICTIM'S HEAD

- Lay the victim on her back, holding her head on your knees to keep it as still as possible.

- Tell the victim to keep her "good" eye still; movement of the uninjured eye will cause the injured one to move as well, which may damage it further.

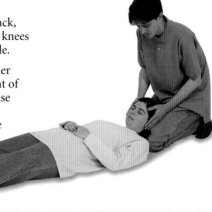

2 GIVE EYE DRESSING TO VICTIM

- Give the victim a sterile dressing or clean nonfluffy pad. Ask her to hold it over the injured eye and to keep her uninjured eye closed.

- Hold the victim's head steady.

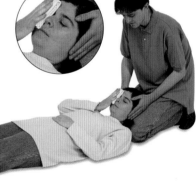

3 TAKE OR SEND VICTIM TO A HOSPITAL

- Ensure that the victim is transported lying down. Dial 9·1·1 or call EMS if you cannot transport her in the position in which she was treated.

Provide support for victim's head

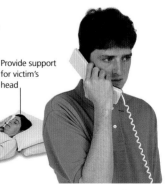

SWALLOWED POISONS

▶ See also p.220

RECOGNITION

- Vomiting that may be bloodstained.
- Impaired consciousness.
- Empty bottles and containers nearby.
- History of ingestion/exposure.
- Pain or burning sensation.

PRECAUTIONS

- Do not attempt to induce vomiting.
- If the victim loses consciousness, make sure that there is no vomit or other matter in the mouth. Open the airway and check breathing (p.252). Be ready to give rescue breaths and chest compressions if needed.
- When giving rescue breaths, use a face shield or pocket mask for protection if there are chemicals on the victim's mouth.

ACTION

CHECK WHAT
VICTIM HAS
SWALLOWED

⬇

CALL 9•1•1 OR EMS

⬇

MONITOR VICTIM

1 CHECK WHAT VICTIM HAS SWALLOWED

- If the victim is conscious, ask what she has swallowed and reassure her.

- Call the Poison Control Center (800-222-1222). Give as much information as possible about the swallowed poison. This information will help doctors to give the victim the appropriate treatment.

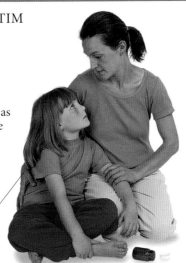

Reassure victim as you find out what she swallowed

2 IF THE VICTIM IS UNCONSCIOUS

- Dial 9•1•1 or call EMS.

- Monitor and record vital signs – level of response, pulse, and breathing (pp.42–43) – until help arrives.

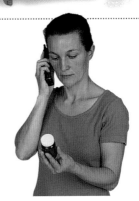

3 IF VICTIM'S LIPS ARE BURNED

- If the swallowed substance has burned the victim's lips, give her frequent small sips of cold water or milk.

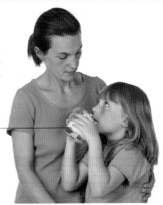

Give victim cool, soothing drink such as milk

OBSERVATION CHARTS

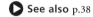 **See also** p.38

Fill in the following charts every time you attend to a victim.

- On the first chart, place a dot opposite the appropriate score at each time interval.

- On the second chart, check appropriate pulse and breathing rates at each interval.
- The completed form should stay with the victim when he leaves your care.

LEVEL OF RESPONSE CHART

DATE.............................VICTIM'S NAME..

OBSERVATION	RESPONSE/SCORE		Time of observation (minutes)					
			0	10	20	30	40	50
Eyes Observe for reaction while testing other responses.	Open spontaneously 4 Open to speech 3 Open to painful stimulus 2 No response 1							
Speech When testing responses, speak clearly and directly, close to victim's ear.	Responds sensibly to questions 5 Seems confused 4 Uses inappropriate words 3 Incomprehensible sounds 2 No response 1							
Movement Apply painful stimulus: pinch ear lobe or skin on back of hand.	Obeys commands 6 Points to pain 5 Withdraws from painful stimulus 4 Bends limbs in response to pain 3 Straightens limbs in response to pain 2 No response 1							
	TOTAL SCORE							

PULSE AND BREATHING CHECK CHART

DATE.............................VICTIM'S NAME..

PULSE/BREATHING	RATE		Time of observation (minutes)					
			0	10	20	30	40	50
Pulse **(beats per minute)** Take pulse at wrist or at neck on adult, or at inner arm on baby (p.42). Note the rate, and whether beats are weak (w) or strong (s), regular (reg) or irregular (irreg).	Over 110							
	101–110							
	91–100							
	81–90							
	71–80							
	61–70							
	Below 61							
Breathing **(breaths per minute)** Note rate, and whether breathing is quiet (q) or noisy (n), easy (e) or difficult (diff).	Over 40							
	31–40							
	21–30							
	11–20							
	Below 11							

INDEX

A

Abdomen
examining for injury 35
hernia 246
pain 245
stitch 247
wounds 142
Abrasions 129, 134–5
Absence seizures 185
Acetaminophen, overdose 222
Aches
abdominal pain 245
earache 243
headache 188
toothache 244
Adhesive dressings 44
applying 49
Adhesive tape 45
securing roller bandages 52
Afterbirth, delivery of 232, 236
Aftercare of victims 36
AIDS
HIV infection 14
human bites 230
Air travel, earache 243
Airway
breathing difficulties 106–16
burns 197
croup 116
hanging and strangulation 108
inhalation of fumes 110–11
obstruction 107
choking 99–102
unconscious victim 107
opening 73
adults 77
children 88
head injury 179
jaw thrust method 167
infants 95
respiratory system 104–5
Alcohol poisoning 223
Allergy 238
anaphylactic shock 123
asthma 115
Alveoli 72, 104
Ambulance stretcher 70
Amphetamines,
overdose 222
Amputation 132
Anaphylactic shock 123
emergency first aid 269
Angina pectoris 124
Animal bites 230
Ankles
bandaging 55, 173
fractures 174

sprains 154
Anus, bleeding from 122
Appendicitis 245
Arms
bandaging 53
slings 60–2
examining for injury 35
immobilizing 51
injuries 160–2
elbow 161
forearm and wrist 162
hand and fingers 163
upper arm 160
muscles 148
traction 151
wounds
amputation 132
bleeding at elbow crease 141
Arteries
bleeding from 128
circulatory system 118
pulse 42
severe bleeding 130–1
Artificial ventilation *see* **Rescue**
breathing
Aspirin
heart attack and 125, 271
overdose 222
Assessing victims 29–33
examining victim 34–5
primary survey 29
secondary survey 30–1
symptoms and signs 32–3
unconscious victims
adults 76, 254
children 88, 258
infants 96, 262
Assessing situation 18
Asthma 115
emergency first aid 267
inhalers 30
Auto-injectors 30, 123
Automated electronic
defibrillators (AED) 74, 82–3
Autonomic nervous system 177
AVPU code, checking level of
response 42, 178

B

Babies *see* **Infants**
Back injuries 165–8
emergency first aid 273
examining for injury 34, 35
pain 168
recovery position 85, 93
treatment 166–7
Bacteria, food poisoning 224
Balance, vertigo 239

Bandages 44, 50–9
applying 49
checking circulation 51
choosing correct size 52
elbow and knee 54
first aid kit 45
general rules 50–1
hand and foot 55
immobilizing a limb 51
roller bandages 44, 52–5
triangular bandages 44, 57–61
tubular bandages 44, 56
Barbiturates, overdose 222
Bee stings 226
Behavior, disturbed 242
Belts, transfer 65
Benzodiazepines, overdose 222
Berries, poisonous 225
Biohazard bags 15
Birth 232–6
Bites and stings 226–30
anaphylactic shock 123
animal bites 230
insect stings 226–7
marine creatures 229
rabies 230
snake bites 228
tetanus 230
ticks 227
Bleeding 127–44
bruising 136
checking for 34–5
childbirth 236
emergency first aid 270
from ear 138
from mouth 140
internal bleeding 122
miscarriage 237
nosebleeds 139
severe bleeding 130–1
shock 120–1
types of wounds 129
vaginal 143
varicose veins 144
see also Wounds
Blisters, burns 196
Blood
blood-borne diseases 250
circulatory system 72, 118–19
clotting 128
composition 119
see also Bleeding
Blood pressure 118
Blood sugar levels 240–1
Boards, moving victims 70
Body temperature 191
fever 239
frostbite 205
heat exhaustion 203

heatstroke 204
hypothermia 206–8
taking 43
Bones
joints 149
skeleton 146–7
structure 148
see also Fractures
Bracelets, medical warning 30
Brachial pulse 42
Brain
absence seizures 185
cerebral compression 179, 181
concussion 179, 180
head injury 179
heatstroke 204
hypoglycemia 241
impaired consciousness 178
meningitis 187
nervous system 177
oxygen deprivation 71, 72
seizures 184–6
skull fracture 179, 182
stroke 183
see also Unconsciousness
Breathing
airway obstruction 107
asthma 115, 267
checking 43
unconscious adult 77
unconscious child 88
unconscious infant 96
circulatory system 72
croup 116
examining for injury 34, 35
fume inhalation 110–11
hyperventilation 114
observation chart 38, 280
opening airway 73
adults 77
children 88
infants 96
rescue breathing
adults 78–9
children 89
infants 96–97
respiratory system 105
Broad-fold bandages 57
Bruises 129
cold compresses 49
treatment 136
Bullet wounds 129
Burns 192–202
airway 197
assessing 192–3
chemical 199, 221
depth 193
dressing 195
electrical 198
emergency first aid 277

flash burns to the eye 201
minor burns and scalds 196
severe burns and scalds 194–5
sunburn 202
swallowed poisons 220
Bystanders 19

C

Calf muscles, cramp 248
Capillaries
bleeding 128
circulatory system 118
temperature control 191
Car accidents see **Road incidents**
Carbon dioxide
hyperventilation 114
inhalation of 110
respiratory system 104
Carbon monoxide 25
inhalation of 110
Cardboard tags 45
Cardiac arrest 82
Cardiopulmonary resuscitation
see **CPR**
Carotid pulse 42
Carry chairs 69
Carry sheets 68, 69
Cartilage 149
Central nervous system 177
Cerebral compression 179, 181
Cerebrospinal fluid 177, 182
Chairs, moving casualty 67
Cheekbone fractures 157
Chemicals
allergy 238
burns 199–200
in the eye 200, 221
Hazchem symbols 22
inhaled gases 221
on the skin 221
pepper spray 201
swallowed poisons 220
tear gas 201
Chest compressions 74
adults 80–1, 256
children 90–1, 260
infants 98, 263
Chest injuries
crush injuries 133
penetrating wounds 112–13
rib cage fractures 164
Childbirth 231–7
miscarriage 237
Children
assessing unconscious victims
88, 258
choking 101, 265
coping with 13
croup 116

nosebleeds 139
recovery position 92–3, 261
rescue breathing 89, 259
resuscitation 86–93, 260
seizures 186, 275
see also Infants
Choking 99–102
adults 100
children 101
emergency first aid 264–5
infants 102
Cholera 249
Circulatory system 72, 118–19
checking circulation
after bandaging 51
unconscious adult 80, 255
unconscious child 90–1, 260
unconscious infant 97, 263
CPR
adults 80–1, 256
children 90–1, 260
infants 98, 263
problems 120–6
anaphylactic shock 123
fainting 126
heart disorders 124–5
internal bleeding 122
shock 120
pulse 42
Cleansing wipes 45
Clips 45
securing roller bandages 52
Closed fractures 150
treatment 151
Clothing
on fire 25
improvised slings 62
removing 40
Clotting, blood 128
Cocaine, overdose 222
Cold
frostbite 205
hypothermia 206–8
temperature control 191
Cold compresses 49
Collarbone, fractures 158
Collars, spinal injury 168
Colles' fracture 162
Coma see **Unconsciousness**
Compresses, cold 49
Concussion 179, 180
Consciousness
checking level of response 42
impaired consciousness 178
see also Unconsciousness
Contusions 129
Convulsions see **Seizures**
Coral stings 229
Cornea 210
flash burns 201

Coronary arteries 124
Cotton padding 45
CPR 73-4
  adults 80–1, 256
  children 90–1, 260
  infants 98, 263
Cramp 248
  stitch 247
Crash helmets,
  removing 41
Cross infection,
  preventing 14–15
Croup 116
Crush injuries 133
Cuts 134

D

Defibrillators 74, 82–3
Dehydration, vomiting and
  diarrhea 247
Delayed reactions 16
Delivery, childbirth 231–7
Diabetes mellitus 240–1
  hyperglycemia 240
  hypoglycemia 241
Diaphragm, hiccups 238
Diarrhea 247
  traveler's 249
Digestive system
  abdominal pain 245
  diarrhea 247
  food poisoning 224
  hernia 246
  vomiting 247
Dislocated joints 153
  shoulder 159
Disturbed behavior 242
Dressings 44, 46–9
  adhesive 49
  applying 46–7
  burns 195
  first-aid kit 45
  gauze 48
  improvised 48
  nonsterile 48
  sterile 47
Drowning 109
Drugs
  administering 37
  assessing a victim 30
  poisoning 222
Drunkenness 223

E

E. coli 224
Ears 211
  bleeding from 138
  earache 243

examining for injury 34
foreign objects 215
internal bleeding 122
vertigo 239
Ecstasy
  heat exhaustion 203
  heatstroke 204
  overdose 222
Elbows
  bandaging 54
  bleeding from joint crease 141
  injuries 161
  wounds 141
Elderly people, hypothermia 207
Electrical injuries 26–7
  burns 198
  high-voltage 26
  lightning 27
  low-voltage 27
Elevation slings 61
Emergencies, action at 18–38
  assessing a victim 29–35, 252–3
  assessing situation 18
  controlling bystanders 19
  electrical injuries 26–7
  emergency first aid 251–81
  fires 24–5
  moving victims 63–70
  multiple victims 21
  telephoning for help 20
  traffic incidents 22–3
  water rescue 28
Emergency Services
  telephoning for help 20
  when to call 74
Emotions, after an incident 16
Environmental injuries 189–208
Epiglottitis 116
Epilepsy 184–6
Epinephrine (adrenaline) 30
  anaphylactic shock 123
  auto-injectors 30, 123
Eyes 210
  chemical burns 200, 221
  emergency first aid 278
  examining for injury 34
  flash burns 201
  foreign objects 214
  pepper spray injury 201
  sterile eye pads 44
  tear gas injury 201
  wounds 138

F

Face
  burns 195, 197
  examining for injury 34
  fractures 156–7
Face shields and masks 45

mouth-to-mouth breathing 78
Fainting 126
Falls, controlling 66
Febrile convulsions 186
Feet
  bandaging
    roller bandages 55
    triangular bandages 58
  checking circulation 51
  cramp 248
  examining for injury 35
  fractures 174
  frostbite 205
Femur 146
  fractures 170–1
Fever 239
  febrile convulsions 186
Fibrin 128
Fibula 146
  fractures 173
"Fight or flight response" 14
Fingers
  frostbite 205
  injuries 163
  torn tendons 154
  tubular bandages 56
  see also Hands
Fires 24–5
  burns 192–202
  smoke inhalation 110
First aid 11–38
  being a first aider 12–13
  emergency first aid 251–81
  giving care with confidence 13
  looking after yourself 14–16
  materials 44–62
  regulations and legislation 17
First aid certificate 11
First-aid kit 45
Fishhooks, embedded 213
Fits 184–6
  emergency first aid 274–5
Flash burns, eyes 201
Food, allergies 238
Food poisoning 224
  overseas travel health 249
Foot see Feet
Forearm, injuries 162
Foreign objects 209–16
  choking 99–102
  in the ear 215
  in the eye 214
  inhaled 216
  in the nose 215
  in the skin 212–13
  swallowed 216
  in wounds 131, 135
Fractures 150–2
  closed fractures 150
  treatment 151

emergency first aid 276
open fractures 150
   treatment 152
   protruding bone 152
stable fractures 150
traction 151
types of
   arm 160–2
   collarbone 158
   facial 156–7
   foot 174
   hand 163
   hip 170–1
   leg 170–4
   pelvis 169
   rib cage 164
   skull 179, 182
   spine 165
unstable fractures 150
Frostbite 205
Fuels, inhalation of 110
Fumes 25
   inhalation of 110–11
Fungi, poisonous 225

G

Gases, inhaled 221
Gauze dressings 48
Gauze pads 45
Germs, cross infection 14–15
Gloves, disposable 45
Glue, poisoning 222
"Good Samaritan" principle 12, 17
Groin, hernia 246
Gunshot wounds 129

H

Hallucinogens, overdose 222
Handling and moving
   victims 63–70
Hands
   bandaging
      roller bandages 55
      slings 61
      triangular bandages 58
   bones 146
   checking circulation 51
   injuries 163
   palm wounds 141
   see also Fingers
Hanging 108
Hazchem symbols 22
Head injuries 179
   cerebral compression 179, 181
   concussion 179, 180
   emergency first aid 272
   examining for injury 34
   scalp bandage 59

skull fracture 179, 182
wounds 137
Headache 188
Headgear, removing 41
Heart
   circulatory system 72, 118–19
   disorders 124–5
      angina pectoris 124
      heart attack 125
      heart failure 124
   emergency first aid 271
   heartbeat 119
   restoring rhythm 74
      defibrillators 74, 82–3
   see also Resuscitation
Heat
   body temperature 191
   heat exhaustion 203
   heatstroke 204
   prickly heat 202
   sunburn 202
Helicopter rescue 64
Helmets, removing 41
Hemorrhage see Bleeding
Hepatitis A 249
Hepatitis B 14
   human bites 230
   overseas travel health 250
Hepatitis C 14
   human bites 230
   overseas travel health 250
Hernia 246
Heroin, overdose 222
Hiccups 238
High-voltage electricity 26
Hip fractures 170–1
HIV 14
   human bites 230
Hormones, "fight or flight
   response" 14
Hornet stings 226
Human bites 230
Humerus 146
   fractures 160
Hygiene
   childbirth 234
   preventing cross infection 14–15
Hyperglycemia 240
Hyperventilation 114
Hypoglycemia 241
Hypothermia 206–8
Hypoxia 106

I

Ice packs 49
Immunization, hepatitis B 14
Impaired consciousness 178
Impalement 132
Improvised dressings 48

Improvised slings 62
Incised wounds 129
Industrial chemicals 221
Infants
   assessing victims 262
   childbirth 231–7
   choking 102, 266
   hypothermia 207
   pulse 42
   recovery position 262
   rescue breaths 263
   resuscitation 94–8, 263
   seizures 186
   unconsciousness 94–98
Infection
   childbirth 234
   cross infection 14–15
   overseas travel health 249–50
   in wounds 136
Information, passing on 37
Inhalation
   foreign objects 216
   fumes 110–11
   gases 221
   respiratory system 105
Inhalers, asthma 30, 115
Injuries, mechanics of 31
Insects
   in ears 215
   insect-borne diseases 250
   stings 226–7
Insulin, diabetes mellitus
   240
Internal bleeding 122
Intervertebral discs 147

J

Jaws
   bleeding from mouth 140
   fractures 157
Jaw thrust 167
Jellyfish stings 229
Joints 149
   injuries
      dislocation 153
      elbows 161
      fingers 163
      knees 172
      shoulders 159
      sprains 154
      wrist 162
      wounds in creases 141

K

Kidney failure,
   "crush syndrome" 133
Knees
   bandaging 54

injuries 172
wounds 141
Knots, bandages 58

L

Labor, childbirth 231–7
Lacerations 129
Legislation 17
Legs
  bandaging 53
  examining for injury 35
  immobilizing 51
  injuries
    amputation 132
    ankle sprain 154
    cramp 248
    hip and thigh injuries 170–1
    knee injuries 172
    lower leg injuries 173
    varicose veins 144
  traction 151
Level of response, monitoring 42
  impaired consciousness 178
Ligaments 149
  shoulder injuries 159
  sprains 154
Lighter fuel, poisoning 222
Lightning 26
Limbs *see* Arms; Legs
Lips, burned 220
"Log-roll," moving victims 167
Low-voltage electricity 27
LSD, overdose 222
Lungs
  airway obstruction 107
  asthma 115
  inhaled foreign objects 216
  penetrating wounds 112–13
  respiratory system 104–5
Lyme disease 250

M

Malaria 250
Marine stings 229
Masks 45
  in rescue breathing 78
Mass gatherings 17
Mechanics of injuries 31
"Medic-Alert" 30
Medication *see* Drugs
Meningitis 187
Menstrual bleeding 143
Migraine 188
Miscarriage 143, 237
Monitoring vital signs 42–3
Morphine, overdose 222
Mosquitoes 250

Mouth 211
  bleeding from 140
  burned lips 220
  examining for injury 34
  insect stings 226
  internal bleeding 122
  knocked-out tooth 140
  sore throat 244
  toothache 244
Mouth-to-mouth breathing
  see Rescue breathing
Mouth-to-nose
  rescue breathing 79
Mouth-to-stoma
  rescue breathing 79
Moving victims 63–70
  arm injuries 161
  equipment 69–70
  hip and thigh injuries 171
  "log-roll" 167
  splints 171
  stretchers 70
Multiple victims 21
Muscles 148
  cramp 248
  ruptures 154
  stitch 247
  strains 154–5
  tears 154
Mushrooms, poisonous 225

N

Nails, checking circulation 51
Narcotics, overdose 222
Narrow-fold bandages 57
Neck
  back pain 168
  examining for injury 34
  spinal injury 165–7
  temporary collars 168
  whiplash injury 31
Needles, sharps containers 15
Nervous system 176–7
  problems 178–88
  spinal injury 165
  structure 176–7
  see also Brain; Unconsciousness
Nose 211
  examining for injury 34
  foreign object in 215
  fractures 157
  internal bleeding 122
  mouth-to-nose rescue breaths 79
  nosebleeds 139

O

Observation charts 280
  using charts 38

Open fractures 150
  treatment 152
Orifices, bleeding from
  ear 138
  mouth 140
  nose 139
  vaginal 143
Orthopedic stretchers 70
Over-breathing, hyperventilation 114
Overdose, drug 222
Overseas travel 249–50
Oxygen
  breathing 72
  circulatory system 72, 118–19
  hypoxia 106
  respiratory system 103, 104

P

Painkillers, overdose 222
Palm wounds 141
Panic attacks 242
Pelvis
  examining for injury 35
  fractures 169
Pepper spray injury 201
Peripheral nervous system 177
Peritonitis 245
Personal belongings 36
Pins 45
Placenta, delivery of 232, 236
Plants, poisonous 225
Platelets 119, 128
Pneumothorax 112
Poisoning 217–29
  alcohol 223
  chemicals on the skin 221
  drugs 222
  emergency first aid 279
  in the eye 221
  food 224
  inhaled gases 221
  plants 225
  swallowed poisons 220, 279
Portuguese man-of-war stings 229
Pregnancy
  childbirth 231–7
  miscarriage 237
Prickly heat 202
Pulse
  checking 42
  observation chart 38, 280
Puncture wounds 129
  animal bites 230
  marine stings 229
  snake bites 228

R

Rabies 250

Radial pulse 42
Radius 146
  fractures 162
Rashes, prickly heat 202
Reactions, delayed 16
Recovery position
  adults 84–5
  children 92–3, 261
  infants 98, 262
  spinal injury 85, 93
Red blood cells 119
Regulations, first aid 17
Relatives, talking to 13
Reports 37
Rescue breathing
  adults 78–9
    with chest compressions 80–1
  children 88–9
    with chest compressions 90–1
  face shields 78
  infants 96–7
    with chest compressions 98
  mouth-to-nose 79
  mouth-to-stoma 79
  pocket masks 78
Respiratory system 103–16
  airway obstruction 107
  asthma 115, 267
  breathing 105
  choking 99–102
  croup 116
  disorders 106–16
  drowning 109
  hanging and strangulation 108
  hyperventilation 114
  hypoxia 106
  inhalation of fumes 110–11
  inhaled foreign objects 216
  inhaled gases 221
  penetrating chest wounds 112–13
  winding 245
Resuscitation
  adults 75–84
    CPR 80–1
    rescue breathing 78–9
    sequence chart 75
  children 86–93
    CPR 90–1
    rescue breathing 88–9
    sequence chart 86
  infants 94–8
    CPR 98
    rescue breathing 96–7
    sequence chart 94
  choking 99–102
  defibrillators 82–3
  priorities 73–4
  recovery position 84–5
  when to call 9·1·1 or EMS 74
Rib cage, fractures 164

"RICE" procedure, strains and
  sprains 154, 155
Road incidents 22–3, 31
  safety 18, 22
Roller bandages 44
  applying 53–5
  choosing correct size 52
  elbow and knee 54
  hand and foot 55
  securing 52
Rupture, hernia 246
Ruptured muscles 154

S

Safety
  emergencies 18
  fires 24
  moving victims 64
  personal 14
  traffic incidents 22
Safety pins, securing roller
  bandages 52
Salmonella, food poisoning
  224
Scalds
  minor burns and scalds 196
  severe burns and scalds 194–5
Scalp
  bandaging 59
  examining for injury 34
  head injuries 180–2
  wounds 137
Scissors 45
"Scoop" stretchers 70
Scorpion bites 227
Sea anemone stings 229
Sea creatures, stings 229
Sea urchin spines 229
Seizures
  absence seizures 185
  in adults 184–5
  in children 186
  emergency first aid 274–5
Sensory organs 210–11
Sexual assault 143
Sexually transmitted infections 250
Sharps containers 15
Shock 120–1
  anaphylactic shock 123, 269
  burns and 192
  emergency first aid 268
Shoulders 149
  dislocation 153
  injuries 159
Signs, assessing a victim 32–3
Skeleton 146–7
  see also Bones
Skin
  allergies 238

bites and stings 226–30
burns and scalds 192–9
chemical burns 199, 221
embedded fishhooks 213
examining for injury 34
prickly heat 202
splinters 212
structure 190, 210
sunburn 202
temperature control 191
Skull 147
  examining for injury 34
  fractures 179, 182
  see also Head injuries
Slide sheets 69
Slings 60–2
  elevation 61
  improvised 62
Smoke 25
  inhalation of 110
Snake bites 228
Soft tissue injuries 154–5
Solvents
  inhalation of 110
  poisoning 222
Sore throat 244
Spider bites 227
Spinal boards 70
Spinal cord
  injuries 165
  nervous system 177
  protection 176
Spinal injury 165–7
Spine 147
  back pain 168
  examining for injury 34, 35
  spinal injury 165–7
    checking for 85
    emergency first aid 273
    moving victims 167
    recovery position 85
Splinters 212
Splints 171
Sprains 154–5
  back pain 168
  cold compresses 49
  types of
    ankle 154
    finger 163
    shoulder 159
Square knots 58
Stab wounds 129
Sterile dressings 44
  applying 47
Stimulants, overdose 222
Stings
  anaphylactic shock 123
  insect 226–7
  marine creatures 229
Stitch 247

Stoma, mouth-to-stoma
 rescue breaths 79
Stomachache 245
Strains, muscles 154–5
Strangulation 108
Stress, looking after
 yourself 16
Stretchers, moving victims 70
Stroke 183
Sunburn 202
Survival bags 45
Swallowed foreign objects 216
Swallowed poisons 220
 emergency first aid 279
Symptoms, assessing a victim 32–3

T

Tear gas injury 201
Teeth
 knocked out 140
 toothache 244
Telephoning for help 20
Temperature, body 191
 fever 239
 frostbite 205
 heat exhaustion 203
 heatstroke 204
 hypothermia 206–8
 taking 43
Tendons 149
 shoulder injuries 159
 strains 154
Tetanus 134, 230
Thermometers 43
Thighs
 cramp 248
 fractures 170–1
Throat
 insect stings 226
 sore 244
 swallowed poisons 220
 see also Airway
Tibia 146
 fractures 173
Tick bites 227
Toes see Feet
Tooth sockets, bleeding 140
Toothache 244
Traction, fractures 151
Traffic accidents 22–3, 31
 safety 18, 22
Tranquilizers, overdose 222
Transfer belts, moving
 victims 65
Transporting victims
 see Moving victims
Travel
 air travel 243
 overseas travel health 249–50

Traveler's diarrhea 249
Triangular bandages 44, 57–61
 folding 57
 hand and foot cover 58
 scalp 59
 slings 60–1
 square knots 58
 storing 57
Tubular bandages 44
 applying 56
Tweezers 45

U

Ulna 146
 fractures 162
Ultraviolet light, flash burns to the
 eye 201
Umbilical cord, childbirth 235, 236
Unconsciousness
 cerebral compression 179, 181
 checking response 76, 87, 95
 choking 100–2
 concussion 179, 180
 diabetes mellitus 240–1
 emergency first aid 252–63
 examining victims 34–5
 impaired consciousness 178
 observation chart 38, 280
 recovery position 84–5
 seizures in adults 184–5
 seizures in children 186
 skull fracture 179, 182
 spinal injury 167
 stroke 183
 see also Resuscitation
Urethra, internal bleeding 122

V

Vaginal bleeding 143
 childbirth 236
 miscarriage 237
Varicose veins, bleeding 144
Veins 118
 bleeding 128
 varicose veins 144
Vertebrae 147
 injuries 165
Vertigo 239
Victims
 assessing 29–33, 254, 258, 262
 controlling a fall 66
 examining 34–5
 handling 63–4
 monitoring vital signs 42–3
 moving 67–70
 multiple 21
 observation charts 38, 280
 passing on information 37

removing clothing 40–1
 treatment and aftercare 36–7
 see also Emergencies
Vital signs, monitoring 42–3
Vomiting 247

W

Wasp stings 226
Waste material 15
Water
 drowning 109
 electrical injuries 27
 hypothermia 206
 overseas travel health 249
 rescue from 28–9
Whiplash injury 31
White blood cells 119
"Wind-chill factor" 206
Winding 245
Windpipe see Airway
Work, first aid at 17
Wounds 127–44
 abdominal 142
 amputation 132
 animal bites 230
 blood clotting 128
 chest 112–13
 cross infection 14–15
 crush injuries 133
 cuts and abrasions 134
 dressing and bandaging 46–59
 emergency first aid 270
 eyes 138
 foreign objects 131, 135
 head injury 179
 impalement 132
 infection 136
 at joint creases 141
 palm 141
 scalp and head 137
 severe bleeding 130–1
 types of 129
Wrists
 bandages 55
 injuries 162

Y

Yellow fever 250

ACKNOWLEDGMENTS

Medical Editor
American College of Emergency Physicians
Jon R. Krohmer, MD, FACEP

AUTHORS

ST. JOHN AMBULANCE
Dr. Tony Lee, Chief Medical Officer
Dr. Lotte Newman, Medical Adviser

ST. ANDREW'S AMBULANCE ASSOCIATION
Mr. Rudy Crawford, Chairman of Medical
and First Aid Committee

BRITISH RED CROSS
Dr. J. Gordon Paterson, Chief Medical Adviser
Dr. Vivien Armstrong, Project Manager

TRIPARTITE COMMERCIAL COMMITTEE

ST. JOHN AMBULANCE
Brian Rockell, Director of Training and Marketing
Richard Fernandez, Publications Manager

ST. ANDREW'S AMBULANCE ASSOCIATION
Brendan Healy, Chief Executive Officer
Christine Cuthbertson, PR, Marketing and Fundraising
Manager

BRITISH RED CROSS
Katrina Thornton, Acting Head of Purchasing
and Supply

AUTHORS' ACKNOWLEDGMENTS
The medical authors extend special thanks to Jim Dorman, Training Manager, St. Andrew's Ambulance Association. In addition, they wish to acknowledge the advice and help of many others, in particular: Carol Lock, First Aid Training Officer, St. John Ambulance; Alex Rose and Bill Gallacher from St Andrew's Ambulance Association; Sir Peter Beale; Anita Kerwin-Nye, National Officer for First Aid, British Red Cross; Lyn Brayne, Miranda Bradley, and Chele Lawrence from the British Red Cross for information on victim handling; Joe Mulligan, Head of Training and Development, British Red Cross; Ken Sharpe, Service and Vocational Development Team Manager, British Red Cross; Dr. Anthony Handley, Chairman of BLS/AED Sub-committee of the Resuscitation Council (UK); Dr. Robert Bingham, Chairman of the Resuscitation Council (UK).

PUBLISHERS' ACKNOWLEDGMENTS
The publishers would like to thank the following for their kind permission to reproduce the photographs: Tim Graham p.5; Matthew Brooke, Ferno (UK) Ltd. for carry chairs, p.69 and ambulance stretcher, p.70.

The publishers would also like to thank:
Caroline Gibson and Sarah Burgess; the British Red Cross for props; Sarah Ashun, Andy Crawford, and Steve Gorton for additional photography; Halli Verrinder for additional illustrations; Karmel Jackson for makeup; Esther Ripley for editorial assistance; Victoria Clark, Gadi Farfour, and Helen Taylor for design assistance; Teresa Pritlove for proofreading; Hilary Bird for the index; the people who appear as models: Sylvia Addison, Norris Allen, Othelia Allen, Alan Austin, Rachel Bancroft, Joe Belcher, Michelle Belcher, Joanna Benwell, Lino Boga-Rios, Claire Bowers, Jonathan Brooks, Venita Choolani, La'Toya Christie, Victoria Clark, Lucy Claxton, Samantha Coote, Steven Coote, Caitlin Cordell, Catherine Cordell, Liam Cordell, Kathy Currie, Jessica Currie, Nigel Currie, Kate Davidson, Sue Davidson, Rowan De Saulles, Peggy Dear, Wahid Din, Kevin Donavia, Chris Drew, Jemima Dunne, Janice English, Richard Fernandez, Gemma Foale, Jackie Foale, James Foale, Jolyon Goddard, Anna Goodman, Victoria Heyworth Dunne, Layla Hopkins, Iona Hoyle, Matt Humphrey, Katie John, Charlie Kenward, Laura Kenward, Crispin Lord, Daniel Lord, Harriet Lord, Philip Lord, Michelle Luc, Sharon Lucas, Joseph Marriott, Tina McDonnell, Julia Miles, Janet Mohun, Jae Sung Ol, John Payne, Gitte Pedersen, Bharti Patel, Aaron Reeve, Jo Reeve, Kate Reynolds, Esther Ripley, Eileen Seed, Glen Snashall, Russell Snashall, Agatha Walcott, Philip Wall, Roger Wall, Edna Walker, Nicole Williams, Sue Williams, Emmanuele Vioulac, Orley Yam, Mark Yeoman.

ST. JOHN AMBULANCE

St. John Ambulance is the UK's leading first aid, transport and care charity. Its mission is to provide first aid and medical support services; caring services in support of community needs; and education, training and personal development to young people.

ST. ANDREW'S AMBULANCE ASSOCIATION

St. Andrew's Ambulance Association is Scotland's premier first-aid training and services provider. We teach vital life-saving skills to over 20,000 people per year. Volunteers provide first-aid cover at public events. We rely on public donations to continue our life-saving work.

BRITISH RED CROSS

The British Red Cross cares for people in crisis at home and abroad. It gives vital impartial support during major emergencies and personal crises, and provides training in first-aid and caregiving.

The red cross emblem is a symbol of protection during armed conflict and its use is restricted by law.